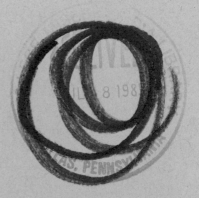

Hospice and Palliative Nursing Care

Hospice and Palliative Nursing Care

Ann G. Blues, Ed.D.

Executive Director
Institute for Health Care Education, Inc.
Portland, Oregon

Joyce V. Zerwekh, C.R.N., M.A.

Coordinator
Hospice Northwest
Northwest Hospital
Seattle, Washington

GRUNE & STRATTON

A Subsidiary of Harcourt Brace Jovanovich, Publishers

Orlando   San Diego   San Francisco
New York   London   Toronto   Montreal
Sydney   Tokyo   São Paulo

Library of Congress Cataloging in Publication Data

Blues, Ann G. (Ann Goben)
  Hospice and palliative nursing care.

  Includes bibliographies and index.
  1. Terminal care. 2. Nursing. 3. Terminal care
facilities. I. Zerwekh, Joyce V. (Joyce Valborg)
II. Title. [DNLM: 1. Hospices—Nursing texts.
2. Terminal care—Nursing. 3. Palliative treatment—
Nursing. WY 152 H828]
R726.8.B55   1983   616'.029   83-12993
ISBN 0-8089-1577-0

© **1984 by Grune & Stratton, Inc.**

Grune & Stratton, Inc.
Orlando, Florida 32887

Distributed in the United Kingdom by
Grune & Stratton, Inc. (London) Ltd.
24/28 Oval Road, London NW 1

Library of Congress Catalog Number 83-12993
International Standard Book Number 0-8089-1577-0

Printed in the United States of America

Contents

v

Acknowledgments

To Lynnell and Walter, who share their soccer, music, long walks, and future plans with me. Their love and enthusiasm have sustained me for the past 18 years.

To Kurt, whose presence in my life has made writing this book possible and whose love and support have made doing it worthwhile.

And perhaps most of all to my mother, Villear Goben, whose belief in me has provided me with the confidence and support always to reach for my dreams.

Special thanks go to the faculties of Centre College of Kentucky and the University of Kentucky, particularly Drs. Joseph Bryant, Paul Cantrell, Charles Hazelrigg, and William Peters. I am grateful also to the many caring people with whom I was privileged to work at the Ephraim McDowell Community Cancer Network, University of Kentucky, Lexington, Kentucky, especially Kathleen Walzer, R.N. My years with the National Hospice Organization have brought me much encouragement and pleasure, and I am indebted to those members of the first Board of Directors, particularly Ina Ajemian, Jo Magno, and Zachery Morfogen for their inspiration and good humor. And to Dame Cicely Saunders, Mrs. Mary Smith, and Dr. Thomas West, who welcomed me to share and learn from their St. Christopher's Hospice experience.

I am constantly supported in my present work through the contributions and good will of the Institute for Health Care Education's Board of Directors and Chairperson, Dr. Thomas Pappas; Kathleen Nance, American Red Cross, Oregon Trail Chapter; Jean Grover, Senior Care; and Dru Duniway, Area Agency on Aging. I am indebted to those involved in problems of the aging in Portland, and the many family members and friends of the elderly who allow me to spend my life doing what I most love, teaching.

—Ann G. Blues

Bravo and garlands go to Elaine McIntosh, Hospice of Seattle Administrator, who has supported the exceptional role flexibility I needed to complete this text, and to Sandy Sennis, who has transformed rough rubble into cleanly typed copy. I celebrate the good hearts and wisdom of the present and past Hospice of Seattle team: Mae Sallee Beals, Colleen Beck, Louise Bonin, Dawn Chang, Lynn Felsinger, Lynn Grotsky, Peter Hunsberger, Irene LaVergne, Dan O'Brien, Polly Purvis, Floyd Scott, Tess Kistler Taft, Lynne Talley, and the volunteer team. We have all grown so much together. I thank my sons, Greg and Joel, who have shared their love and laughter and have prevented me from taking myself too seriously.

Finally, my deep gratitude goes to Adeline Leraas and Katherine Ness at St. Olaf College Department of Nursing for nurturing in me an acute sensitivity to the patient experience; to Emily Campbell at the University of Wisconsin School of Nursing for her clear clinical vision that sharpened mine, and to the Religious Society of Friends (Quakers), which has fostered my understanding of the unity and sacredness of life.

—Joyce V. Zerwekh

Foreword

One of the saddest moments in medicine comes when the physician knows there is no longer anything that can be offered to the patient. Until recently, there has been no alternative but for the physician to say, "There is nothing more we can do for you," and to leave the patient alone to face death and dying. Although a social survey done in 1970 in Connecticut showed that 67 percent of the people interviewed expressed a desire to die at home, only 20 percent of the people were actually able to do so. The rest usually end their lives in hospitals or nursing homes, where very often heroic measures are employed to "save" or prolong their lives even when it is known that cure is not possible.

The hospice concept as an alternative mode of care for the terminally ill came into the consciousness of Americans because of the work of Dr. Cicely Saunders at St. Christopher's Hospice in London, and the work of Dr. Elisabeth Kubler-Ross, who has written several books on death and dying. With the establishment of the first hospice program in New Haven, Connecticut, made possible by a grant from the National Cancer Institute, people became increasingly aware that patients whose lives are nearing the end can be helped to die painlessly, peacefully, and with great dignity. After this, the hospice movement started to grow by leaps and bounds in the United States.

The hospice concept, known commonly as "hospice," advocates that when the quantity of life can no longer be increased, the quality must be the maximum possible. In order to achieve this, hospice addresses the problems that are unique to the dying patient—pain, loneliness, and loss of control. Hospice, therefore, often palliates when cure is no longer possible. In addition, hospice recognizes that human beings are not just physical bodies but a composite of physical, social, psychological, and spiritual elements. In order to address all of the needs of a dying patient, therefore, a hospice team must be interdisciplinary in nature. Hospice also recognizes that human beings are not isolated but are surrounded by family members or other significant people. For this reason, hospice deals with the patient and the family members as a unit of care.

Because of the rapid growth of the hospice movement in the United States, it is very important that both consumers of hospice care and potential providers of health care should have a thorough understanding of the hospice concept. It is for this reason that this book on palliative care/hospice care programs is so timely and of such great importance. Ann Blues and Joyce Zerwekh are highly qualified to write a book such as this one. Dr. Blues is one of the founders of the hospice movement in the United States. Her professional background as a health educator eminently qualifies her to write about quality care. Her past position on the board of directors of the National Hospice Organization and her role as the President of the Board in 1980 have given her a comprehensive perspective of the hospice movement in the United States that very few people have. Ms. Zerwekh's patient care experience provides the clinical expertise necessary to complete this very useful text.

I recommend this book to all those who feel the need for better care for the dying.

Josefina B. Magno, M.D.
Director, Institute for Hospice Studies
Washington, D.C.

Prologue

How little the real sufferings of illness are known and understood. How little does anyone in good health fancy him or . . . herself into the life of a sick person. —Florence Nightingale

The needs of the dying person do not differ so much from those of the healthy man or woman. Who, well or ill, does not want love, security, physical comfort, and the self-respect that comes from meaningful activity? It is not, therefore, the needs that are so different in those with longer or shorter futures, but rather the circumstances of their lives.

For the dying person, many basic needs are denied, or at best lowered in priority. Love is often replaced by awkward silence, meaningful self-help by dependence, self-respect and dignity by submission to futile attacks on a disease.

More frightening than any treatment is the thought of dying alone, unaided. For dying is a social activity, as is being born. News of someone being "found dead" saddens us. We shudder at the implication that someone was alone or neglected in this final experience, that no helping hand was there, no recognition given to the passing.

The dying patient and his or her family need us to apply relevant, appropriate skills to meet their needs. These skills may at times parallel and at other times diverge from those necessary to research, diagnosis, and cure. With proper matching of the skills of curing and caring we can diminish the isolation, guilt, and unnecessary suffering so often experienced by the terminally ill.

Our hope is
that in watching we should learn not only how to free patients from pain and distress, how to understand them and never let them down, but also how to be silent, how to listen and how just to be there. —Dame Cicely Saunders

I shall live a year, barely longer. During that year let as much as possible be done. —Joan of Arc

Preface

This textbook covers a broad spectrum of knowledge necessary to the comprehensive care of the dying person and his or her family members. Although the book emphasizes the integral role and unique responsibilities of the nurse, it is also intended to serve as a helpful source for health team members of other disciplines.

The book itself is an interdisciplinary achievement, for it combines understanding gained from long-term hospice program development with extensive experience in hospice nursing practice and education. The text addresses both care for the dying person and family and ways of sustaining the programs that make that care possible.

Because our goal is to teach not only the concept of hospice but also its practice, we have included in this text a variety of useful examples and resources for application.

In addition, each chapter begins with a series of true–false discussion questions designed to begin an open dialogue on the issues discussed in the chapter. The reader can use these questions for self-evaluation both before and after reading the narrative. The "correct" answers are included at the back of the text, but beware of considering these answers absolute—the issues are complex and the answers debatable. We invite you to explore and draw conclusions for yourself.

Ann G. Blues
Joyce V. Zerwekh

Contributors

Alma Stanford, B.S.N. (coauthor, Chapter 14) is currently Hospice Coordinator for the Providence Medical Center, Seattle, Washington. She is a board member of both the National Hospice Organization and the Washington State Hospice Organization.

Lynn Talley Walters, B.S.N. (author, Chapter 12) is currently Clinical Coordinator for the Hospice of Seattle, Seattle, Washington. She is a member of Sigma Theta Tau.

Hospice and Palliative Nursing Care

1

Hospice Philosophy of Appropriate Care

Answer the following questions True (T) or False (F). Answers appear on the last page of this chapter.

1. *A patient should never be locked into either the cure or the care system.*

2. *Palliative care is a passive method of helping a person accept the inevitable course of his or her illness.*

3. *Pain has either a physiological or psychological basis that can best be eliminated through aggressive curative therapy.*

4. *Patients should be treated as if they can be cured until the last possible moment and then allowed, in the last few hours of life, to die comfortably.*

5. *It is unethical to admit that a patient may die when any curative therapy—even if it is ineffective—can still be maintained.*

6. *If after a period of symptom control the patient feels stronger, the medical team should press for a return to vigorous curative therapy.*

7. *The choice of what is appropriate care should always be within the "informed control" of the patient.*

8. *Patients should be permitted, barring extreme circumstances, to die where they wish.*

9. *Incorporating some of the patient's possessions, foods, and routines into the environment of the in-patient facility can offer the patient contentedness and security.*

10. *No teaching hospital can provide the humane, patient-centered, palliative care that is appropriate for the dying.*

One woman, with a year's history of unrelenting pain from a carcinoma of the pancreas, drew her pain as a small rodent boring into the side of a tree trunk. A few traces of green at the top were described to be as "her life, trying to get through." A friend wrote to us, after her death: "It was nothing short of a miracle. When I last visited her in a previous hospital she was like a demented animal—consumed with pain, incoherent of speech and quite vicious. I was very frightened, not knowing how to cope and felt unable to face another visit. Words cannot describe my reaction when I saw her in St. Christopher's—restored to the dignity of a calm, rational human being again despite her physical suffering. From then on I was able to remain with her for hours at a time, instead of minutes, holding conversation and discussing things of interest dear to her heart and of your special interest in her. By so doing, I too have gained in spiritual strength. I can only thank you for making my friend's last days bearable when once they were unendurable."

T HE POINT of the above story and perhaps of this chapter can be summed up quite simply: the statement "There is nothing more to be done" should never be applied to the dying patient. Even though there is a time when the medical effort may turn primarily from the arresting of the disease to the relief of symptoms, this stage of treatment, called palliative care, may be every bit as aggressive and determined as curative care. Its aim should be to relieve the patient and his or her family of physical, emotional, spiritual, and social distress and thus to free them to concentrate on the matters of living.

A PHILOSOPHY OF MODERN CARE

As our society has evolved in the past hundred years, many forces have come together to depersonalize care of the dying. Until the end of the last century, many Americans were living in large multi-generation homes and had close and longstanding ties to their families and neighbors. Whenever

---

*From Saunders, C.M. Patient care; An introduction. *Topics in Therapeutics. 4* Pitman Medical, London, England, 1978, p. 74. With permission.

someone became very ill there was a ready-made support system, and doctor, minister, and relatives called on the family as needed. There were few medical institutions, and in general patients had little choice but to be cared for at home while a disease ran its natural course.

Certainly, no one would advocate a return to 19th-century medical and nursing practices. Nevertheless, it is quite true that frequently a physician or nurse of the last century would put an arm around a patient's shoulder because there were no other remedies available to ease the person's pain. Today that arm may not be offered; instead, a drug may be administered. The problem is not the use of the drug, which may secure the patient's physical comfort. The problem is the missing closeness between helping professional and patient. Combined physical and emotional therapies bring the greatest relief.

A philosophy of care that combines the most modern techniques with loving concern for the person seems a rather obvious choice for professions dedicated from the earliest time to the relief of suffering. Yet the generally agreed purpose of medical care in technically advanced countries is to cure people. Medical professionals are trained to use complex technical support facilities for the express purpose of curing people. Vast improvements have been made in the general level of health and in the care available for the young and middle-aged with controllable infectious diseases. The decline, since the early 1900s, in the incidence of the major communicable diseases has resulted in more people living longer and to a higher incidence of chronic illnesses such as cancer, heart disease, and stroke in the older populations (Dobihal, 1974). Because we have not yet found the remedies for these chronic diseases, health care givers "are seeing increasing numbers of patients for whom they are not really trained to care—the so-called terminally ill patients. These are patients with diseases that can neither be cured or controlled (despite all appropriate curative therapeutic efforts) and that can be expected to progress and cause death" (Hadlock, 1980, p. 133). These patients may suffer not only from inappropriate curative care but also from uninformed and inept palliative care.

So, we have not defeated death; we have simply changed the common causes of death. In those cases where stroke, heart disease, and cancer—the primary pathological causes of death—are characterized by a debilitating course and overwhelming symptoms, cure-motivated care, with its emphasis on aggressive, eradicating therapies, is often inappropriate. However, in our death-denying system, medical care frequently persists in distressful therapies, and relief from symptoms and anxiety is offered only secondarily. As Herman Feifel (1977) notes, medical advances have lengthened the time between the diagnosis of a fatal malignancy and death, and the patient has more time to develop unrelenting pain, fear, unwanted dependency and even feelings of dehumanization.

In part, our reluctance to administer palliative care may reflect our inability to admit the inevitability of death. In a popular old children's verse, death was seen as a natural part of the human cycle:

Solomon Grundy,
Born on Monday,
Christened on Tuesday,
Married on Wednesday,
Took ill on Thursday,
Worse on Friday,
Died on Saturday,
Buried on Sunday,
This is the end of Solomon Grundy

—Anonymous

But we have come to disguise the reality of death with euphemisms—people do not die, but "pass away" or "meet their Maker." Physicians—even those who recognize the effectiveness of the palliative care system—have often held out for a curative regime long past its usefulness. Over and over, patients have received an excessive "dose" of that curative regime who are admitted to palliative care programs only in the last 48 hours of life.

The physician, J. Englebert Dunphy, who urged his colleagues on many occasions to "care" for their patients, has described what he believes to be the most appropriate care for the dying patient. Although Dunphy supports the belief that life should be saved whenever there is hope that the patient may be returned to "a state of tolerable well-being," he holds that "there is no moral responsibility for prolonging life by any specific medical treatment when it is clearly evident that this course only preserves an existence in a state far worse than death" (Dunphy, 1976, p. 317). There can be infinite debate on the benefits of sustaining hope of cure compared with the advantages of recognizing the need to accept that life is coming to an end. There is no need to resuscitate or prolong a life by forced feedings or antibiotics, Dunphy continues. "It is inhuman to drag the dying patient to radiation therapy, to transfuse him repeatedly or give him massive toxic and nauseating chemotherapy.... That is the science without the humanity of medicine" (Dunphy, 1976, p. 318).

Shakespeare expressed it perfectly in *King Lear*. The King, broken and ill, is dying. As he loses consciousness there is an attempt to revive him but Kent, who has been most true to him, cries,

Vex not his ghost: O, let him pass! he hates him much
That would upon the rack of this tough world
Stretch him out longer

—(act V, scene III).

THE CURE AND CARE SYSTEMS

Cicely M. Saunders in her book *The Management of Terminal Disease* has identified the two systems of care in Figure 1-1—the cure and care systems. Saunders points out the large areas of overlap between these two systems and the need to be ever alert to the possibilities each system offers a particular patient. Each system should be available as the patient needs it. Whenever there is reasonable doubt about restoring the patient to health or tolerable existence, curative or controlling treatment must be continued. Saunders (1978) emphasizes that "as active treatment becomes irrelevant, the movement may be mainly towards 'Care', but no patient should become locked irretrievably in what is (or may become) for him the wrong system (pp. 1–2). What is appropriate may change, and the hospice team needs always to be alert to this possibility.

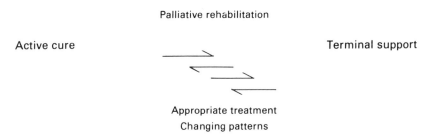

Palliative rehabilitation

Active cure   Terminal support

Appropriate treatment
Changing patterns

Figure 1. The cure and care systems. The overlapping arrows indicate that skilled control of the problems of advanced and terminal diseases does not necessarily have to wait until all other treatment is abandoned; its successful use may indeed make that treatment more effective. (Adapted from Saunders, C.M. *The management of terminal disease.* New York: Oxford University Press, 1983. With permission.)

Hospice is a program of palliative and supportive care which recognizes the physical, psychological, social and spiritual needs of dying persons and their families. This care is provided by an interdisciplinary team of professionals and lay volunteers. It is available without regard to the patient's ability to pay on a 24-hour-a day, seven-days-a week basis. Hospice care continues into bereavement. Palliative care is that which provides the most modern and sophisticated treatment to relieve the symptoms and distress of the disease process.

It is not uncommon for patients, after a period of individualized palliative care, to appear stronger. They may ask to visit children, become involved in a project, or wish to participate in a famliy event. This renewed vigor may trigger the physician's desire to reinstate more aggressive curative therapies. Such a decision should be carefully reviewed with the patient, who may value the brief "wellness" that makes possible participation in something that both gives fulfillment to life and helps facilitate acceptance of death.

In other cases, increased strength may encourage patients to reevaluate their interest in more active programs of therapy. Indeed, it is not unheard of that a patient's renewed tolerance to treatment causes a switch to a highly effective cure-oriented treatment and a remission. It should always be made very clear to patients and families that both the cure and the care systems are available and that one can move freely between them if it is generally agreed to be appropriate. (Schmale & Patterson, 1978, pp. 16–17).

Attention to such a comprehensive and ambitious task as good palliative care must be the continuing priority of a variety of caregivers who are able to be both specialists and generalists in an interdisciplinary setting. At the core of such care is the recognition of patients as valued, loved, supported human beings with a right to dignity and control in their dying.

WHEN IS PALLIATIVE CARE APPROPRIATE?

For which patients is palliative care appropriate? The answer seems clear: the incurable patient, the person who cannot be cured by aggressive therapy. In fact, however, the answer is far from clear. The problem is that it is impossible to apply the term *incurable* with absolute certainty. Patients seen by one specialist and diagnosed incurable may be considered candidates for aggressive therapy by another.

An essential component of appropriate care is conscientious assessment of the individual patient. Knowing when aggressive curative therapy is no longer effective is not a simple matter. Before instituting palliative care, the following questions should be answered in the affirmative.

- Has every possible conventional curative therapy been used in an effort to eradicate or control the disease?
- Are symptoms that indicate a terminal stage actually related to progressive disease and not to other conditions that are not terminal? K.C. Calman (1978) cautions that "sinister symptoms" are sometimes quite simple; for example, a patient may have bronchitis not pulmonary metastases, gallstones instead of liver metastases, or a prolapsed intervertebral disc rather than a disseminated abdominal lymphoma.
- Can palliative care relieve symptoms so as to add substantially to the patient's quality of life?
- Are the patient and his or her family informed and active participants in the decisions that are being made regarding choice of treatment?
- Has a complete assessment been performed by a physician and a

multidisciplinary team in order to document the course of the disease and the patient's specific problems?

- Does this assessment include attention to the patient's psychological, spiritual, and social needs?

It is only when these foregoing questions have been competently answered in the affirmative that an appropriate course of action can be chosen. Thus the decision of what is appropriate care must be arrived at jointly by physician, interdisciplinary team, patient, and family. And decisions are not always based on purely physiological factors. For example, a young man may decide to avoid further surgery so that he will be able to continue as an assistant coach for his 9-year-old son's soccer team in the regional tournament. Another man may not be content unless he is convinced that every possible—even experimental—treatment is being tried. The choice should always be, to a great extent, within the "informed control" of the patient.

THE ELEMENTS OF PALLIATIVE CARE

Proper care of the dying patient does not end with a willingness to withdraw extraordinary forms of treatment. Skilled nursing care, relief of pain and distressing symptoms, supportive family counseling, and bereavement care all help permit death with dignity and relative comfort. This book addresses the major elements of hospice care for the dying, including the following:

- *Symptom control:* a thorough but noninvasive *assessment,* individually titrated drugs regularly administered to control pain and retain alertness, and constant attention to *sources and therapies for any discomfort*
- Treating patient and family as a unit of care
- Available *home and inpatient* care, 24 hours a day, seven days a week
- Physician-directed medical services, nurse-directed nursing care, and *interdisciplinary* attention to the patient's physical, psychological, spiritual, and social suffering
- *Volunteers* to help the family maintain a normal daily life
- Continuing *bereavement care* for the family and support throughout mourning

Palliative care is far from passive hand-holding. John Hinton has recently reaffirmed the importance of hospice expertise in alleviating pain and other distress. Hinton (1980) concludes that "continued physical distress has such a major influence on patients' psychological states that its presence can well swamp the effects of other elements of terminal care" (p. 2). In the groups

Hinton (1963) sampled in the 1960s, 8 percent of patients who were free of physical distress showed moderate depression, but 35 percent of those who still experienced physical distress were either moderately or more severely depressed.

The care system as defined by Saunders comprises the best and most skillful medical and nursing care combined with concern for the whole patient. It is in fact the "efficient, loving care" that Saunders repeatedly articulates.

If at all possible, patients should be permitted to die where they wish. In some cases homes may be a good place—a comfortable and secure place—to die (Barzelai, 1981). Home, however, is not always practical or even possible. A patient may live alone and have no close relatives or friends, community support services may be lacking, or the home itself may not be physically adaptable to patient-management needs. And in some cases symptom management may be sufficiently complex to require hospital nursing attention and equipment. In these cases, an institution can strive to provide as home-like an environment as possible. A personal, warm environment into which patients can bring some of their belongings can provide a feeling of familiarity. In more than a few cases patients have come to enjoy their institutional surroundings as safer, less lonely, and even more pleasant than their own homes. For others, of course, the unhappiness of being removed from the familiarity of their homes is overwhelming.

A very important criterion for judging the appropriateness of care is patient–family opinion of that care. A study conducted by Hinton compared patients' views of their palliative treatment, in four different settings: (1) an inpatient hospice, (2) the hospice home-care program, (3) a teaching hospital, and (4) the Foundation Home, a large, converted house that provides an informal atmosphere for people with progressive cancer. According to Hinton (1980), "there was a tendency for the groups who were found to be more settled emotionally to give more praise for their care. Patients looked after by the Hospice staff tended to express the greatest approval" (p. 2). Assessments by the staff and spouses yielded parallel results.

One interesting finding of Hinton's study was that although home-care hospice patients were less emotionally calm than hospice inpatients, they were still highly approving of their care. Even though they were less tranquil than inpatients, they liked their care at home best. Patients may prefer treatments and settings that do not isolate them from the support of those they love.

It should be noted that patients' praise for staff was quite as high in the teaching hospital setting as in the hospice programs. Hospital patients, who were in radiotherapy wards, described the "nurses' kindness and how much the staff tried to help" (Hinton, 1980, p. 5). This should serve as a reminder that staff helpfulness can compensate for the shortcomings of any setting. Thus there are not settings that, by virtue of physical environment alone, are unsuitable to care for the dying. C.B. Roehrig expresses the belief that an ICU setting can provide an excellent opportunity for applying both the humanistic and scientific talents necessary to unique needs of the dying patient (1981). The bases of patients' praise of staff were promptness of attention, gratitude for efficient care, and a feeling of being made welcome. "I feel one of the family.... I've never seen anything like it" (Hinton, 1980, p. 6).

Adequate care of the dying is then bound up in understanding the needs of patients and families. Let us ask ourselves, as D. Shepherd (1976) suggests, "how we may achieve a broader understanding of death and dying. Let each of us ask how, as individuals, we relate to patients with terminal illness and whether our relationship is near the ideal and, if not, let us take steps now to learn more about the one experience that we have in common with our patients" (p. 35).

REFERENCES

Barzelai, L.P. Evaluation of a home-based hospice. *Journal of Family Practice,* 1981, *12*:2, 241–245.

Calman, K.G. Physical aspects. In Saunders, C.M., *The management of terminal disease.* London: E. Arnold, 1978.

Dobihal, E.F., Jr. Talk or terminal care? *Connecticut Medicine,* 1974, *38,* 365.

Dunphy, J.E. Annual discourse on caring for the patient with cancer. *New England Journal of Medicine,* 1976, *295,* 317.

Feifel H. (Ed.). *New meanings of death: Death in contemporary America,* New York: McGraw-Hill, 1977.

Hadlock, D.C. Hospice care: Its implications and influence on current health care concepts. *Long-term Care & Health Services Administration,* Summer, 1980, p. 133.

Hinton, J.M. The physical and mental distress of the dying. *Quarterly Journal of Medicine,* 1963, *52,* 1–21.

Hinton, J.M. *What do patients think of hospice care?* Paper presented at International Conference, St. Christopher's Hospice, 1980, 1.

Roehrig, C.B. Internist, physician, friend. *Internist,* 1981, *22:3,* 3–16.

Saunders, C.M. (Ed.). *The management of terminal disease.* London: E. Arnold, 1978.

Saunders, C.M. Patient care: An introduction. *Topics in Therapeutics 4,* Royal College of Physicians of London, Pitman Medical. Pub Ltd. London, 1978, 72–74.

Schmale, A.H., Patterson, W.B. Comfort care only: Treatment guidelines for the terminal patient. In Garfield, C.A., *Psycho-social care of the dying patient.* New York: McGraw-Hill, 1978.

Shepherd, D.A.E. Terminal care: Towards an ideal. *Canadian Medical Association Journal,* 1976, *115,* in Ajemian, I., Mount, B.M. (eds.), *The Royal Victoria Hospital Manual on Palliative/Hospice Care,* Arno Press, N.Y., 1980, pp. 34–35.

1. T	6. F
2. F	7. T
3. F	8. T
4. F	9. T
5. F	10. F

2

Honesty Tempered With Hope

Answer the following questions True (T) or False (F). Answers appear on the last page of this chapter.

1. *Most patients are willing to talk about death if professionals seem comfortable in discussing it.*

2. *Informing the patient and family should be an ongoing process, not restricted to a single conference.*

3. *Physicians who continue to tell patients that they are improving when in fact they are dying are preventing depression in both patient and family.*

4. *Patients need simple answers; they could not understand most medical diagnoses and therapies even if these were explained to them.*

5. *What sometimes seems to be insensitivity on the part of a professional who is dealing with a dying patient may actually be awkwardness and discomfort.*

6. *It is possible to be too honest and to tell the truth at the wrong time to someone who is dying.*

7. *There is a possibility that learning of a terminal prognosis will cause a patient to give up.*

8. *One of the chief advantages of sharing the truth with patients is that they are freed to talk about their feelings, wishes, and concerns.*

9. *The wishes of the head of the family who does not want the truth told to the patient should always be honored.*

10. *If a patient consistently avoids discussing his or her prognosis, the care team should devise a way to make the truth evident to the patient.*

*Truth and hope are not mutually exclusive, and the informed patient is
frequently better able to fight for his life because he knows the real battlefield.
Surely most of us wish to take some responsibility for our dying as well as for
our living!**

MOST PROFESSIONALS now believe that patients are entitled to
explanations of their illnesses that are understandable and convincing, yet the
problem of what a seriously ill or dying patient should be told (and how and
when) is one that constantly exercises the minds of those with clinical
responsibility. If medical–nursing care is to become the cooperative team
venture we idealistically project, the doctor, nurse, support team, patient, and
family should have rapport; truth should be shared so that the patient's
problems and concerns can be fully discussed and addressed.

CHOOSING HONESTY

There is no formula for dealing honestly with the dying patient and his or
her family. The most important thing to realize is that there are many options;
silence, denial, or blunt truth are not the only alternatives. The character of
the patient and the personalities of the physician or nurse will greatly influence
the time and manner of telling. It is very difficult to assess the patient's ability
to handle the impact of truth when it is unpromising of cure, and only a naive
and extremely inexperienced person would claim the ability to do this easily
and accurately. Many professionals have seen patients of apparent strength
and iron will who, when told their illness is grave, turn their faces to the wall.
And sometimes the patient judged helpless and demanding will receive similar
news with philosophical fortitude. It is important to understand that there is
also a group of patients who cannot handle any kind of distressing news with
emotional stability. Emotional disturbance and mental illness occur in the
general population; thus, dying patients may be emotionally or mentally
disturbed as well. The additional stress of an unfavorable prognosis may

_____

*From Saunders, C.M. *The Management of Terminal Disease,* London: Arnold Ltd., 1978.

precipitate an emotional crisis. The most frequent response, however, is probably relief at having been told straightforwardly but kindly the facts of one's illness. However bleak these facts may be, clear knowledge dispels the corroding uncertainty about what is happening or may happen.

According to Saunders (1965), "there are many different truths just as there are many ways of imparting them" (p. 12). To choose the most effective time and response, one must be aware of what the patient really wants to know.

The question may not be so much, Do you tell the patient? as, How do you tell your patient? And perhaps the question, What do you let your patient tell you? may be even more important. The process "frequently lies in a relationship rather than in words. Indeed one might question whether those who have no relationship to offer should use words at all" (Saunders, 1978, p. 30). The greater need may be for someone who tries to be aware of what the patient is thinking and takes the time to wait for a question.

Many patients would be willing to talk about death if staff could bring themselves to discuss the problem with them. Patients frequently have many more unresolved questions than they ask. Seldom does a first or second visit or conversation elicit genuine and deep-seated fears and doubts. It is only through waiting and talking at a number of levels that one learns what patients or family members are facing and what their thoughts about this are. The thoughts may be quite different from day to day as the illness demands interpretation and re-evaluation, and as family and social circumstances alter. The help needed at each stage may be quite different. In terminal illness, each bit of "losing ground" physically may seem to be a major defeat unless it is anticipated and put into perspective or controlled.

Keeping the communication network open and checking for possible misunderstandings when new information is given will often eliminate the need for those sudden, terrifying moments of truth that both teller and hearer dread. Patients need to be included all along in relevant information and reasonable decision-making situations. This on-going process by which the patient and relatives remain "on the inside" of what is going on greatly minimizes the chance that the patient and/or family will be dealt a single, disastrous blow for which they are unprepared. Information developed through multidisciplinary team communication can be explained and reinforced by nurses, technicians, counselors or other persons to whom the patient addresses questions and listens (Kastenbaum, 1978).

THE PATIENT-PHYSICIAN RELATIONSHIP

Patients do not always receive a great deal of help in dealing honestly with their diagnosis. Physicians may feel that the idea of death is too much for the patient to tolerate or that because the patient will deny it anyway there is little use in divulging it. Or physicians may fear that the information will precipitate a suicidal depression. Perhaps more important, when their patients are near death, physicians' own coping mechanisms may be sorely strained. Once they have made the decision to withdraw aggressive therapy, they may experience an overwhelming sense of futility and failure. As a result, medical teams of house staff and physicians often tend to curtail their bedside visits; such visits become increasingly brief and perfunctory. The truth is that physicians are sometimes more afraid of death than are the seriously or the terminally ill. Studies by W.D. Kelly and S.R. Friesan (1950) have indicated that while most cancer patients want to be told about their disease, many physicians do not want to tell them. It will be interesting to see if in the future the increasing attention to this problem in medical schools and professional journals will alter physicians' attitudes.

The doctor–patient relationship is fundamentally a human encounter in which truth is indispensable. Every person is of unconditional value, not because of unique assets or accomplishments, but because of his or her human existence. The individual liberty of each patient should be respected, and this respect implies that everyone has the right to choose alternative courses of action and to participate in them.

It seems that in this generation most patients are ready to have an increasing share of information; indeed, they are demanding it. It will serve their needs and ours better by discussing with them more openly what is happening. The realization of dying often overlays a feeling of loss of trust in the medical process. Death exists despite modern medicine—the patient may feel betrayed. "The doctor said he got it all—he was wrong." Or "the doctor said I was going to get better and now this is happening." The patient may then try another doctor, another treatment, another hospital. Frequently patients select unconventional forms of therapy that have little or no effect and isolate the patient from good continuing medical care.

Physicians often cite the Hippocratic Oath as justification for not revealing distressing prognosis; the oath vows to keep the patient "from harm and injustice?" This stricture has frequently been interpreted as an admonition not to tell patients about their condition or prognosis for fear of causing them undue distress. It also allows the physician, as the sole knowledgable person, to maintain control over the patient and his or her disease.

Fallibility

Perhaps medicine should be more aware of its limitations. People are born; they have lives that are either better or worse, fulfilling or disappointing, troubled or untroubled; and they die after few or many years. In this flow of existence, medicine does what it can to control illness and disease. Sometimes medicine's influence on life is dramatic, at other times it has little effect, but in any event it neither guarantees to control cure nor the life of the patient. Failure to share this fallibility with patients and their families is a serious omission.

No one would suggest that it is an easy thing to discuss death with the patient who faces this prospect. To some this may seem like opening a Pandora's box. But having seen the physical and emotional relief individual patients and their families experience when this communication is begun, it seems far better to continue to work toward understanding. For one of the authors of this book, the following comment by a patient has become symbolic of the terminal patient's desire to know his or her prognosis. After his conference with medical staff, this patient said, "I feel better now, braver. I know where it is I'm going, and who will help me get there. It's a lot better than stumbling along alone in the dark"(Patient, Personal Communication, 1978).

In response to a question during Grand Rounds at Washington University–School of Medicine Jewish Hospital of St. Louis concerning guidelines for telling patients that they may die, Kübler Ross (1972) said, "I could tell after a while whose physician the patient was by the degree of comfort experienced by the patient.... I do not believe the variable is whether or not they have been told. The variable is how comfortable the physician is in facing the dying patient. We had, at our institution, one surgeon who was particularly effective in this area. I think that he conveyed belief that he would stay with them until the end" (p. 178).

Truth and Control

Part of the physician's reluctance to reveal the whole truth may stem from what some physicians call the anguish of control and the desire not to share this responsibility with the patient. Patients may feel hopeless and isolated, it is true, if physicians do not appear to be in control of the situation. Yet, as David Peters (1979) writes "Laetrile, watercress diets, coffee enemas, diets, all give the patient two things. They give him hope, and they give him control over his own body. He is doing something actively for himself, to himself. If the medical profession gives up hope, doesn't want to give away control, the patient is going to find hope somewhere else, control somewhere else"(p. 36).

Some physicians may escape their responsibility by denying that a patient's death appears imminent. They may claim "heavy patient load" or "home obligations" to explain their reluctance to spend time with the patient. Others may employ anger as a defense against anxiety, particularly if such anger can be channeled toward the "enemy," the disease. This phenomenon, called displacement, lets the physician blame the patient's death on external circumstances such as overwhelming disease, patient delay in seeking help, or hospital bureaucracy. Displacement allows the physician and often the nurse to confront the death without relating it to personal failure. Since society may erroneously equate death with medical failure, this defense may protect the physician or nurse, both of whom see all too many deaths, against constant blows to their self-esteem (Artiss & Levine, 1973, p. 107).

THE LANGUAGE OF TRUTH

Explanations, to be understandable, must deal with medical and pathological concepts in terms that the intelligent layman can comprehend. The professional must resist the temptation to hide behind a terminological barrage. This is true whether it is a question of giving a diagnosis in a hopeful situation or of confirming a poor prognosis.

What often seems to be professional evasion or even insensitivity may stem from a very real awkwardness in handling a painful disclosure. A college professor described the conference confrontation with his physician one hour before he was discharged:

He did then do essentially what I had asked him to do, that is, to level with me regarding the diagnosis. It was a very hard thing for him to do. If he could have found any way of avoiding telling me, he would have. It was a terribly painful thing for him to have to lay it on the line. But he did. The way in which he did it was kind of staccato, impersonal, matter of fact. This is what the symptoms are, this is the progression of the symptoms. How long do I have to live? Six months to three years.

The only break in his facade was when I asked him to clarify. He had prepared a little speech. But any time I asked him for a little bit more information or a judgment on those facts, I could almost see his shell coming back (Anonymous, 1972, p. 506).

Ways of Telling a Difficult Truth

Howard P. Hogshead (1978), who considers the sensitive delivering of bad news an art, has given suggestions that may aid both the teller and hearer in handling the information. Hogshead emphasizes the need to say nothing that is untrue. He urges us to keep communication an ongoing experience, telling each piece simply, as it occurs, in comprehensible language. He suggests allowing pauses to allow for questions, as well as asking questions to see if what you are saying is clear. One should not argue with denial, Hogshead says. When patients are ready, they will "hear" what they need to hear. Saunders (1978) also implores us never to "assault another person with a truth which [she or he] is not yet ready to handle" (p. 5).

Perceptions in the sick may be less acute, and feelings and emotions may be flattened. Normal modes of reacting to the truth may be influenced by preoccupation with disease. It is important to remember that patients may not react either consistently over a period of time or consistently with their own values to the idea that they are dying. It is important to be aware of these changes in mood and perception and to adjust dialogue to them accordingly.

The decision of what, how, and when to tell a patient his or her prognosis must be based on individual needs and strength. G.W. Milton (1973) discusses the self-willed death. As a general rule, Milton suggests, it is desirable to give patients details of their prognoses. Often enough, however, the truth affects patients adversely. We must carefully and sensitively consider our disclosures, but ultimately patients are responsible for their own response. Milton compares the attitude of self-willed death to the syndrome associated with the primitive practice called "pointing the bone." In this ceremony, a victim, who is aware of the spell being cast, is condemned to death. Victims believe so strongly there is no escape from the spell that they simply give up living. Indifference, withdrawal, and silence finally lead to death.

A similar syndrome can be seen in patients who receive a terminal diagnosis (as well as in some people who are put in nursing homes) and can lead to early and unexplainable death. Milton cautions us to be alert for the patient who, even though she or he has often been cheerful, seems to change overnight. Such patient "lies inert in bed.... He does not seem to be terrified, but is vague, evasive, and shows blank indifference. If asked whether he has any pain, his eyes will avoid contact and he will answer 'No, no pain... everything is fine.' He eats little, does not sleep well, but complains from neither. He does not lament his fate.... He gives the impression of being indifferent" (Milton, 1973, pp. 1435–1436).

Maintaining Hope

It is worth repeating that the real issue is whether or not the hope that is essential to the dyng patient is maintained. No matter how realistic the circumstances of the disease and the impending death, no matter how mature both patients and those around them are in discussing the extent of the disease, no matter how paradoxical it is to say—every person must be granted the privilege of hope. Even to the end, most patients and their families hope for the discovery of a new drug or treatment. This hope should not be forcibly taken away. Such hope is not entirely contrived. There are many times when we do not know precisely how the disease is progressing, or what effect therapies will have.

Yet there is an even deeper level of hope. It is the hope of conciliation with persons from whom the patient has felt estranged. Still deeper is the hope that in the end we may be at peace with ourselves and our God or sense of life's purpose. This is best expressed by Worcester (1961): "It is the patience and the courage and the endurance which must be allowed." Such fulfillment allows the patient his finest form of courage. Death, in such cases is often preceded by a perfect willingness to die. This is most frequently seen when the patient has had good care and when family and caregivers have an opportunity to come to terms with the reality of the illness and to prepare themselves for the changes that will come about when the patient dies. Seeing this adjustment relieves the patient of feelings of guilt and the anticipation of disaster that death, if sudden and unexpected, will cause.

A precise and uncompromising prognosis—in months, days, or weeks—need not be given. A physician, perhaps, needs to say, "You are not a statistic.... You have this illness, but I don't know how much time you have left, so live life everyday as fully as you can. I will always be here to help you. No matter how far (your cancer) progresses, I will not abandon you" (Peters, 1979, p. 34).

Lipton (1978) has found that parents are very comforted to know more about the ending and that hopes "do not entirely hinge upon whether or not the child is saved. Hope he concludes "is also attached to . . . the assurance that the parents can have some control over the end" (p. 59).

When A Child Is Dying

Particularly difficult is the situation of the dying child. The parents may have had forewarning of the seriousness of the disease. Often, however, the disease is leukemia, and the symptoms are not so severe and may have been clearly visible only briefly. The ongoing building of understanding is particularly important in this situation. Foley & McCarthy describe various methods of medical management: Some are vague in communicating with families about diagnosis and prognosis. Others discuss the prognosis realistically but focus families' attention on lengthy and comfortable remissions. Still others emphasize the breakthroughs in research. The experiences of these investigators indicate that describing leukemia and its prognosis honestly and describing the hope of remissions and comfort measures is the most helpful approach in dealing with young patients and their families. "We tell parents," they state, "the seriousness of the situation and offer every suppport possible."

REASONS FOR TELLING THE TRUTH

Patients frequently cope far better with a series of gentle disclosures than professionals predict. In a study of how patients respond to and cope with the information that they are dying, Barney Glaser and Anselm Strauss (1978) carefully studied patients and family members who had varying levels of awareness of the imminence of death—no awareness, suspicion, pretense, total awareness. Although these researchers do not make value judgments about honesty, they interpret their evidence as supportive of the desirability of awareness in most circumstances. They report that people say they want to know and that most fare better after they do know.

Richard A. Kalish (1978) has done some research in which he controlled for socioeconomic differences and found ethnic–cultural variations among groups on the issue of whether a friend should be told she or he is dying. An affirmative answer was given by 60 percent of black respondents, 49 percent of Japanese Americans, 37 percent of Mexican Americans, and 71 percent of "Anglos." There was little sex difference. With respect to age, 59 percent of younger adults, 56 percent of the middle-aged, and 42 percent of the older persons interviewed replied affirmatively. The study also revealed that people are more likely to want to be told that they are dying than to feel that others should be told.

The Need to Talk

Perhaps the most compelling reason for being honest with a patient is addressed by Peters, who at a time when he was fighting cancer himself wrote *From Both Ends of the Stethoscope.*

> The patient always find out the truth, and it is a cruel deception to lie to the patient but you would be surprised how often that is done. The patient may have some things he wants to get done, some very important things in his life, and when he has been deceived you'll alienate him from his doctor and his family because he won't be in on the deception. It is a fatal mistake—a bad one to make. Once you connive you're on the road to everlasting connivance, and it's a bad road (Peters, 1979, p. 36).

Kalish (1970) has listed many sources from which patients may receive input about their conditions other than from the physician. Among these sources are overheard comments; direct statements from other staff, family, or clergy; changes in visitors' behaviors; medical routines and physical status; and self-diagnosis, including reading medical books, record, and charts.

Patients do sometimes learn of their diagnosis by overhearing a discussion. If we are so concerned that patients may not be able to bear the truth, how can we tolerate the possibility that they may hear it in such insensitive ways? These messages, which may be vague or confused, can often cause patients needless apprehension and anxiety. They may then turn to the nurse for clarification.

Those who feel that they cannot acknowledge this new information about the extreme seriousness of their conditions are then left to wonder about changes and are deprived of the explanations of palliation that will correct the discomfort they envision. Not knowing will cause the patient to fantasize about what will happen. More often than not this imagination, free to run wild, will be worse and lonelier than the truth, no matter how painful the latter is. Instead of protecting the patient, as we intended to do by not talking openly, we actually are isolating him or her. Early in the disease process, the patient may be in a mood of high hope to fight the disease, but with second or third hospitalizations the optimism wanes and isolation grows. Friends don't talk about it, the patient doesn't want to burden the family, and the doctor doesn't want to upset the family. Often, therefore, at a time when there is really a need to talk, people are not talking.

The Need to Tell One's Story

One of the most common needs of dying patients is the need to tell what they are feeling. Within many patients who are dying, there is a powerful need to tell their own story. This drive to share with others the feelings and experiences associated with dying may serve an emotionally cathartic function. It may also signify a gesture to immortality in leaving a legacy of information for those who remain behind. Here, it is more important that we *listen* honestly than that we talk. We should be more concerned about how we understand and comprehend than about what we say. One of our most important functions may be to develop in patients enough trust that they choose us to receive their story. For listening well is neither automatic nor necessarily easy. Receiving the story, however, has profoundly important benefits for the staff as well as for patients. In dealing with truth, patients will go through many different stages—alternative moods of withdrawal and warmth, helplessness and self-control, inhibition and expression of emotion. All of these stages are evidenced in the way they feel and talk. It is only with people who have dealt honestly with them throughout the course of the disease that they can do this.

The Effects of Honesty

The physician, nurse, and counselor can also encourage patients to ask questions to which they want answers. When a patient discovers the spread of a symptom, for instance, it is usually a fearful experience. One patient said, "When I discovered the second lump growing in an area which had had maximum therapy of Cobalt 6, I knew it was the beginning of the end." Honesty, therefore, can correct overreaction and overemphasis of something that may or may not be a recurrence. It can negate myths and misconceptions and lessen fears that often are far worse than the reality.

The patient may not be ready, for example, to discuss the entire prognosis but may be able to ask questions and respond with respect to concerns about specific symptoms. Talk of symptoms can of course be a way to avoid more difficult questions, but it can be carried on in such a way as to bring deep reassurance. Attention to a person's symptoms—with an attitude of sensitivity and dedication rather than of pity or indulgence—will relay to the person the message that the discomfort is understood and that something will be done about it.

Other questions concerning anticipated symptoms or the course of the disease process may follow, such as "Will I have pain?" "Will I become unsightly?" "Will it happen in my sleep?" Thus the real questions are gently addressed, and the fear is drained out of the person even as they are articulated (Saunders, 1965).

By honestly answering whatever is genuinely asked, we may help a patient achieve that feeling of security that can enable him or her to face *any* future. Honesty allows the possibility that time may be well used. The time of terminal illness may be one of growth and shared preparation. However, if patients are not informed, and if the circumstances of their lives are hidden from them, that time of lying may mar the memory of good relationships and undermine the health of survivors. Playwright Robert Anderson whose first wife, Phyllis, died in her thirties after a 5-year struggle against breast cancer, writes as follows that the complicated ruses, deceptions, explanations become stressful to maintain. Later the family may feel they have deprived their loved one of the opportunity to share dying with someone (Brody, 1977).

At the time the death becomes a probability, a family can understand that reality, and if the dying patient's family knows she or he will die, grieving frequently begins for that death. This grieving can be helpful if it includes the patient, because the patient is able to settle affairs and to see the value that she or he has to others. If patients do not know what is happening yet see the grief of others, they either undervalue or handle it in suppressive ways. If at the time others are grieving, patients are not—even if this is because they do not know the seriousness of their disease—they may anger others or create distance between themselves and those they love by seeming to act inappropriately. If they do suspect the truth but, because of the lack of openness, do not recognize that others know, they will grieve alone.

HONESTY IN ACTION

The nineteen cancer patients surveyed by Geoffrey Gorer (1965) who died in ignorance of their disease were survived by bereaved families who exhibited much regret and bitterness. Good marriages were thought to have been reduced to "unkindness and falsity by this deception." On the other hand, Hinton (1963) found that the great majority of 102 dying patients in a general ward knew that death was more than likely imminent although no one had told them their prognosis. These two studies, when looked at side by side, present a very disturbing picture. The truth from which the patient is being "protected" is the truth that forces him or her to live in isolation (Saunders, 1965). This results more often than not in a withdrawn and depressed dying person and a family that lacks the communication and support necessary to ease the burden of the impending loss.

Bereavement studies at Harvard have shown that sudden death is far more devastating to survivors than a death that is anticipated and gradual (Darkes, 1978). Colin Murray Parkes (1978) also cites comments by the husband of a longterm resident at St. Christopher's. This man spent eight years visiting the ward and summed up his experience and the experience of St. Christopher's by saying, "By the end of about a week, when they know they won't have any more pain, they begin to live quite happily and face what is to come" (p. 45). Content that everything possible was being done, this couple honestly shared the experience of each stage of the wife's dying.

Whose Responsibility is Honesty?

Patients who suspect the truth but who have not discussed their prognosis with the physician present a serious dilemma for the nurse. By the terminal stage, the nature of the physician–patient relationship has generally been formed: it is either honest or it is not. If it is not honest, the patient, who may need the physician most during this time, may not be able to communicate this need. The patient may even project failure of cure onto the physician. It is therefore appropriate for the team to support honesty. Thus, if the physician is unable to deal honestly with the patient, it becomes the obligation of the team—the nurses, specifically—to address the issue.

Professional Honesty and Patient Denial

It is important to keep in mind that in some cases, although the patient is told the truth, she or he reports otherwise out of denial. Thus the patient may be deprived of the relief afforded by getting feelings out into the open even when medical or nursing personnel are willing to talk. Denial, which may occur in any stage, is the most prominent defense mechanism used by dying patients. They are frequently silent or uncommunicative. Patients may block themselves off from information, thereby jeopardizing their relationships with team members, family, and friends. At this point they begin to feel isolated and rejected, and such feelings are often quite realistic because people give up trying to get through.

The care provider cannot assume that because patients ask no questions, they have none to ask. They may be afraid, because the whole subject has been conveyed to them as too dangerous or frightening. With time, security that needs will be met and a confidence in the care team's concern develops. At this point, any member, nurse, physician, counselor, or volunteer may be suited to hear the first question. Again, this is where the true multidisciplinary team can function so efficiently to keep all those in direct contact with the patient synchronized in information giving. The physician in a supportive team situation may, if she or he prefers not to confront the patient's questions, allow another, such as the nurse or the minister, to do it.

Honesty and the Family

It is also equally important that family be dealt with honestly. Often family conversations are best held in the presence of the patient so that each family member is aware that others know the serious nature of the illness. It relieves each of the burden of believing they shoud tell one another. They can be supportive to one another, and there are fewer differences in the ways family members interpret what is happening. They are able to face learning about the new stages and processes of the disease together. By informing husband, wife, and family members together, each can serve as an advocate and share in decisions.

Often, the nurse can be of the greatest help by supporting information sharing. If the family is aware of the patient's condition—and most are—their real worry is not so much whether the patient will die but the manner of his or her death. The security that the nurse can provide the family through constant attention to detail and assurances for a death that will be as comfortable as possible is immeasurable. Efficiency, when personally applied, is very comforting. The peace of mind brought by the relief that the patient is in the hands of a nurse with substantial experience and training in relief of symptoms is great.

If the family is to be supported through the hard times of terminal illness, it may be necessary to achieve a closeness that is ordinarily unusual outside the family unit or the unit of close friends. It may be appropriate to hold a person's hand or to put an arm around a person who is in deep distress. The honesty one needs to be able to do this will also help one take the necessary detached view of what is really going on.

The effect on patient and family of honest discussions depends on several factors: (1) proper timing, (2) effective communication, (3) an individualized and caring presence, (4) a good and positive attitude toward management, and (5) a hope for control of symptoms resulting in a degree of comfort. The physician and the nurse must, therefore, both reflect compassion as well as honesty. It is optimism tempered by good judgment, not a promise of things that are unobtainable, that maintains a warm, hopeful, compassionate attitude between health care providers and the family.

THE NURSE'S RESPONSIBILITY TO HONESTY

The nurse can provide the physician with valuable information about the patient's attitude, doubts, fears, and ability to understand and cope, thus helping the physician in the task of telling the patient about his or her condition at the appropriate time and in the most sensitive way. The nurse can also provide insights into the ways in which the family will react—with support, denial, or anger. Nursing assessment may be able to predict reactions of fear on the part of the family members that could cause them to change physicians or treatments or to move to other geographic areas. Such reactions should be anticipated, so that the patient does not get caught in the center of a whirlwind debate over "what is best for" him or her.

Remember, too, that it may be the patient who is refusing to deal with the truth, not the doctor. When patients and families have been given a bad prognosis by their physicians, they will sometimes turn to the nurse for contradictory evidence or for proof that the patient is actually getting better. It is wise to find out, if possible, exactly what the patient has been told—preferably in advance of a talk with the patient and to listen carefully to the patient's questions, which may reveal concerns other than the issue of death. Aggressive attention to the progress that can be made in promoting quality of life may turn patients' thoughts from a fatal diagnosis and help to maintain their trust and confidence in the care team. A team or a nurse–physician conference may let the physician know about a patient's denial or about questions the patient is asking. Such a conference may be all that is needed to stimulate physician–patient communication.

The Nurse's Right and Obligation to Disclose the Truth

If communication between patient and physician remains poor, the nurse's role as listener and reliever of fears and anxieties becomes even more important. Rod R. Yarling (1980), in an inquiry directed to the National Joint Practice Commission of American Medical Association (AMA) and the American Nursing Association (ANA), has developed an ethical analysis of the nurse's moral and legal right and obligation to disclose the truth to terminal patients. The article's main points are discussed briefly here, but the reader would be well advised to examine the original article.

Yarling begins by presenting a hypothetical case of a middle-aged woman who has not been told that she has a malignant tumor of the colon that has metastasized. Both the patient's physician and her family have decided not to tell her the truth of her condition. The oncology nurse, of whom she is asking repeated questions, is instructed by the physician to reveal nothing. The head nurse, though aware of the seriousness of the dilemma, advises that it is probably best to abide by the physician's wishes. The oncology nurse is extremely uncomfortable about acting against her own judgment of the patient's best interests and about lying to this woman, who has come to trust her.

Disclosure of Information

In his extensive discussion of this situation, Yarling (1980) raises two basic issues:

- What are the rights of the patient to information about his or her condition in a case of terminal illness?

- Is the disclosure of diagnostic and prognostic information to terminal patients a right and obligation solely of the physician or is it a right and obligation also of the nurse?

Yarling addresses these issues in a series of four points, which are summarized in the next few paragraphs.

Point 1: Patients' legal rights to information.   At this writing, in many states, patients may exercise a legal right to their records only by instituting a law suit against the hospital or doctor involved in their care and by having the records supoenaed for evidence. In the remaining nine states, access to medical records may be limited to the patient's attorney or patients may have access to their own records under particular circumstances. Thus in general, patients do not have the legal right to routine access to their records or to any other mode of information regarding their diagnosis and prognosis.

Point 2: Patients' moral rights to information.   Denying a patient information about his or her terminal disease is equivalent to denying that person the freedom of self-determination. Lying to a patient seriously undermines the patient–professional relationship, which is based on trust. The patient does have a moral right to truthful information, according to Yarling, if she or he requests that information.

Summarizing the first and second points, patients generally do not have a legal right to information; therefore no one can claim a corresponding legal obligation to provide them with information. According to Yarling, patients do have a moral right to information; therefore someone has a corresponding moral obligation to provide it to them.

Point 3: Moral obligation.   Moral obligation, Yarling says, rests on anyone who

- is possessed of information about a patient's prognosis
- has the competence to disclose it
- is requested by the patient to do so

Nurses who fulfill the foregoing conditions find themselves in a dilemma in which *moral responsibility to the patient requires that they give honest answers to questions that they are capable of answering; their traditionally defined responsibility to the physician requires silence and lies; and their legal status is clearly unclear.*

Point 4: The nature of the information.   It is assumed by many that only the physician ought to make the disclosure of a limited prognosis. Certainly the determination of a diagnosis requires medical knowledge. According to Yarling, however, the decision to disclose information is also a psychological and moral one, and the action of telling the patient requires psychosocial skills. Because of this need for combined skills, the position that the decision should be only a medical one is difficult to sustain.

That the information is in the best interests of the individually assessed patient and that the decision to disclose it is not primarily medical but is rather moral has, Yarling points out, direct implications for the qualifications of the decision-maker. The effects of the disclosure which might be anxiety, depression or withdrawal will alter a person's physical state. Neither the physician nor the nurse can claim, by virtue of profession alone, a privileged position with respect to making the judgment.

Clearly, Yarling says, the best possible solution is for those most closely observant of the patient from medical, spiritual, and psychosocial points of view to undertake a careful analysis, reach a consensus, and give the patient a unified message. But if the physician, with or without team input, decides to withhold information that the patient is requesting, the nurse is put in a situation of triple jeopardy: First, the nurse must go against what she or he perceives as morally correct for the patient. Second, the nurse is placed in a position of having to lie, not out of conviction, but out of loyalty to the physician or the institution or—more commonly—out of concern for the security of his or her job. Third, given the nurse's necessarily frequent interaction with the patient, it is the nurse who must live day after day with the deception.

Summary and Guidelines

The professional's moral right to disclose is determined by the following three factors:

- Competence to provide an accurate description of the disease process and possible therapies
- Collaboration with the care team and family
- Rapport with the patient

Either a physician or a nurse who meets these qualifications through shared professional knowledge, team support, communication skills, and sensitivity to patient needs has the moral right to answer questions truthfully. Each should be responsible for assessing how much she or he knows about a patient's physical and psychological status and for acting accordingly. "Collaboration and communication among those responsible for a patient's care are essential to safe, efficient, high quality care" (Yarling, 1980, p. 509).

The preceding analysis indicates that the nurse who responds honestly to the terminal patient's question about his or her condition with accurate information, sensitivity, and the full knowledge of professional colleagues and within a context of trust and support (rapport) is on firm moral ground. At this time there are no clear legal precedents for determining the nurse's liability. Thus Yarling (1980) recommends that the nurse placed in the position we have described make a vigorous, albeit nonthreatening effort to convince the physician who does not wish to disclose an unfavorable prognosis to a patient that the nurse instead should be allowed to undertake this responsibility.

CONCLUSION

There are many truths and many ways of stating each. It is best, through listening, to try to learn the particular truth the patient needs in order to answer his or her most immediate doubt. Truth may be offered in the simplest and kindest way possible and always with the openness that allows the patient to disregard it if it is still too hard a fact to face. If honesty is built into the professional–patient relationship all along, the traumatic "moment of truth" can be softened, and the patient becomes a partner in the course of the treatment and in its results.

Listening is extremely important, perhaps more than telling. One must be alert to understanding the real source of the patient's distress, alert to changes in the character of the patient's relationships, which often result in real or feared isolation. Listening can also enable the professional to discover the anxiety the patient may be experiencing with increasing pain. By listening, the professional can learn about the uniqueness of each patient and thus help the person in more meaningful and relevant ways. The professional can help counteract the common tendency of patients to experience diminished self-esteem and can understand more quickly what factors underlie a particular patient's physical, spiritual, psychological, and social problems.

Rather than impose a "need to be honest" on each person, it is best to wait until patients are secure in their courage to handle the truth. Nearly always that time will come if the opening is gentle. If one is sensitive to patients' coping power, one will sense when they are ready for more information. By this time, if patients ask for the truth, they are seldom unable to receive it. And having encountered the fact of their imminent death, most often they can get on with the business of living out their lives with usefulness and peace of mind.

REFERENCES

Anonymous. Notes of a dying professor. *Nursing Outlook,* 1972, *20,* 506.

Artiss, K., Levine, A. Doctor–patient relations in severe illness. *New England Journal of Medicine,* 1973, *288,* 1210–1214.

Brody, J.E., Holleb, A.I. *You can fight cancer and win.* New York: McGraw-Hill, 1977, pp. 203–204.

Foley, G.V., McCarthy, A.M., The child with leukemia. *American Journal of Nursing,* 1976, *76,* 1115–1122.

Glaser, B.G., & Strauss, A.L. Awareness of dying. Chicago: Aldine, 1965.

Gorer, G. Death, grief and mourning in contemporary Britain. Cresset Press, London. In Saunders, C.M., Telling Patients, *District Nursing,* September, 1965.

Hinton, J.M. The physical and mental distress of the dying. *Quarterly Journal of Medicine,* 1963, *32,* 1–21.

Hogshead, H.P. The art of delivering bad news. In Garfield, C.A., *Psychosocial care of the dying patient.* New York: McGraw-Hill, 1978.

Kalish, R.A. The quest of the dying process. *Omega,* 1970, *1,* 57–59.

Kalish, R.A. A little myth is a dangerous thing: Research in the service of the dying. In Garfield, C.A., *Psychosocial care of the dying patient.* New York: McGraw-Hill, 1978.

Kastenbaum, R. In control. In Garfield, C.A. *Psychosocial care of the dying patient.* New York: McGraw-Hill, 1978.

Kelly, W.D., & Friesan, S.R. Do cancer patients want to be told? *Surgery* 1950, *27,* 822–826.

Kübler-Ross, E. Discussant, Wessler, S., Avioli, L. On death and dying, *Journal of the American Medical Association,* 1972, *221,* 174–179.

Lipton, H. The dying child and the family: the skills of the social worker, in *The Child and Death,* Zahler, O.J.Z., (ed.): St. Louis, C.V. Mosley Co., 1978, pp. 52–71.

Milton, G.W. Self-willed death or the bone pointing syndrome. *The Lancet,* 1973, *1,* pp. 1435–1436.

Parkes, C. Psychological Aspects. In Saunders, C.M., *The management of terminal illness,* London: Arnold Ltd., 1978.

Peters, D. From both ends of the stethoscope. *San Diego Physician,* October 1979, pp. 30–37.

Saunders, C.M. Telling patients. *District Nursing,* September 1965, p. 12.

Saunders, C.M. *The management of terminal disease,* London: Arnold Ltd., 1978(a).

Saunders, C.M. Terminal care. In Garfield, C.A., *Psychosocial care of the dying patient,* New York: McGraw-Hill, 1978(b).

Worcester, A. *The care of the aged, the dying and the dead.* Springfield, Illinois: C.C. Thomas, 1961.

Yarling, R.R. Ethical analysis of a nursing problem: The scope of nursing practice in disclosing the truth in terminal patients. Supervisor Nurse, reprinted in *Hospice Education Program for Nurses,* DHHS Publ. No. HRA, Md., 1981, pp. 81–127.

1. T	6. T
2. T	7. T
3. F	8. T
4. F	9. F
5. T	10. F

3

Understanding the Patient Experience

Answer the following questions True (T) or False (F). Answers appear on the last page of this chapter.

1. *The course of grief normally progresses in strict order, from disbelief to anger to depression to acceptance.*

2. *The physician needs only one session with the patient to explain a terminal prognosis.*

3. *The dying person loses the capacity to make choices and needs others to take over this function.*

4. *The dying person commonly fears pain and choking as death nears.*

5. *The dying person needs to have medical language translated into everyday language.*

6. *Dying people generally understand the physical changes to expect as their disease progresses.*

7. *It is common for the terminally ill to develop new styles of communication as death draws near.*

8. *It is the nurse's responsibility to move a patient from denial into open awareness.*

9. *Expressing grief over loss of a limb uses different coping mechanisms from those used in expressing grief over loss of life.*

10. *Most dying people would learn well if classes were arranged for them explaining details of their disease and diagnostic tests.*

*It turns out you can live a lifetime in a day; you can live a lifetime in a moment;
you can live a lifetime in a year.... I don't think people are afraid of death. What
they are afraid of is the incompleteness of their life.**

THIS CHAPTER describes the process of learning to know people who
are dying, to understand their experiences, and to help them with common
struggles. Caregivers must be willing to see the dying person as a fellow
traveler in life, passing down the same final path that will confront us all one
day. Caregivers need to learn how to listen attentively, how to handle the first
encounter with a terminal diagnosis, how to encourage realistic hope, and
how to empower the dying person by encouraging strong identity, active
decision making, and learning. The patient is best understood and continuity
is facilitated when a primary nurse and a primary physician each develop
strong ongoing relationships with and accountability to the patient, listen
carefully to him or her, and develop a plan of care accordingly.

LISTENING AND UNDERSTANDING

The dying person has often lived through a time of illness, progressive
debilitation, and the tremendous emotional strain that accompanies any
life-threatening situation. Most have experienced extensive diagnostic testing;
aggressive treatment that may have included surgeries, radiation, drugs, and
medical regimens they have endured with difficulty; and progressive dependency on a long parade of professional and nonprofessional workers. Their
medical experience is too often a dehumanization process that robs people of
their identity. The only way to know people's identity is to listen to them tell
you who they are. *There is no greater gift you can give a person than to sit
down and listen to his or her story.* This attention is one of the most magical
aspects of the hospice movement, where it has become an integral element of
care.

---

*From Rosenthal, T., *How Could I Not Be Among You?* New York: G. Braziller, 1973.

Table 3-1. *Elements of Attentive Listening*

- Being comfortable with silence.

- Using a warm yet clearly audible tone of voice.

- Using open questions that give the patient a broad opportunity for response.

- Avoiding interruptions.

- Using encouraging nonverbal behaviors with which the patient is comfortable. Eye contact, touching, nodding, and physical closeness may encourage some people, whereas others may withdraw; individual reaction must be determined.

- Being aware of both verbal and nonverbal messages transmitted by the patient.

- Offering the patient an accurate summary of these messages.

- Encouraging the patient to validate or change this summary.

Active listening enables the patient to express his or her perceptions and feelings and demonstrates the listener's concern and respect for the person. Understanding and trust develop over time. Some patients may choose not to express themselves, but regularly "setting the stage" even if the "play" never goes on will build trust over time.

Table 3-1 lists the essential elements in listening attentively and encouraging verbalization. These elements become the foundation for an ongoing helping relationship wherein the dying person is heard, has a continual opportunity to reflect on his or her experience, and knows that feelings and perceptions can be expressed and acknowledged.

A TERMINAL DIAGNOSIS

At some point, patients note that their disease is assuming increasing power in their lives, progressively draining energy and impairing normal activity. Physicians become aware that there is no longer any reasonable hope of curing or controlling the spread of disease, and patients' conditions are expected to deteriorate despite the best treatment. People in this situation are terminally ill and dying.

Telling the Patient

There is no common definition of the state we label *terminal,* when a person is recognized as dying. Physicians vary in their judgment of the situation and in what they tell patient and family. It is always desirable to ask the patient early in the course of illness or diagnosis, "How much do you want to know if the news is bad? What do you want your family to know?" An explanation of terminal status should emphasize that comfort and support are now the goals. This is in contrast to the familiar traditional statement, "There is nothing more we can do for you now."

A patient should have several conversations with the physician to clarify the doctor's conclusions, ask questions, and explore personal implications. Many times the news will be so overwhelming that a person will respond with emotional shock, and perhaps forget all or part of what the physician has said. Thus there should be several sessions with the physician until the facts are clear and understood by the patient. In reality, it is the nurse who does most of the followup exploration with the patient after the physician initially presents the news. This is true because of the nurse's more ready presence at the patient's side when or if the patient is ready to begin open discussion and conscious planning.

Many people want to know how much time they have left, especially if they want to use the time well. This is a question that cannot be answered with certainty. A wise professional offers a prediction that covers a broad range of expectancy based on the typical course of the particular illness, and always leaves room for exceptions. A dying person is often left in the paradoxical situation of needing to get his or her "house in order" while leaving room for life and unexpected "stays of execution."

Some people are not told that they are terminally ill even when it has become increasingly obvious to everyone that their condition is deteriorating. In these cases, the focus of attention rests in trying one more treatment, changing medication, or calling in another specialist. This situation is more likely to develop if the team providing care are involved in high technology medicine or if they consider each patient death a personal failure. It then becomes the paradoxical burden of the patient or family to confront professionals with obvious reality, and to make their wishes known. One may hope that nurses will increasingly function as patients' advocates in this process. *Those who are not informed about their life-threatening situation are wrongly denied their right to choose the way they will end their lifetime. They live out their final moments with last words unspoken and tensions unresolved.* They are abandoned to the false illusion of a technological solution to ultimate human mortality. The focus is on a medical answer until the last resuscitation fails.

Note that although modern thinking favors honesty and disclosure, some dying persons *do* choose not to confront their deaths openly. They should of course be allowed to follow the approach that gives them comfort.

Facing Losses that Precede Death

The dying person faces an overwhelming series of changes and losses of self. Many fear these "little deaths" more than death itself.

Loss of body functions is often progressive but may also come suddenly. Nothing can be taken for granted: walking, eating, breathing, sleeping, going to the bathroom, and countless other activities may be compromised. The boat is being taken over by a mutiny and the course charted is unknown. The person becomes progressively more dependent on others for performance of basic functions. Body parts are often lost (mastectomy, amputations, colostomy) or dramatically altered in appearance due to illness or therapy. The exterior surface of the body is changed due to problems such as fluid retention, muscle wasting, hair loss, pallor, or jaundice. One of my patients lost over 100 pounds in one year. In a deodorized society, the bad smells of a deteriorating, malfunctioning body can be one of the greatest burdens of all.

Equally dramatic may be the loss of social or interpersonal functioning brought about not only by change in physical capacity to perform roles but by fear and withdrawal or overprotection by others that progressively isolates the person. Friendships, sexual relationships, marital relationships, parental relationships, work and community functions are all impaired by reduced physical capacity. Too often these are given up in despair, rather than modified within the continuing capacity of the person to be involved. Friends can share new, slower satisfactions and meanings; intimacy and sensuality can be enhanced, not lost, until the moment of death; parents and children can share simple experiences (a hug, a picture, a tape recording) that can remain with the survivors for a lifetime; and mechanisms for social usefulness can often be worked out with those interested.

The losses described may often be reflected in nursing diagnoses of disturbance in body image, self-esteem, role performance, and personal identity. The patient responds with grief to these losses with the process and coping mechanisms described in the following section on normal grief. Nursing therapy focuses on listening, encouraging expression of grief, maintaining the person's dignity in performing functions that she or he can no longer manage independently, and creative problem-solving with patient and family to enhance remaining abilities and develop alternatively satisfying roles and choices.

Case Example: Diminished Body Image and Role Performance

A 26-year-old woman is admitted to your home health agency for terminal care. She has been told, two weeks earlier, that her two-year battle against osteosarcoma is over. The physician has no more therapy to recommend. The patient has lost her right arm at the shoulder. Her left anterior chest wall is covered with visible tumors, and new lumps seem to appear here and in the axilla every day. She has extensive lung and pleural metastases. Pain is controlled after your recommendation to start methadone 5–10 mg. through her Hickman catheter every 4 to 6 hours. She is receiving one liter daily of dextrose and saline at her request "because I have so much left to do." She is living with her sister while her husband and four-year-old daughter live thirty miles away.

List all the ways you can think of that might enhance this woman's body image and her role performance in the remaining weeks. Just brainstorm without being limited by thoughts of all the possible obstacles to the ideas you generate.

Normal Grief

Grief is the human reaction to loss that occurs regularly throughout life with the identity changes that occur developmentally; with separation from and loss of loved people; with changes in home, work, and environment; with deteriorating health; and in the face of one's own death. The components of the experience are the same, but vary in intensity from, perhaps, mild disorganization and anger when moving to a new neighborhood to the engulfing emotions of losing one's own life or that of a loved one. Responses to grief are quite individualized, and they are not seen in discrete sequential stages; rather most people tend to shift back and forth in their use of coping mechanisms. The common initial reaction to loss or news of impending loss is shock and denial; emotions are numbed, and affect may be flat. Some people die too quickly to move beyond this phase. On the other hand, denial may be prolonged in certain individuals. Our culture tends to deny death and grief. Prolonged denial in the dying person is exhausting to patient and caregiver and prevents release of energy for communication or creative resolution of issues. For most people, awareness of reality emerges, though denial continues to be used as an intermittent or concurrent protective device. Awareness brings intense sadness and crying, anger, guilt, bargaining, and— ideally—resolution. People respond to loss as they have responded to prior losses. Those who have avoided expressing grief before will often go this path again. Those used to weeping and raging and talking about their suffering are likely to proceed to a level of acceptance that allows them hope and conscious decision making. Individual response to grief is profoundly influenced by cultural heritage. Patterns of coping with death and dying that are traditional in particular ethnic subgroups are affected significantly and sometimes unpredictably by encounter with the American mainstream.

When the nursing diagnosis is *grieving,* nursing therapy focuses on grief counseling, teaching patient and family to recognize normal grief process in themselves and others, and affirmation of all healthy behavior. Grief counseling fosters expression of thoughts and feelings, and such expression allows movement toward resolution and acceptance of loss. This must be done with great sensitivity to personal, cultural, and familial history. Individual patient counseling to assist movement through normal and dysfunctional grief is explored more fully in Chapter 10.

HOPE

There are two kinds of hope in a person who has been diagnosed as dying. There is hope for longer life, despite contrary medical facts, and there is hope for good quality of life in the time remaining.

Length or Quality of Life

Human beings cling ferociously to their hopes for long life. "It can't be true" is a natural reaction to hearing a terminal prognosis. Even as the individual moves through grief to a resolution, she or he may confuse us by expressing hope for cure at one moment, then calmly making funeral plans at another moment. *Everyday reality for most dying people is living somewhere between acceptance of death and hope for improvement and longer life.* As has been noted, some will never outwardly acknowledge their own dying and place continual hope in long life, perhaps buying a day at a time as they fail.

Remember that medical predictions are not infallible; they do not leave room for the workings of the unknown. The power of mind and spirit over body cannot be disregarded. The respected medical practice of Carl Simonton and the counseling practice of Stephanie Matthews-Simonton have demonstrated dramatic improvements in those people diagnosed terminal who commit themselves to dramatic change in lifestyle to emphasize wellness, positive thinking, and active use of imagination (Simonton, 1978). Conscious choice of a sick role over a healthy role is significant in determining when and how death occurs. Every once in a while, a patient who has the "terminal" stamp from a competent physician simply refuses to die on schedule.

As dying becomes more certain, the definition of hope changes to hope for good quality of life in the time remaining. Good quality of life includes relief from fear, symptom relief, and the power to choose how to live at the end of a lifetime. Many people choose to make the experience as normal as possible and to maintain "business as usual" in their personal lives for as long as they can. Some choose to live more intensely, or more consciously.

Fear

Dying is a fearful experience. People fear the gradual loss of themselves as has been described: changed body image and function, weakness and deterioration, loss of roles and relationships. They fear the gradual slipping away of identity until death itself takes identity as it is known in this life. Fear of the unknown is great and may be alleviated by information and planning, though death itself remains the ultimate unknown. Loss of personal power in the dying process is a major source of fear, as will be discussed in the next section. The most frequent fear expressed by the patients in one large, home hospice program is that of uncontrolled suffering: pain, choking, strangling, seizures, violent upheaval at the time of death. Other fears expressed most commonly include the experience of death itself, fears about the reactions of other family members, and fears about the well-being of those who will survive. Not surprisingly, these patients express great need for around the clock availability of health professionals to help with problems, and they want ongoing information about changes in their condition and what they mean (Schubert, 1982).

When the nursing diagnosis is *fear,* therapy focuses on realistic hope to maximize function and relationships, to maintain identity and respect, to know what is happening to oneself, to retain control of one's own life and make choices, to have physical symptoms well controlled and help nearby, and to have good times. The rest of this chapter develops some tools that the nurse can use to turn such hopes into realities.

EMPOWERING THE DYING PERSON

The ideals of Western society encourage the development of an individual's sense of power, but institutional power and hierarchical authority often discourage people from feeling powerful in their everyday life. "Recent research has shown that as many as eighty per cent of us will comply with an unreasonable request without objecting" (Alberti, 1975). As a result, large numbers of people withdraw from self-assertion without ever developing a clear identity with definite opinions. "It's safer to be passive, childish, always waiting for the cue from others, but then you have become a shadow" (Newman, 1977). With a nursing diagnosis of *power deficit,* the approach focuses on ways of encouraging the development of identity and decisions.

Methods to Strengthen Identity

The end of a lifetime is the last chance to follow that ancient admonition, "Know yourself." We can assist patients to know themselves by helping them identify the values and strengths on which they can build. Ask patients what they believe in, what values have guided their lives; ask what they like most about themselves. Encourage them to describe their proudest moments, and to look at the qualities that have contributed to their best image of themselves.

Encourage patients to explore their past, with an active effort to forgive themselves and others and to unbind themselves from immobilizing past resentments and preoccupations with failures of others and of self. People may choose to write letters of forgiveness or apology, to meet with people to reconcile past resentments, to role-play statements of forgiveness with a helping person, or to confess past guilts and to seek assurance of ultimate forgiveness from clergy.

One of the most useful ways to facilitate a strong sense of identity is to encourage people to verbalize their life stories. You can encourage patients to explore their life stories by asking them about the generations before them, about their parents, their own childhoods. Suggest that they recall the landmarks of growing up, the milestones of their adult lives. Ask what they would like to do again, what they consider their greatest blessings, what in their lives remains unresolved.

One useful technique for self-discovery is to begin a journal or diary. In a journal, people can actually write down their life review. They can go through their life history and include key people and events. Some may choose to record the events of everyday life and possibly to examine the quality of the experience and what might be changed. Some people may wish to include a place in the journal for feelings and reactions, but they should avoid criticizing and analyzing themselves. Exploring feelings by writing spontaneously without self-judgment can significantly foster self-awareness. You may want to look at Ira Progoff's *At a Journal Workshop* (1975) to see if the approach Progoff describes may be useful for your patients.

Some people may choose to use a tape recorder, or to deliberately organize photograph albums so as to review the past and capture the present. Recordings, albums, and journals can be a meaningful legacy for survivors.

Meditation helps many people toward a greater consciousness of each moment in life. Those who make this a regular discipline find that they are better able to pay attention to life and to let the distractions float by. Those who meditate can develop a broad awareness of themselves in an existence filled with the wonder of daily life and appreciation of its blessings. See Chapter 7 for a brief description of basic meditation and relaxation practices.

Discovering others

Some patients may develop a growing openness to others as well as to themselves. There can be a willingness to reach out in joy and sorrow, love and anger. That willingness replaces the masked ball, where we all move around each other [in masks and] as caricatures, extending pleasantries and often bearing hidden resentments. It takes great courage to be known as we really are, and to know others unmasked. Practice begins with actively listening, not interrupting, and nurses can serve as facilitators for those who want to improve their relationships with family and friends.

Decision Making

The ending of a lifetime brings the opportunity and necessity for many decisions. Those who have made an effort to know their own minds will find it easier to know their preferences at the end of a lifetime. Most people are able to be actively involved in choices about life and treatment until they are very close to death, yet few possess the tools to make those choices. If we do not encourage and support dying people in making their own decisions, these decisions will be made for them by the course of their illness and at the convenience of strangers and institutions. There are a great many decisions that a patient can make. They range from what form of treatment to choose to how to live one's remaining everyday life. Table 3-2 contains just a partial list of choices the dying may need and wish to make.

Table 3-2   *Choices for the Dying*

- Should I take this diagnosis seriously or disregard it and try to go about business as usual?
- Should I ask for other opinions?
- Should I try nonconventional therapies?
- Should I accept treatment to prolong my life?
- What side effects of treatment am I willing to put up with?
- With whom will I discuss my decisions?
- Should I continue my daily life without change as long as I am able?
- What parts of my life are most important to me?
- What people do I want to be with?
- Do I want to make changes in the way I am living?
- Do I want to live more consciously?
- Do I want to change relationships with people?
- Do I want to deepen my spiritual life?
- Where do I want to die? What resources need to be found to care for and comfort me?
- What support can those I love offer me?
- What are my final wishes regarding ceremonies, my body, and my possessions after death?
- What unfinished business do I have? Do I want to finish it?
- What legacy can I leave my loved ones?

Active choice involves first deciding what one really wants, and then figuring out how to get there. Encourage dying people who are beginning to develop awareness of their prognosis to express *goals desired.* Encourage them to write a list of everything they want, even the most ridiculous things. Over days or weeks, you can help patients sort out and revise until they arrive at a list of perhaps ten or fewer items that can be accomplished in the near future. Help people formulate goals that can be achieved despite the limitations of finance and infirmity. Those people with very limited energy will need special assistance to determine priorities and set achievable short-term goals. Those with more energy and a longer prognosis can realistically identify broader goals.

Case Example: Mother with Hodgkin's Disease

A 40-year-old divorced mother with Stage Four Hodgkin's Disease identified the following realistic short-term goals:

- Ask to see a doctor at the University before taking all the drugs they say I should have.
- Spend more time with Connie and Ellen (friends).
- Ask the junior high school if they could find a counselor who knows how to help kids if their mother is dying.
- Read to Howard and Keith (her children) every night before bed, like we used to.
- Take a hot bath every night.
- Find out what vegetables might grow on the porch, since I don't see how I'm going to get out in the garden this year.
- Ask Aunt Lucy to see if she would come and live with us for a while.
- Maybe Mark (friend) could start giving me regular backrubs.
- Write to the Memorial Society for literature.

It is especially valuable to guide the person to focus on those day-to-day choices of pleasant moments that bring joy. Assist patient, family, and friends to identify simply energizing activities, like those in Table 3-3, that best fit the individual's own life situation.

Table 3-3.   *Energy Sources*

Walking in the woods	Eating good food
Visiting the zoo	Being free to set one's own schedule
Working in the garden	Having a good cry
Painting a picture	Cooperating
Pounding nails	Doing something with a friend
Being with friends*	Having a good argument
Enjoying peace and quiet*	Being courageous
Dancing	Enjoying a good sleep*
Reading a good book	Sharing laughter*
Taking a vacation	Seeing a good movie
Communing with God*	Listening to a good concert
Being accepted by others*	Going to a sports event
Cooking	Having someone seeking my advice
Playing ball	Swimming
Hugging someone*	Driving in the country
Being in pleasant surroundings	Walking on the beach
Forgiving myself*	Sewing
Listening to music*	Writing
Meditating	Repairing something
Making love	Singing
Making an important decision	Helping someone
Loving and being close to others*	Soaking in the tub
Drinking wine*	Smelling a flower*
Having a good backrub*	Touching someone*

Source: Adapted from Savary, L., & Berne, P. *Prayer ways. San Francisco: Harper and Row, 1980. With permission.*
*Require minimal energy output

Setting goals is the first step, but achieving them is more difficult. The patient can be assisted in developing *plans of action* to reach each goal; identifying *obstacles* that might be encountered along the way and ways of dealing with them; identifying ways that she or he might create obstacles (*sabotage* the plan) rather than face the risk of success; and determining a *timeline,* or helping the patient to manage his or her time (Miller, 1981). Some people find it useful to identify the way they are actually using each hour of the day, perhaps recording their activities over several days, and comparing the result with a list of the activities they value most. As energy wanes and disease and treatment dominate time, it becomes more and more important for the nurse to help the patient to clarify priorities and decide to delegate some activities to other people in order to pursue those that are most highly valued.

Remember that active decision making at the end of life requires going against a more passive, childlike role that may have brought security in the past. In particular, the sick role conventionally demands submission to medical authority. The patient must make the switch from the enforced dependency of the sick role to the greater autonomy of the dying role in which the final tasks of life must be resolved (Williams, 1982). The health professional should of course be a partner and consultant to the patient as she or he completes these final tasks, not an authoritarian taskmaster.

If people are to gain renewed confidence in helping themselves and making active choices, they often will need support in asserting themselves. Three basic techniques used in assertiveness training to facilitate self-assertion are (1) modeling assertive behavior for the client, (2) encouraging the client to role-play critical situations in which she or he can practice assertive behavior, and (3) supporting the client's testing of assertion in reality and providing an opportunity for review of this test afterward (Alberti, 1975).

Case Example: Grandfather Asserted Himself

Casey McIntire, a 76-year-old widower, lived with his 50-year-old daughter, Dorothy, and son-in-law. He had had a colostomy for a diagnosis of colon cancer 1½ years beforehand. The tumor extended into the retroperitoneum and bladder. He was suffering extensive lower extremity edema and draining fecal material through a Foley catheter when his daughter urged Casey to consult with an oncologist performing a new type of aggressive combination chemotherapy.

On the day that stool first appeared in his urine, Casey informed the staff nurse of his decision to seek no more therapy. Yet he knew his family wanted him to fight, "Maybe I'll have to do what Dorothy wants. She's so afraid to think of me passing on." The nurse offered to role play Dorothy as he tested various words to explain his choice. He also explored with the nurse the best timing for discussion with Dorothy. The nurse returned two days later to see if the plan worked. After tears and anger, Dorothy and her husband had accepted those words that Casey had been practicing, "I can't take those drugs to make you feel good. I have to do what's best for me."

Getting Information

Lack of knowledge and lack of opportunity to learn continues to be a major problem for the consumer throughout the entire health care system. Consumers are demanding more information, but they are not equipped to make optimal use of it. Lacking an understanding of normal anatomy and physiology, a particular disease and its course, treatment possibilities, treatment risks and benefits, and normal human reactions to illness and loss, the dying person is limited in his or her ability to make choices. It is therefore essential that nurses, the professionals most frequently at the patient's side, become skilled in teaching strategies to promote learning by people under high stress. Knowledge reduces fear of the unknown and empowers people to take control of their own lives and their own care. At the same time, fear can inhibit the acquisition of information. Learning occurs at the patient's own pace.

The Oncology Nursing Society and the American Nurses Association Division on Medical Surgical Nursing have published standards for the outcome of nursing practice that focus on the teaching role. These standards state that the client and family must possess knowledge about the disease and therapy in order to attain self-management, participation in therapy, optimal living, and peaceful death (Oncology Nursing Society, 1979).

A teaching relationship begins with attentive listening to assess the person's knowledge, concerns, and motivation for understanding and self-care. Learning objectives are stated not in terms of what the nurse teaches, but rather in terms of how the learner behaves following the teaching, in terms of his or her *own* goals. Thus the outcomes of the teaching relationship are measurable; see Table 3-4 for criteria put forth by the ONS and ANA.

The teaching process must be modified for the dying person to allow for his or her high level of stress and fear, intermittent denial, exhaustion, and ongoing battle with physical symptoms. *One-to-one discussion with trusted caregivers is the most reliable teaching method.* Patients need to gradually absorb information and clarify the implications for themselves. Threatening information is often explored bit by bit. Repetition is essential as the patient draws courage to put the pieces together. Often the patient's condition and the treatment options are in a stage of flux. Physicians speak in terms of this therapy or that procedure affecting the results of this blood test or that scan. Patients can be at a loss to understand the implications of medical jargon for their living and dying. With ongoing change in status, *nurses can sift through and interpret medical information to make it relevant to the experience and decision of the patient.* They can translate medical language into human terms. They can equip the patient to ask relevant questions and they can clarify information from the physician and other specialists.

Table 3-4. *Outcome Criteria for Patient–Family Teaching*

Client and family should be able to—

- Describe the state of the disease and therapy at a level consistent with their intellectual and emotional states

- Participate in the decision-making process pertaining to the plan of care and life activities

- Identify appropriate community and personal resources that would provide information services

- Describe appropriate actions for highly predictable problems, oncological emergencies, and major side effects of disease or therapy

- Describe the schedule when ongoing therapy is predicted

- Describe plans for integrating valued actitivies into daily life

Source: Oncology Nursing Society, American Nurses' Association Division on Medical–Surgical Nursing Practice. *Outcome standards for cancer nursing practice.* Kansas City: American Nurses' Association, 1979. With permission.

Case Example:

A 48-year-old, single, high school history teacher had a modified radical mastectomy with two positive nodes. She underwent a course of Cytoxan, Methotrexate, and 5FU. There were no signs of disease until almost four years later, when she presented with right upper quadrant pain. Workup revealed widely metastatic disease, involving the liver, parietal skull, two anterior ribs, left femoral head, and cervical and thoracic spine. The patient was treated with radiation to the ribs and lumbosacral spine.

Currently, this woman is receiving Tamoxifen po bid., and every three weeks intravenous cycles of Cytoxan, Adriamycin, and 5FU. The chemotherapy dose that causes tumor response is also causing significant bone marrow depression. The patient has twice been placed in protective isolation for severe neutropenia, and she continues to have a low grade fever of unknown origin. The doctor has told her that it is his goal for her to go back to work. When she asks how she is responding to treatment, he speaks in terms of lowered billirubin and calcium levels and says "we'll see after the next treatment." The patient is to be readmitted if her fever goes over 101° F. She is puzzled about how to plan for her future and has asked for clarification and information in a family conference with the nurse and social worker next week.

What are the issues here? How might you proceed to increase this woman's understanding and ability to make decisions? What would you do at the family conference? How else could you encourage her personal power?

Group learning experiences can be valuable for those extraverted people who have previously coped with stress in their lives by seeking out others in mutually supportive ways. Such patients may welcome attending group teaching sessions on a wide variety of topics while they are in the hospital. Community groups such as Make Today Count or Can Surmount provide patients an opportunity for acquiring information about life-threatening disease, therapy options, and coping skills while offering each other emotional and social support.

Written materials are always valuable teaching tools, but their use must be geared thoughtfully to an assessment of the patient's previous experience with learning by means of the written word. Some people who are not oriented toward the written word do well with simple, straightforward written summaries that reinforce facts or instructions presented orally. Such sum-maries should be individualized, and the person should not be given pamphlets and information sheets if the nurse judges that general information might confuse or distract from practical understanding. Many patients appreciate the use of informational sheets and pamphlets to reinforce learning; they should never be used, however, without opportunity for one-to-one discussion. An increasing number of books and pamphlets are available for readers to increase the understanding of those with life-threatening illnesses. A few of these resources are included in the list of references at the end of this chapter. Some people will appreciate the opportunity to read personal accounts of others with terminal diagnoses.

REALISTIC EXPECTATION

Readers who are hoping for great transformations in people they want to help must be reminded that people generally die in the same style that they have lived. When a person copes by silence or by doing business as usual or by never giving up hope for a long life, those choices are valid options and demand respect from those of us who believe in freedom to choose. Given time and energy, some dying people may wish to make deliberate plans for the end of their lifetime. Whatever their choice, we help most by standing by to offer aid in whatever way they will allow, on their own terms.

REFERENCES

Alberti, R., & Emmons, M. *Stand up, speak out, talk back.* New York: Pocket Books, 1975.

Duda, D. *A guide to dying at home.* Santa Fe, New Mexico: John Muir, 1982.

Krementz, J. *How it feels when a parent dies.* New York: Knopf, 1981.

Kübler-Ross, E. *Death: The final stage of growth.* New Jersey: Prentice-Hall, 1975.

LeShan, E. *Learning to say goodbye: When a parent dies.* New York: Avon, 1981.

McCloskey, J.C. How to make the most of body image theory in nursing practice. *Nursing,* 1976, *76*, 68–72.

Miller, G.P. *Life choices.* New York: Bantam, 1981.

Miller, W. *When going to pieces holds you together.* Minneapolis: Augsburg, 1976.

Moldow, D.G., & Martinson, I.M. *Home care for dying children: A manual for parents.* Minneapolis: University of Minnesota Press, 1979.

Newman, M., & Berkowitz, B. *How to take charge of your life.* New York: Harcourt Brace, 1977.

Oncology Nursing Society, American Nurses' Association Division on Medical–Surgical Nursing Practice. *Outcome standards for cancer nursing practice.* Kansas City: American Nurses' Association, 1979.

Progoff, I. *At a journal workshop.* New York: Dialogue House, 1975.

Savary, I., & Berne, P. *Prayerways.* San Francisco: Harper and Row, 1980.

Schubert, V. *Anticipatory guidance for family caregivers to manage the last few days at home.* Presented at Hospice of Seattle Advanced Symposium on Care of the Terminally Ill, Seattle, February 26, 1982.

Simonton, O.C. *Getting well again.* New York: Bantam, 1978.

Williams, C. Role considerations in care of the dying patient. *Image,* 1982, *14,* 8–11.

1.	*F*	*6.*	*F*
2.	*F*	*7.*	*F*
3.	*F*	*8.*	*F*
4.	*T*	*9.*	*F*
5.	*T*	*10.*	*F*

4

Assessment and Goals of Care

Answer the following questions True (T) or False (F). Answers appear on the last page of this chapter.

1. *Assessment of functions should be limited to those measurements that are necessary to determine specific palliative measurements or to understand the course of the dying process.*

2. *Frequent blood drawing for complete blood counts and chemistries is essential to conscientious management of terminal patients.*

3. *A comprehensive psychosocial evaluation of the patient and family is possible at first assessment.*

4. *Assessment of the cultural dimension and support network should include inquiry about coping during earlier periods of stress.*

5. *Spiritual assessment focuses primarily on past and present church or temple attendance.*

6. *Anger, denial, powerlessness, and isolation are common hospice psychosocial diagnoses.*

7. *Hospice care patient goals are determined by listing for the family the capabilities of the agency.*

8. *Negotiating goals when family members are in conflict involves bringing about a compromise that incorporates each member's position.*

9. *Anticipatory guidance can minimize crises during the downhill course.*

10. *Some people will choose not to contract for hospice care if they perceive that that decision implies giving up the option of curative care.*

The ultimate truth is one, but it is given to man only as it enters, reflected as in a prism, into the true life relationships of human persons. We have it, and yet have it not, in its multicoloured reflection.*

EFFECTIVE CARE of the terminally ill and their families is based on a comprehensive assessment and goal-setting process that seeks to reflect the multidimensional nature of both patient and family. The process is ongoing, as each encounter improves our vision of the whole person and situation. The first encounter generally occurs with admission into the hospice program. From the beginning, the patient's choices and priorities are paramount considerations.

ADMISSION

The patient who is referred for hospice care and meets admission criteria must decide during first encounters whether to choose hospice care. In so doing, the patient is effectively choosing where to live and die.

Referral

Anyone should be able to make a hospice referral: the patient, friends, family, relatives, physician, or health and social service professionals. No referral should be seriously considered, however, until patient and/or family have been given a clear description of services available and goals, and until they have given their consent to at least an initial evaluation by the hospice team. Some will be unnecessarily threatened by the description of a team "to help the dying" and will be better served by description of "a group to help those with life-threatening illnesses" or "to provide practical emotional and physical help for those with advanced illnesses."

Admission criteria generally include patient–family consent to care;

---

*Buber, M. *Pointing the Way*. New York: Harper and Brothers, 1957.

46

physician approval; limited life expectancy, when cure is no longer considered a realistic outcome (a 6-months prognosis is commonly identified); determination by staff that medical, nursing, and/or psychological needs require skilled intervention; and determination of a reimbursement mechanism. For home care, the presence of a primary caregiver in the home who will take responsibility is usually essential. However, some people choose hospice help to stay at home alone as long as possible, although eventually physical distress and the safety hazards imposed by immobility will necessitate that they leave home or find help. Often such patients will acknowledge their need only when crisis compels.

Initial Evaluation and Decision

The initial contact with a hospice team member involves patient and team member "eyeballing" each other and coming to some conclusions about what each brings to the situation. Nursing assessment and determination of goals begin at this time. The nurse's primary tool at this meeting is active listening followed by reflection of his or her understanding of the patient-family experience (see Chapter 3). The nurse is attentive to the likelihood of limited patient energy and focuses on concerns that require immediate help. She or he provides concrete specific information to patient and family about the hospice services available and about how the particular patient and family might make use of them. The capabilities of nursing are conventionally poorly understood and underestimated in our society, so the nurse needs to be explicit and not too humble about exactly what she or he can offer. Examples from outcomes achieved with other cases can be very helpful to help prospective patients and families understand those services for which they are contracting.

The decision to choose hospice care is complex. It is made on the basis of people's awareness of their own needs and their perception of the hospice program as having the ability to respond to those needs. To the degree that people understand the hospice program as a program to care for the dying, they will have to ask themselves whether they must "give up," and, by accepting such care, seek palliation only. Indeed, each hospice program must choose whether to be involved with those who have end-stage, life-threatening illness but are ignorant or in denial of their dying, or actively choose to fight for life. The following two cases show how some of these questions arise in the choice of hospice help.

Case Example: Rejection of Hospice Help

Mr. and Mrs. Chang are lawyers. Following multiple myocardial infarctions and an unsuccessful coronary artery bypass, Mr. Chang, age 54, is in congestive heart failure that is not responding to diuretics. His primary nurse refers his wife to the hospital hospice team. The hospice nurse's first contact is with Mrs. Chang in the hospital lounge. Mrs. Chang describes her husband as a "strong, proud man" who had risen rapidly in his profession until his first MI five years ago. She is working full time, and there are two adult children in another city. Mr. Chang expects his wife to stay at his side in the hospital. She sleeps in the chair.

After the nurse introduces herself, Mrs. Chang notes that she has seen a television program describing the hospice movement. The nurse proposes a tentative plan of help to include emotional and spiritual counseling, improved control of the presenting symptoms of dyspnea and persistent chest pain by consulting with the primary physician and nurses, and teaching the couple how to manage the disease and prevent symptomatic crises. Mrs. Chang congenially denies that her husband is "bad enough for hospice." "Maybe later," she says. Her goal is to have no one "upset" her husband. Hospice care is postponed—perhaps forever—because of the Changs' chosen coping style. The hospice nurse leaves her office number and receives Mrs. Chang's permission to "drop in" again in a few days.

Case Example: Acceptance of Hospice Help

Mrs. McCarthy's 14-year-old daughter Janine has battled cystic fibrosis all her life. The tertiary care center where she has received her treatment is 150 miles from her father's farm. She must be alone during treatment except when her mother comes twice a week on the bus to stay for an afternoon. Janine has a tracheostomy that requires suction of purulent, blood-tinged sputum. She has an extensive drug regimen of bronchodilators, steroid, antibiotics, and cough suppressants. Janine tells the social worker, whom she has known for five years, that she never wants "to come back to this place. I want to go home and stay there and die if I must. I want to be in my own room with Mom and Dad and Ruthie around." The physician agrees to a hospice referral. He thinks Janine may live a month or two but could die at any time.

The nurse's admission interview is a tearful bedside conference with the mother and daughter. Both Janine and her mother want Janine to be home "when she passes over," but Mrs. McCarthy is fearful she can't handle it. She agrees to hospice help with a clear goal "to find out what I need to know to keep Janine happy and comfortable. I'll try it for a couple of weeks, if a nurse can come tell me I'm doing it all right." The nurse agrees to this goal.

Inpatient or Home Care

We look toward a future when a full hospice continuum of home care, outpatient care, day care, hospital, and skilled nursing facility hospice programs will be available, just as a broad range of locations for birthing is now coming into being for the pregnant woman. Currently, however, few communities offer such a range of possibilities. Ideally, hospice programs undertake to coordinate care wherever the patient is. A growing number of hospices offer a full range of inpatient and home care services, which federal Medicare reimbursement for hospice care now mandates. Realistically, a person choosing home hospice care may have to choose between conventional hospital or nursing home facilities for help with acute symptom crises or when family caregiving resources are exhausted. Similarly, full-fledged home hospice care may not be available to the person in an inpatient hospice program. Many hospital hospice units or hospice teams that provide special care wherever the patient is in the hospital still operate under the utilization review and regulations of an acute care facility. Thus a dying person must be discharged if his or her dying does not necessitate complex technical care (IV's, oxygen, injections, dressings, etc.). A lingering, nontechnological, inpatient hospice death is usually possible only in hospice programs within skilled nursing facilities or in separately administrated inpatient hospices.

Most people are periodically admitted to inpatient facilities for management of acute needs. When they are nearing death they should be able to make an informed decision about whether to die at home, or in a hospital or skilled facility, or in an inpatient hospice program. Each proposed hospital discharge is a turning point when critical decision making can be facilitated by the hospice team.

Discharge planning involves the patient and those expected to offer home support and care in the process of determining the patient's anticipated needs and how they can be met. The professional inpatient team provides a data base to determine home care strategies. A conference among patient, family, and health team is extremely useful for hearing all points of view and setting realistic goals. An important nursing function is practical planning with *anticipatory guidance,* in which likely problems are anticipated and the patient and family are helped to prepare for various contingencies (see Chapter 7 for a discussion of issues the patient-family must address in coping with lingering and downhill courses of illness at home). It is essential before discharge to determine whether patient and family have safe knowledge of essential nursing measures and palliative approaches and whether they have arranged the home suitably and obtained essential medical equipment, organized caregivers, and learned how to get help for questions and emergencies. Many people are not prepared in these areas and when they are not, plans for discharge should be questioned. Suppose, for instance, that a patient and his wife have avoided help in learning catheter care and how to give medications. They deny that the patient is becoming progressively more bedridden, and they have no one available to help the wife, whose "bad back" limits her ability to lift and bend. In this situation, the hospice team might point out the limitations of the home-going plan to husband and wife and explore other options with them.

Often people cope amazingly well at home in a familiar environment. The living room sofa can serve as a bed, and an empty egg carton makes a good pill sorter. People must have the final choice of what they will face. Hospice staff inform them of what support the team can muster and assist them if they wish to mobilize family and community resources. (See Chapter 9 for a discussion of creating a positive environment wherever the patient and family decide that death shall occur.)

ASSESSMENT

Attention to the humanity of the dying person and of his or her close network of family and friends is central to assessment. Development of rapport leads us to focus first on the patient's and family's perceived needs and priorities. These are given first attention during admission, only then does comprehensive assessment proceed. For example, an initial visit to the bedside of a patient who is terrified of strangling or suffocating will lead us to thorough cardiopulmonary assessment and the initiation of pharmacological, relaxation, and teaching approaches to manage the patient's struggle; other assessment must wait until he is calm. Or we may be called to the home of a patient who is concerned about the exhaustion and stress her daughter, who is primary caregiver, is experiencing. Once we have addressed this issue and begun some action to alleviate the problem, we can turn to physical assessment of the patient.

The whole philosophy of assessment in hospice care is different from that used in cure-oriented care. To begin with, as we have seen, the patient provides the leads in the initial baseline assessment. In addition, assessment should be comprehensive; it should cover physical, emotional, social, cultural, and spiritual dimensions. Too often, dying people will tell you that their physical exams have become superficial, or almost nonexistent: "They just draw my blood and renew my prescriptions." It is important to keep in mind, however, that assessment is limited by the patient's energy. Some areas may not be examined if they are expected to cause the patient distress or undue energy expenditure in the process. Careful judgment must be used in deciding what body functions to monitor regularly and whether monitoring that is intrusive or painful serves a palliative purpose.

Assessment of Physical Changes

History-taking and physical examination must be performed with a concern for what specific information and what diagnostic measurements are actually useful in determining specific palliative measures or understanding the course of the illness. The intrusive and/or invasive nature of any physical assessment must be evaluated for each patient. For example, a patient was described by hospital staff as being verbally very abusive. Hospice staff respected the patient's right to "stop being poked and prodded and needled like some animal." The patient soon came to trust the hospice staff, and he shifted the focus of anger from medical staff to his terminal prognosis. Eventually, the patient even let staff listen to his chest and make some appropriate symptom management suggestions.

Especially in situations where patients feel they are being intruded upon or are experiencing significant discomfort, good judgment as to what should be checked with regularity is crucial. For example, it may be desirable not to take blood pressure routinely but only with a specific purpose. In a case of known symptomatic hypertension, such a purpose might be to determine need for medication change, to determine whether dizziness may be due to postural hypotension, or to determine how close a person is to death. Similarly, procedures such as neurological or rectal examinations may not need to be performed routinely but only when patient report of symptoms indicates a need to investigate. For instance, a patient reporting possible seizure activity and transient left-sided weakness requires immediate and thorough neurological assessment to determine palliative management. Or, a patient with a sudden severe left lower quadrant abdominal pain who cannot remember his last bowel movement should have a thorough examination to determine a differential diagnosis and identify the appropriate palliative approach. *Complaints should be investigated to determine the best palliative measures specific to the cause.* Too often new symptoms in the dying person are disregarded as somehow "par for the course." An exception to this kind of thorough investigation may be appropriate when a person is within hours or days of death.

The importance of laboratory work or other diagnostic procedures performed to increase medical documentation of patient status, but not for any purpose that would lead to improved patient quality of life, should be periodically reconsidered. For instance, a hospice team questioned weekly blood drawing to determine hematocrit and platelet count for a young leukemic patient. A careful review revealed that these tests determined when to transfuse packed red blood cells, a procedure that enabled the young man to have more energy until the end of his life, and when to transfuse platelets, which lessened the fear of hemorrhage.

Physical assessment begins with the eliciting of subjective information from patient and family as they report their experience with physical changes. McCorkle and Young (1978) have devised a useful tool that measures patient-family perception of the severity of ten common symptoms acknowledged to be distressing to cancer patients. This device does not include anxiety, cough, and dyspnea as symptoms, although other observers indicate these are common problems in cancer patients, because the patients themselves did not recognize and report them as among their major concerns. In these investigators' population of 45 cancer patients, of greatest concern—and in order of frequency of report—were bowel problems, appearance, appetite, insomnia, fatigue, mood, mobility, pain, concentration, and nausea.

McCorkle and Young's symptom distress scale can be adapted and utilized by nurses or hospice programs to provide a quick determination of patient—family experience with common symptoms. The scale (Fig. 4-1) can be used easily as a paper and pencil checklist by the person who is oriented toward written expression, has energy, and functions with clear mentation. For some patients such use may be inappropriate and intrusive; however, it can still serve the nurse as a patient-family interviewing guide that quickly

Figure 4-1. Symptom scale.

Each of the following categories lists 5 different numbered statements. Think about what each statement says; then place a circle around the one statement in each category that most closely indicates how you have been feeling lately. The statements in each category are ranked from 1 to 5, where number 1 indicates no problems and number 5 indicates a maximum number of problems. Numbers 2 through 4 indicate that you feel somewhere in between these two extremes. Please circle one number in each category.
(Hospice of Seattle, scale based on McCorkle, 1978, instrument).

Nausea (1)
(sick to my stomach)

1	2	3	4	5
I seldom feel any nausea at all.	I am nauseous once in a while.	I am often nauseous.	I am usually nauseous.	I suffer from nausea continually.

Nausea (2)
(sick to my stomach)

1	2	3	4	5
When I do have nausea, it is very mild.	When I do have nausea, it is mildly distressing.	When I have nausea, I feel pretty sick.	When I have nausea, I feel very sick.	When I have nausea, I am as sick as I could be.

Appetite

1	2	3	4	5
I have my normal appetite.	My appetite is usually, but not always, pretty good.	I don't really enjoy my food as I used to.	I have to force myself to eat my food.	I cannot stand the thought of food.

Insomnia

1	2	3	4	5
I sleep as well as I always have.	I have occasional spells of sleeplessness.	I frequently have trouble getting to sleep and staying asleep.	I have difficulty sleeping almost every night.	It is almost impossible for me to get a decent night's sleep.

Pain (1)

1	2	3	4	5
I almost never have pain.	I have pain once in a while.	I frequently have pain—several times a week.	I am usually in some degree of pain.	I am in some degree of pain almost constantly.

Pain (2)

1	2	3	4	5
When I do have pain, it is very mild.	When I do have pain, it is mildly distressing.	The pain I have is usually fairly intense.	The pain I have is usually very intense.	The pain I have is almost unbearable.

Fatigue

1	2	3	4	5
I am usually not tired at all.	I am occasionally rather tired.	There are frequently periods when I am quite tired.	I am usually very tired.	Most of the time, I feel exhausted.

Bowel

1	2	3	4	5
I have my normal bowel pattern.	My bowel pattern occasionally causes me some concern and discomfort.	I frequently have discomfort from my present bowel pattern.	I am usually in discomfort because of my present bowel pattern.	I am in continual discomfort because of my present bowel pattern.

Concentration

1	2	3	4	5
I have my normal ability to concentrate.	I occasionally have trouble concentrating.	I often have trouble concentrating.	I usually have at least some difficulty concentrating.	I just can't concentrate at all.

Appearance

1	2	3	4	5
My appearance has basically not changed.	My appearance has gotten a little worse.	My appearance is definitely worse than it used to be, but I am not greatly concerned about it.	My appearance is definitely worse than it used to be and I am concerned about it.	My appearance has changed drastically from what it was and I am very concerned about it.

Breathing

1	2	3	4	5
I usually breathe normally.	I occasionally have trouble breathing.	I often have trouble breathing.	I very frequently have trouble breathing.	I always have severe trouble with my breathing.

Figure 4-1 (continued)

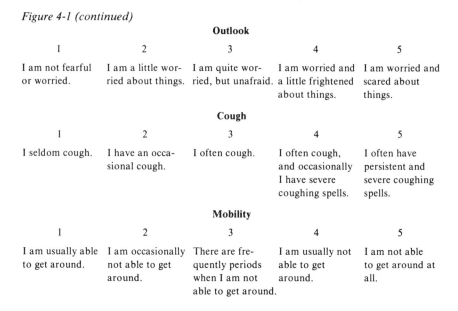

Outlook

1	2	3	4	5
I am not fearful or worried.	I am a little worried about things.	I am quite worried, but unafraid.	I am worried and a little frightened about things.	I am worried and scared about things.

Cough

1	2	3	4	5
I seldom cough.	I have an occasional cough.	I often cough.	I often cough, and occasionally I have severe coughing spells.	I often have persistent and severe coughing spells.

Mobility

1	2	3	4	5
I am usually able to get around.	I am occasionally not able to get around.	There are frequently periods when I am not able to get around.	I am usually not able to get around.	I am not able to get around at all.

identifies those symptoms that are most troublesome. A modification of McCorkle and Young's symptom distress scale can be seen in Figure 4-1.

In Table 4-1 the reader will find a systematic guide to priority physical assessment by nurses of the dying. Data must be gathered with clinical discrimintion; the primary hospice nurse must choose the categories to focus on and the information to determine regularly. Often the dying person has diminishing contact with a physician for diagnosis of changes; thus the eyes, ears, and hands of the nurse must be particularly sensitive to pick up any problems that can be reversed or minimized palliatively. The guide is designed to gather both *subjective* and *objective* information in major physiological categories where malfunction is likely.

Psychosocial Assessment

Assessment of the whole person reflects attention to individual coping, family and social network, cultural considerations, and the spiritual dimension. For each of these psychosocial assessment areas, this section presents a series of questions designed to encourage broad, in-depth exploration by the nurse investigator. Inquiries directed to the patient must be highly individualized. As in physical examination, the choice to gather information must be scrutinized for intrusiveness and relevance to palliative goals as the latter have been chosen by the patient. Psychosocial assessment begins at first contact, but it can move toward comprehensiveness only as a relationship develops.

Table 4-1. *Priority Physical Assessment for the Dying*

I. Cardiovascular-respiratory function
A. Known disease, drugs, therapies affecting function
B. Subjective data
1. Patient report of common symptoms: Note character, onset, duration, frequency, factors precipitating and relieving
    a. Dyspnea, orthopnea, cough, sputum description, problem expectorating secretions
    b. Chest pain, "palpitations"
    c. Lower extremity pain with rest or activity; other changes in sensation; changes in color or temperature; swelling
2. Reported impact of functional disability
    a. Patient knowledge of disability and treatment
    b. Effects on activities of daily living and life style
    c. Changes in body image, social role
    d. Emotional response
C. Objective data
1. Characteristics of sputum
2. Indices of peripheral circulation: mental status, lower extremity circulation, urine output
3. Chest inspection, palpation (percussion)
4. Lung and heart auscultation
5. Inspection of neck for venous engorgement, carotid palpation
6. Vital signs
D. Evaluate whether the following measures and others should be discontinued or continued as helpful to palliative goals.
1. Intake and output, daily weights
2. EKG
3. Bone marrow biopsy
4. X-rays, scans, arteriography
5. Blood work, particularly CBC, blood gases, electrolytes, enzymes

II. Gastrointestinal function
A. Known disease, drugs, therapies, affecting function
B. Subjective data
1. Patient report of common symptoms: Note character, onset, duration, frequency, factors precipitating and relieving
    a. Diet history
    b. Oral discomfort
    c. Anorexia or weight loss
    d. Dysphagia, dyspepsia
    e. Nausea or vomiting
    f. Abdominal discomfort
    g. Flatulence, distention
    h. Characteristics of stool; bowel habits and patterns; incontinence
    i. Anal discomfort
2. Reported impact of functional disability
    a. Patient knowledge of disability and treatment
    b. Effects on activities of daily living and life style
    c. Changes in body image, social role
    d. Emotional response
C. Objective data
1. Inspection of mouth
2. Abdominal inspection, palpation, auscultation for bowel sounds
3. Characteristics of stool, vomitus, GI drainage, stomas, wounds
4. Digital rectal examination if patient reports related symptoms
D. Evaluate whether the following measures should be discontinued or continued as helpful in palliative care:
1. Calorie counts and weights
2. Endoscopy
3. X-rays, scans, analyses of digestive products
4. Lab tests of blood and urine: Bilirubin, enzymes, proteins, ammonia

III. Genitourinary and gynecological function
A. Known disease, drugs, therapies affecting function
B. Subjective data
1. Patient report of common symptoms: Note character, onset, duration, frequency, factors precipitating and relieving
    a. Urinary incontinence
    b. Retention, difficulty starting stream, oliguria
    c. Dysuria, frequency, urgency, hematuria
    d. Possible manifestations of uremia:

(continued)

55

Table 4-1 (continued)

nausea and vomiting, behavioral and cognitive changes, neuromuscular irritability
 e. Suprapubic, abdominal, testicular, perineal, low back, costovertebral angle pain
 f. Menstrual changes
 g. Breast changes
 h. Vaginal–urethral–peripheral lesions discharges
 i. Changes in sexual functioning
 2. Reported impact of functional disability
  a. Patient knowledge of disability and treatment
  b. Effects on activities of daily living and life style
  c. Changes in body image, social role
  d. Emotional response
 C. Objective data
  1. Characteristics of urine
  2. Characteristics of urethral, vaginal, wound drainage
  3. Suprapubic, inguinal, and perineal inspection; palpation as indicated; presence of costovertebral angle tenderness
  4. Breast inspection, palpation
 D. Evaluate whether the following measurements should be discontinued or continued as helpful in palliative care:
  1. Intake and output (I & O)
  2. Urinalysis, microbiology
  3. Cystoscopy, X-ray, biopsy, arteriograms
  4. Blood drawing to determine indices of uremia (azotemia, hyperkalemia, metabolic acidosis)

IV. Fluid and electrolyte status
 A. Known disease, drugs, therapies affecting function
 B. Subjective data
  1. Patient report of common symptoms:
  a. Decreased or increased intake of fluid or food
  b. Decreased or increased output: Urine, feces, vomitus, perspiration, other body discharge
  c. Swelling
  d. Weakness, dizziness, impaired mentation, nausea

 C. Objective data
  1. Patient–family estimate of I & O
  2. Abdominal girth, presence of pitting edema
  3. Lying, sitting, standing blood pressure; venous filling
  4. Moisture of mucous membranes, skin turgor
  5. Changes in cardiac rhythm
  6. Level of consciousness
  7. Muscle weakness or irritability
  8. Hypoventilation, hyperventilation
 D. Evaluate whether the following measures should be discontinued or continued as helpful in palliative care:
  1. 24-hour accurate I & O
  2. Serial weights
  3. Serum electrolytes, pH
  4. Blood gases

V. Muscoloskeletal function
 A. Known disease, drugs, therapies affecting function
 B. Subjective data
  1. Patient report of common symptoms: Note character, onset, location, duration, frequency, factors precipitating and relieving
  a. Pain, tenderness
  b. Weakness, endurance
  c. Limitation of movement
  d. Deformity
  e. Inflammation
  2. Reported impact of functional disability
 C. Objective data
  1. Use of supportive devices
  2. Posture, gait, handedness
  3. Endurance
  4. Motor function while performing activities of daily living
  5. Muscle atrophy, wasting; palpation of masses; spasm
  6. Range of motion of joints
  7. Muscle function
  a. Flaccidity, hypertonicity, contracture
  b. Muscle strength and coordination while performing activities of daily living

VI. Neurological function
A. Known disease, drugs, therapies affection function
B. Subjective data
  1. Patient report of common symptoms:
    a. Weakness, dizziness, poor coordination
    b. Defective memory or thinking
    c. Problems with speech
    d. Loss of consciousness
    e. Pain, numbness, unusual sensations
    f. Seizures, tremors
    g. Thoughts
  2. Reported impact of functional disability
C. Objective data
  1. Mental status (Cohen, 1981)
    a. Level of consciousness
    b. Physical appearance, grooming
    c. Psychomotor behavior
    d. Mood and affect
    e. Intellectual performance
    f. Speech
    g. Thoughts
  2. Aphasia, dysarthria
  3. Bilateral muscle strength
  4. Integrated motor function: watch ADL's
  5. Balance, gait, proprioception
  6. Unintentional movements

  7. Sensory changes
  8. Visual changes, pupillary check
  9. Bowel or bladder control
  10. Bulbar function
  11. Changes in vital signs with increasing intracranial pressure.
D. Evaluate whether the following measures are indicated as helpful in palliative care:
  1. Brain scan
  2. Angiography, spinal x-rays
  3. Lumbar puncture

VII. Skin status
A. Known disease, drugs, therapies affecting function
B. Subjective data
  1. Patient report of common symptoms:
    a. Tenderness, burning, itching
    b. Warmth or coolness
    c. Sensitivities, allergies
  2. Reported impact of impairment
C. Objective data
  1. Personal hygiene
  2. Color, temperature, turgor
  3. Wounds, ulcers
  4. Rashes
  5. Odors and excretions
  6. Factors predisposing to breakdown: emaciation, malnutrition, immobility, incontinence, diminished peripheral circulation.

The following questions pertain to *individual coping.*

• Who is this person? What has been his or her life experience prior to illness?
• What is the person's knowledge and perception of problems, current illness, and prognosis?
• How is the person dealing with the present crisis?
• What have been the person's past strategies for coping with difficulty?
• Is there any history of psychiatric problems?
• What is the person's mood and affect?
• What has been the impact of physical disability on the person's daily living, life style, body image, social role, emotional response? (This question appears also in Table 4-1 on physical assessment.)

The next set of questions pertains to the person's *support, or family and social, network:* nuclear family, relatives, friends, lover, co-workers, and members of the same social groups. This book emphasizes the needs of the family as well as the patient, and it defines "family" as the close network of relatives and/or friends who have strong emotional ties and reciprocal relationships with the patient. Quite often, unfortunately, such resources are limited in terminal illness when patients have taken pride in their independence and thus have maintained a restricted social network.

The following questions explore the patient's support network.

- Who are the family members and significant others in the patient's immediate supportive network?
- What kinds of relationships does the person maintain within this network? What are common interaction patterns?
- How has the person used the network in earlier times of crisis?
- What are the resources and limitations of the current network?
- What are the needs of individuals in the network?
- What are the supportive capabilities of the extended community network: neighborhood, church, social organizations, community services?

Refer to MacElveen, 1979 for further discussion of social network assessment.

An individual lives and dies as part of a cultural system. Paxton, Ramirez, and Walloch (1976) have identified comprehensive cultural assessment as part of a holistic nursing model. The following questions, adapted from these writers' discussion, take account of *cultural considerations* in assessing the person in relationship to his or her culture:

- What is the degree of the person's belief in and adherence to an ethnic–cultural system separate from the American mainstream?
- What are individual and family beliefs about cause and cure relating to the illness and, in general, about health, illness, death, and male-female roles?
- Are folk practitioners and/or remedies being used or considered?
- What cultural behaviors are valued and tabooed?
- Is there a desire for special religious ceremonies?
- Do medical–nursing practices conflict with cultural or religious persuasion?
- What are cultural preferences about food, music, recreation?
- How does socioeconomic status affect patient and family needs?

Nurses usually acknowledge the *spiritual dimension* as integral to a person's life but have been hesitant to ask questions about belief and practice, lest patients feel intruded upon or threatened by nurses' own beliefs. The hospice movement is in the forefront of the recognition of spiritual concerns. Chaplaincy is an integral aspect of overall caregiving, and all team members take responsibility for the spiritual care of patients. Ruth Stoll (1979) has developed a "spiritual history guide" that can be incorporated into the psychosocial nursing assessment. Her questions are to well phrased that they are presented here vertabim.

Concept of God or Deity

- Is religion or God significant to you? If yes, can you describe how?
- Is prayer helpful to you? What happens when you pray?
- Does a God or deity function in your personal life? If yes, can you describe how?
- How would you describe your God or what you worship?

Sources of Hope and Strength

- Who is the most important person to you?
- To whom do you turn when you need help? Are they available? In what ways do they help?
- What is your source of strength and hope?
- What helps you the most when you feel afraid or need special help?

Religious Practices

- Do you feel your faith (or religion) is helpful to you? If yes, would you tell me how?
- Are there any religious practices that are important to you?
- Has being sick made any difference in your practice of praying? Your religious practices?
- What religious books and/or symbols are helpful to you?

Relation Between Spiritual Beliefs and Health

- What has bothered you most about being sick (or in what is happening to you)?
- What do you think is going to happen to you?
- Has being sick (or what has happened to you) made any difference in your feelings about God or the practice of your faith?
- Is there anything that is especially frightening or meaningful to you now?*

Spiritual assessment is generally best undertaken following the nurse-patient understanding gained from initially pursuing other dimensions of the psychosocial assessment. Often just one or two of Stoll's queries will open up a discussion of the person's spiritual identity. Some patients may, at this time, state clearly that they do not want to discuss spiritual–religious matters.

Diagnostic Conclusions

The nursing assessment process includes both data collection and clinical analysis of data in order to identify problems. In 1973, the first National

---

From Stoll, R. Guidelines for Spiritual Assessment. *American Journal of Nursing,* 1979, *79,* 1574–1577.

Table 4-2. *Nursing Diagnoses Accepted by the National Group for Classification*

Activity intolerance	Health maintenance, alteration in
Airway clearance, ineffective	Home maintenance management, impaired
Anxiety	Injury, potential for
Bowel elimination, alteration in: constipation	Knowledge deficit
Bowel elimination, alteration in: diarrhea	Mobility, impaired physical
	Noncompliance
Bowel elimination, alteration in: incontinence	Nutrition, alteration in
Breathing pattern, ineffective	Oral mucous membrane, alterations in
Cardiac output, alteration in: decreased	Parenting, alteration in
Comfort, alteration in: pain	Powerlessness
Communication, impaired verbal	Rape–trauma syndrome
Coping, ineffective individual	Self-care deficit
Coping, ineffective family: compromised	Sensory perception, alteration in
Coping, ineffective family: disabling	Sexual dysfunction
Coping, family: potential for growth	Skin integrity, impairment of
Diversional activity, deficit	Sleep pattern disturbance
Family processes, alteration in	Social isolation
Fear	Spiritual distress
Fluid volume deficit, actual	Thought processes, alteration in
Fluid volume deficit, potential	Tissues perfusion, alteration in
Gas exchange, impaired	Urinary elimination, alteration in patterns
Grieving, anticipatory	Violence, potential for
Grieving, dysfunctional	

Source: Kim and Moritz (1982) and "National Nursing Diagnosis Group Forms Association."

Conference on Classification of Nursing Diagnoses was called to begin to state and classify nursing diagnoses. Since then regular conferences of the National Group for the Classification of Nursing Diagnoses have developed and approved a standardized language, classification, and beginning list of nursing diagnoses. Table 4-2 lists diagnoses identified as of April, 1982.

These diagnoses are used to discuss physical symptom management of each diagnostic category. These few psychosocial nursing diagnoses which have been classified are referred to occasionally in this text but, in the authors' opinion, they remain too vague and nonspecific to be cited as expert

Table 4-3. *Psychosocial Diagnoses Common to Hospice Patients*

Anger	Financial concerns
Ambivalence	Grief reaction
Expression of hostility	Unexpressed
Physical abuse; fighting	Immobilizing
Confusion, disorientation	Coping mechanism used: _____
Contradictory patient goals	Immaturity, ineffective coping
Denial, lack of understanding	Isolation
Closed awareness, avoiding issues	Cultural, language
Needs downplayed	Lack of social supports
Ignorance of feelings	Personal reticence
Ignoprance of disease	Emotional withdrawal
Reduced mentation,	Lack of goals, no future planning
impaired decision making	Exhaustion,
Dependency, powerlessness	overextension of caregivers
Patient loss of personal power	Self destructive behavior
Dependent family or friends	Suicidal thoughts
Depression, hopelessness	Stress-related symptoms
Fear	Unfinished business remaining

diagnostic conclusions. Table 4-3 presents the hospice psychosocial diagnoses developed at Hospice of Seattle. These diagnoses were determined from clinical evaluation of data gathered in ongoing psychosocial assessments.

GOAL SETTING

Following assessment with identification of problems and nursing diagnoses, goals of care should be defined. Hospice care goals should be individualized and formulated on a continuing basis by an ongoing process of negotiation.

Negotiation

At the first visit to the dying person and/or to the person's relatives, the nurse should identify how the program can be of help. The nurse's suggestions of possible goals should be determined by the resources of the team and based on assessment that has been as comprehensive as patient circumstances allow. The nurse should use language that, to the best of his or her ability to judge, is understandable and will be heard, as determined by the patient-family's level of stress and awareness of the dying process.

Patient Goals	Family Goals
1. Achieving comfort	1. Keeping patient home
2. Staying at home	2. Keeping patient comfortable
3. Retaining independence	3. Maintaining family integrity
4. Increasing strength	4. Learning home nursing care
5. Maintaining family integrity	5. Other
6. Fighting illness	

Merged Goals

Nursing Goals for Patient-Family

1. Maintaining daily activities
2. Completing unfinished business
3. Addressing spiritual issues
4. Managing symptoms
5. Choosing home versus hospital versus nursing home
6. Determining amount of help desired
7. Exploring issues and feelings
8. Making decisions
9. Planning for changes, emergencies, death

Figure 4-2. Three sets of goals that must be merged, those of the patient, the family member, and the nurse (Based on unpublished work by Elizabeth White and Lynn Talley, 1982, based on study at Hospice of Snohomish, Everett, Washington.

Patients, family members, and friends will each have their own points of view and goals, some of which they will choose to express and some of which will be hidden for a while. The nurse must observe interpersonal dynamics carefully in order to understand interaction patterns and needs expressed. Initially, the nurse should seek to identify clear goals that the patient—and, ideally, a family member—find comfortable. The nurse can synthesize patient goals, family member goals, and the whole range of possible hospice team goals into his or her articulation of goals about which the patient and family feel comfortable. Figure 4-2 summarizes the individual goal statements of 58 patient-families at the Hospice of Snohomish County, Washington, and contrasts them with a list of issues and goals that the hospice nurse believed were important. The nurse must bring these three sets of goals together for a workable focus. The following case example illustrates such a merging of goals.

Case Example: Goal Negotiation

Carolyn Lane's husband, Roger, was dying slowly from a brain tumor. Carolyn's friend read about the local hospice, and Carolyn contacted the hospice staff with the stated goal of having "someone to talk to about all this."

During the initial assessment process, Roger Lane denied any particular worries: "We're doing all we can here. I have complete trust in the doctor. You come for the wife if she wants you." Carolyn described her own high stress state; for example, awakening in the morning with fingernails pressing into her palms and her body drenched in sweat. She had many questions regarding her husband's volatile emotions, progressing immobility, and multiple medications. Her stated desire was that hospice staff teach her what she needed to know to care for Roger, as well as lend her a sympathetic ear.

In outlining the possibilities for assistance, the nurse indicated that hospice staff could help Caroline reduce stress and could provide emotional support for Roger. As neither husband nor wife agreed to the latter two goals, the nurse affirmed that she would focus on their stated priority goals: teaching nursing measures and symptom management to Carolyn and providing her with supportive listening.

It is more difficult to merge goals when two or more family members have conflicting goals that are mutually exclusive. First of all, it is essential that the nurse avoid the pull to take sides in a power struggle. Similarly, the hospice team must be alert to the divisive forces that may attempt to pit one team member against another. Team members must work to maintain a calm presence that continually refocuses and centers the helping goals on maintaining comfort and dignity for the dying person. The hospice goal is not to tackle the healing of a fragmented family system at this time. Those family members who request help to change the quality of their own lives should be assisted through the anticipatory grieving and bereavement process but referred outside the hospice program for family or individual counseling.

During a crisis of conflict in the family, the nurse and/or counselor should try to bring those affected into a family conference that is best facilitated by one or two hospice team members with experience in family mediation. Such a conference creates a structure for face-to-face dialogue in which each person can stand his or her own ground while acknowledging the right of another person to a differing viewpoint. "A dialogical meeting with an opponent recognizes the importance of both parties in the relationship, which promotes the possibility of an answer emerging between them" (Arnet, 1980, p. 133). The hospice team then facilitates a respectful hearing of each point of view. It is useful to re-state and summarize each position. Often this effort of really listening to each other brings a realization of common ground. It is then possible to make an effort toward resolution that incorporates each person's position. Remember that the goal of such hospice mediation efforts is not to do family therapy or to right all the old wrongs. It is to keep the peace so that the patient can die as she or he chooses. As warring family members work to reach mutual goals, they must be continually reminded of this purpose. Even if family members refuse to confer, the hospice team uses threads of this mediation process to negotiate workable goals. In the following case example, such threads were woven into family-centered hospice goals despite ongoing family feuding.

Case example: Goal Negotiation Amidst Conflict

Marjorie Worzek was referred to the hospice team by her physician. She was dying of pancreatic cancer and very frightened. She was 72 years old and a widow; her two children hadn't seen each other for years. During the initial assessment process, Mrs. Worzek stated that her primary goal was to go home and be cared for by her children. She described herself as overwhelmed by waves of despair, and stated clearly her goal to work through spiritual issues. She had some nightmarish visions of how she might die, and she told the nurse she wanted to talk about "what really might happen and what we should do." She also complained of immobilizing sacral pain radiating into the right buttock, unrelieved by the prescribed Percodan tab i every 6 hours prn. The nurse initially defined four mutually agreed upon goals of care: discharge planning, addressing spiritual issues, anticipatory planning for death, and improved pain control.

Separate interviews with the son and daughter, however, revealed different opinions. The son, Darrell, believed strongly that Marjorie belonged in a nursing home "where they can care for her properly." He described feelings of animosity toward his sister Candy: "We hate each other's guts. We always fought as kids, and I've avoided her successfully for the last ten years. I don't see any reason to change now." He was also very concerned about his mother "becoming a doper" and stated a goal of getting her off "dangerous drugs." He wanted to get a second opinion, in the hope that another doctor might try a different treatment for his mother: "Candy's too ready to give up. I think we need to fight this thing." Candy, in contrast, wanted her mother to have a "good death" at home "if that's what Mom wants. Darrell's always been so selfish. I don't see why we should listen to him now." Candy had had experience with counseling and asked for help for herself. She was currently experiencing insomnia and frequent headaches.

The nurse negotiated a mutually agreed upon teaching goal with Darrell: "to explain more about the hospice philosophy of pain control and what you can expect with this disease." The nurse then contracted to help Candy consider the possibilities of her mother's home care and to refer her to the team social worker for counseling to support her through the stress of her mother's dying. Fortunately, both Candy and Darrell, albeit somewhat skeptically, agreed to confer together with the hospice social worker and nurse.

At the conference, both Mrs. Worzek's children expressed their opinions strongly and emotionally. They did agree at the beginning, however, that they both wanted "what is best for Mom," and the facilitators needed to remind them of this shared purpose as they tried to work out compromises during the session. Darrell was surprised to learn that the nurse thought Candy was capable of learning all the nursing measures necessary for his mother's care. He agreed to talk to his mother "in private" the following day, to express his opinions, and then go along with her wishes. He and Candy agreed that if their mother wanted to home, they should undertake a two-week trial period. Candy acknowledged her own stress level and admitted that she was committed to caring for her mother at home, but fearful that she might "break down on the job." At the same time, she was resistant to hearing from the social worker that her mother's insurance would probably pay for a licensed private-duty nurse in the home: "I really want to do it all by myself. I don't think Mom would want a stranger." Darrell, however, thought that hiring a private-duty nurse would be a realistic move. Candy slowly agreed: "Well, maybe one 8-hour shift a day would be all right. Maybe at night."

Candy and Darrell got into one disagreement after another during their mother's dying. Their mother did go home and received nursing care from both Candy and Darrell as well as from private-duty nurses' aides. Candy and Darrell were always totally opposed on the issue of the palliative use of drugs, and this conflict required frequent mediation. The hospice team helped the brother and sister to unite reluctantly in their common focus "to give Mom our best." After her death, they both felt good about their involvement but returned to opposite coasts of the United States with no stated intention of seeing each other except to tie up estate matters and avoid "locking horns" in the process.

Changing Goals

The process of setting goals begins with the first assessment, and it is ongoing with each encounter. Goals change during the variable course of dying. Glaser and Strauss (1968) describe a variety of potential courses, which they define as "dying trajectories": slow, lingering death in a custodial institution; lingering in the hospital; lingering at home; a rapid, expected, downhill course; and a rapid, unexpected, downhill course. Each trajectory can be shaped and influenced by patient, family, institutional, and professional caregiver decisions.

The lingering course of death permits the identification of goals of care for stable periods. Ideally, such goals may include development of a strong trusting relationships between nurse and patient, planning in anticipation of a coming downhill course, life review, working out the highest possible quality of life in the time remaining, self-development, and spiritual growth (see also Chapter 3). In contrast, some patients and families perceive no need for help when they are not in crisis and ask staff to back off completely: "Don't call me, I'll call you when I need you again." Some choose limited counseling, to focus on specific issues. Others allow an occasional nursing contact that focuses on maintaining physical well-being. It is noteworthy that the existing health care medical expense and reimbursement systems generally do not recognize the terminally ill person's need for such help during stable periods. These systems are oriented to crisis and deterioration as indicators of need for nursing intervention.

The first step in goal-setting during periods of downhill course and crisis involves emotional and physical crisis intervention. Central processes in crisis intervention include active listening, encouraging the expression of feeling, guiding the understanding and acceptance of reality, identifying effective coping strategies, and linking the patient-family to a helping network. Many physical crises can be side-stepped for those patients and families who have allowed us to teach them problems to expect and how to prepare in advance to manage these problems (see Chapter 7). For those with unanticipated physical changes and deterioration in status, the goal is to restore equilibrium using the principles of palliation described in Chapters 7, 8 and 9. The nurse should beware, however, of managing life-threatening changes with merely palliative means when the patient is not ready to die. She or he should ask, is more aggressive therapy appropriate? Similarly, he or she should assist with value and goal clarification when resuscitative measures are being considered for a patient with advanced, irreversible pathology who is accepting of death. Once the presenting problem is resolved and an even keel restored, the nurse can help the patient and family map out options for future care and can give them an idea of what they can expect to experience. Some patients and families will choose full awareness and extensive teaching, in order to anticipate events and control them. Others, at the opposite extreme, will seem to lead their lives from crisis to crisis, with no sense that events can be prevented or controlled. Such people may be uninterested in the nurse's efforts to teach them to prevent the next crisis, yet they may actively seek help when the next wave of trouble comes. Nursing goals are continually adapted to the events of the downhill course.

REFERENCES

Arnet, R.C. *Dwell in peace.* Elgin, Illinois: The Brethren Press, 1980.

Buber, M. *Pointing the way.* New York: Harper and Row, 1957.

Cohen, S., & Harris, E. Mental status assessment: Programmed instruction. *American Journal of Nursing,* 1981, *81,* 1493–1518.

Glaser, B., & Strauss, A. *A time for dying.* Chicago: Aldine, 1968.

Kim, M.J., & Moritz, D.A. (Eds.). *Classification of nursing diagnoses.* New York: McGraw-Hill, 1982.

MacElveen, P.M. Assessing social networks in health and illness. In Popiel, E.S. (Ed.), *Social issues and trends in nursing: Chautauqua 77.* Thorofare, N.J.: Charles Slack, 1979.

McCorkle, R., & Young, K. Development of a symptom distress scale. *Cancer Nursing,* 1978, *1,* 373–378.

National Nursing Diagnosis Group Forms Association. *American Journal of Nursing,* 1982, *82,* 1040.

Paxton, P., Ramirez, M.C., & Walloch, E.C. Nursing assessment and intervention. In Branch, M.F., & Paxton, P.P. (Eds.), *Providing safe nursing care for ethnic people of color.* New York: Appleton-Century-Crofts, 1976.

Stoll, R. Guidelines for spiritual assessment. *American Journal of Nursing,* 1979, *79,* 1574–1577.

1. T		*6. T*	
2. F		*7. F*	
3. F		*8. T*	
4. T		*9. T*	
5. F		*10. T*	

5

The Hospice Team

Answer the following questions True (T) or False (F). Answers appear on the last page of this chapter.

1. *The interdisciplinary team comprises nurses from all specialties working as supervisors to those in the social professions.*

2. *Team members need to understand, among other things, the skills and knowledge of each other's professions.*

3. *Teamwork is a natural phenomenon that maintains itself without effort on the part of team members.*

4. *If the leader understands the team purpose and function, the team will function efficiently.*

5. *Team leadership is usually best determined by status of the members' professions.*

6. *Most teams have both stated and implied norms for behavior.*

7. *At the core of all interdisciplinary team function is good communication.*

8. *Communication seems to occur best in teams of at least ten persons.*

9. *One team member can improve his or her team's ability to function.*

10. *The roles of caregiver and administrator are by definition adversarial.*

Team members must develop a sensitivity to and respect for each other that values differences as well as similarities. *

INTERDISCIPLINARY TEAMS have not developed without good reason. The health care system and the knowledge base necessary to provide competent care have increased in both volume and complexity. New specialties and new professional groups have developed to meet the multiple and diverse needs of patients and their families. It is being recognized that when these many groups and individuals ply their separate skills but fail to share their plans or decisions with one another, the result may be disastrous for the patient.

In a hospital that had "coordinated patient-care services" and many on-paper interdisciplinary teams, an elderly farmer with cancer, a survivor of numerous treatments, specialties and departmental shufflings, described his discordant experiences crudely, but clearly. "If the people who built my house," he said, "had communicated as badly as this staff does, every time I turned on a light switch my toilet would flush."

The idea of a health care team is a noble one: a group of individuals, each with different knowledge and experience, come together and pool those resources for the benefit of the patient and family. The underlying assumption is that the patient and family are a complex and interrelated system of physiological, psychological, social, and spiritual systems and that no single person can address all of the patient's or the family's needs.

In the ideal team situation a psychologist might say, "We can't take Mrs. Myer's concern about her symptoms too seriously; she is preoccupied with all bodily changes." However the aid could return with the comment, "She didn't act that way before she heard she was going to start chemotherapy; I think her illness isn't all that's worrying her."

Or a physician might say, "Mrs. Murdstan couldn't be in much pain; she is usually sleeping when I look in at 4 p.m." And a nurse could respond, "The

*Lowe, J.I., Herranen, M. Interdisciplinary team concepts, in *Hospice: Education Program for Nurses,* Proj. Dir. Henry, D.M., DHHS Publication HRA 81-27, 1981, p. 1043.

narcotic you have prescribed to be given as she requests it needs to be reevaluated. She waits until the pain is intense to ask for it, then it's such a large does, it puts her under. Could we discuss a smaller dose, regularly administered?" The physician might then respond with an individually titrated, regularly monitored and administered medication.

Many write about the interdisciplinary, or multidisciplinary, team, but few such teams really exist. Newer or remodeled hospitals frequently have included team meeting rooms on every floor. But how often have these areas become overflow storage rooms, lounges, or libraries? And when they have been used for meetings, such "health team conferences" comprise mostly nursing staff. Physicians are quick to say that they are too busy, even though they would like to attend (Epstein, 1974). Some may be convinced that they do not need other than medical consults. Others may seek to avoid the threatening prospect of submitting their judgments to the critical appraisal of the rest of the team. And for their part, some nurses may prefer their unchallenged authority; they may not wish to have to justify their judgments and responsibilities to physicians.

Yet some teams are functioning far better these days than was ever imagined possible ten years ago. Usually the common denominator in the effectiveness of these teams is the belief of the members—physicians, nurses, counselors—in the right and the responsibility of each member to share.

The hospice care team is really very special because it comprises more than a group of people. It includes the professional staff, with their many talents and philosophies; it includes the patient; and it includes the patient's family. In short, the team comprises a whole society of caring persons who are related to one another in their focus on and concern for the patient-family. The team is committed to the philosophy of hospice; it is also committed to the care of its own members. No team member can be denied his or her role on the team, and that role must be acknowledged. Roles may change as team members develop new skills or as the needs of the dying person foster new sensitivity, knowledge, and strength.

TEAMWORK

Teams do not necessarily function just because they exist. Lowe and Herranen (1981) point out that teamwork is based not on an administrative decision, but on multiple professions working together to deliver comprehensive health care (p. 424). Teamwork, they suggest, is a continuous process. Since teams are constantly changing, they require constant evaluation. Moreover, team members must share a basic "philosophy and framework for working together in order to achieve the stated goals/tasks" (Lowe & Herranen, 1981, p. 1043). There are, of course, exceptions such as the serious crisis in which the goal is so clear and important that those of many different values and philosophies cooperate well.

There should be a consensus among team members as to how the group will examine its process, level of achievement, and methods of improvement.

Most important, the effective interdisciplinary team is made up of people who understand the importance of their unique knowledge and who are able both to accept the contributions of other members and to carry out decisions. An underlying precept for the successful functioning of a team is that no *one* person possesses all the expertise, time, and compassion necessary for the care of patients and families.

Five elements of team function are common to interdisciplinary teams. In order to understand why a team does or does not function well, one must be able to analyze these elements.

Group Purpose

The overall purpose of the hospice team is its raison d'être: to care for the dying patient. Specific goals can be outlined by defining the tasks to be accomplished. In analyzing goals it is essential to understand (1) how they are evaluated, (2) who sets and evaluates them, and (3) how committed the team is (as individuals and as a group) to the goals. Frequently as the composition of a team changes, there is less agreement, commitment, and clarity about the team's exact purpose. Individuals joining or being assigned may have different expectations or purposes for their involvement. Or as a program changes and grows, the goal of the team may need to change. For example in its early stages the team may spend the majority of time on development while later groups will be involved with converting plans to functioning services. Whereas the original team may have been excellent at generating and conceptualizing patient care programs, they may be less effective at implementation.

Roles

Another element of team function is the roles individuals play in responding to stated goals and purposes (Lowe & Herranen, 1981). Each person has an idea of how she or he should act and, to a lesser extent, a concept of how every other team member should act. These perceptions are based on many things including education, professional position, perceived importance of one's own skills, past team experiences, and a variety of social concepts. People relate quite differently to different groups and hierarchies, according to their perceived roles and stature in each group.

Rubin and Beckhard (1972) have pointed out that there can be vast differences between the way individuals perceive their own rules and the way others see them. Such differences lead to role ambiguity (not knowing what is expected), role conflict (expectations are not compatible), or role overload (multiple obligations cannot be met). The way these problems of role function operate in a palliative care team can be understood by examining the view of the nurse's role in patient care decisions held by the nurse, the physician, the chaplain, and the volunteer. It is quickly evident that unless there is a fair amount of consensus in this area, stress, disillusionment, or even anger may develop.

Leadership

Most groups have a leader who has been designated either by assignment, by election, or by informal assumption of the role. Sometimes a formal leader is supplemented by several actual leaders who keep the project moving and make most of the decisions. Leaders are often appointed because of professional stature. It is equally—perhaps more important—that they want to lead, are clear about and committed to the group's stated purposes, and have the necessary leadership skills and interpersonal sensitivities to get the job done under agreeable conditions.

The way a group is directed by its leadership is interdependent with the stated and implied rules it has for its functioning. New members of some groups soon discover that there are acceptable and unacceptable ways of getting something done; they are informed about—"the way we do things around here." Some groups allow disagreement and openly discuss problems. Others express only positive feelings and will not tolerate dissension. Such "norms" are powerful determinants of group members' behavior. Norms are most obvious when violated. For example, the offender may be met with silent disapproval or a joking reprimand or may eventually be isolated from communication.

Communication

The subtlest behavior norms have a great effect on patterns of communication. At the heart of all interdisciplinary team activity is good communication, both vertical—in the giving and receiving of orders—and horizontal. All team members must be able to share their observations, frustrations, questions, and decisions and to receive feedback from those who, through different experience and education, can expand their levels of knowledge.

What appears to be good communication may sometimes reflect only that certain team members are consistently talking with others. People who are threatened by such openness have great difficulty functioning as part of a team. It is helpful to note whether team members talk both at meetings and less formally, if all team members talk, and if volunteers and the patient-family are included appropriately.

Communication seems to occur best in groups with between five and seven members; expression of differing viewpoints is facilitated, and everyone seems able to participate. In larger groups the processes become more formal.

Some people dominate while others are silent, and subgroups form to increase the feeling of group membership for nondominant members.

Decisions and Actions

The basic tasks of a group are the decisions it makes and actions it takes upon those choices. In patient care, decisions are made in a variety of ways: by one caregiver, by a caregiver and the patient-family, by several team members in consultation, or by the team in consensus. Team members are most likely to get behind and work for an idea or project they themselves have helped create. Clearly, people should have the confidence and support to make daily decisions in their own fields without having a team discussion. On the other hand, a complex problem like recurring pain should not be dealt with by any one team member without hearing the opinions of those involved in the patients' physiological, spiritual, social, and emotional welfare. It is essential also that the team be informed once decisions are made so that contradictions of effort do not occur. Teamwork is an effort—and it takes common sense, sensitivity, and a healthy self-image.

DEVELOPING A HOSPICE TEAM

Teams providing hospice care develop slowly, and the process is never complete. The amount of work required to create and maintain a functioning hospice team is usually greatly underestimated. Part of the challenge offered by working on a hospice team reflects the differences between the hospice philosophy of care and the traditional approach. Beckhard (1974) has used many of these functions we have described to illustrate these differences. Whereas such functions as purpose and leadership are quite clear on the traditional surgical team, they are often nebulous on hospice interdisciplinary teams. The purpose of the surgical team is specifically to operate and to heal; the hospice team's purpose—the comprehensive care of patient and family—varies constantly because it is dependent on ever-changing needs. The tasks, unlike surgical tasks, are thus often unclear. The roles of those who perform these tasks must clearly be both overlapping and flexible in order to evolve in ways that keep individual patient needs at the center of team function.

It is in decision making that we find what may be the one of the greatest differences between the traditional medical model and hospice. For instance, on the surgical team there is a clear hierarchy for decision making; in hospice, decision making is a group process or it is delegated first to one or two team members and then to others, depending on a matching of their skills and expertise to patient-family needs. Communication, rather than being a simple chain of command, is an open, ongoing, and honest flow of information in order to effect informed choices (Beckhard, 1974).

THE COMPOSITION OF THE HOSPICE CARE TEAM

According to the National Hospice Organization (1979) the core members of care team include but are not limited to:

- Patient/family unit
- Primary physician and hospice physician
- Administrator
- Nursing director and staff; patient care coordinator
- Clergy
- Social worker
- Volunteers

Many other professionals interface with this core group as necessary, in order to meet individual patient–family needs throughout illness and bereavement.

The Patient-Family Unit

There are at least two important reasons why the patient and family should be included in a very real sense as team members. First, it is they who are experiencing the impact of illness, feeling the exact physiological and emotional changes, and developing expectations regarding the effect the care plan will have on their lives.

Second, research has indicated that patients and families involved in decisions and plans for their care are far more committed to and supportive of such treatment (Hayes-Bautista, D., 1976).

Many health care professionals are still quite uncomfortable about including patients and families in discussions and decisions even though they may articulate a belief that this should be done. The staff position of "patient advocate" has developed at least partially to remedy this omission. However, it is the responsibility of every team member to listen carefully to patient–family concerns, to interject those concerns into team decision making, and to keep the patient and family informed about choices and outcomes.

Whereas patient–family participation has traditionally been a matter of "educating" patients and families as to the correctness of the choices made by the professionals, in palliative care the patient–family's opinions should lie at the very center of decisions. (See Chapter 4 for a complete discussion of joint goal setting.)

Primary Physician and Hospice Physician

The primary physician frequently remains the physician in charge and does not transfer clinical responsibility to a hospice physician. In this type of program, the hospice medical director serves as an administrator, spokesperson, and educator. She or he establishes standards of medical service, develops and executes organizational plans, and educates and advises on matters in the medical community. The extent to which the medical director coordinates the entire hospice team and patient management varies from one program to another.

In other programs hospice physicians are responsible for the clinical management of patients and the coordination of therapies and services. Primary or community physicians refer their patients to the hospice program and the hospice physician. This may occur where there is a hospital-based hospice unit and home care program. In this case, hospice physicians are reimbursed for services. Hospice medical directors serving in an administrator—educator—advisor role have frequently been volunteers or paid a moderate yearly stipend as consultants although this may change with newer reimbursement criteria.

Administrator

The administrator may or may not be an active part of the care team, but she or he is always an influence on the care given. The financial resources of a hospice, whether meager or immense, must be secured, budgeted and well managed in order for any program of care to survive. Some caregivers erroneously dismiss the importance of the administrator without considering that a good administrator frequently is all that keeps the program afloat. Administrators must be responsible for directing all aspects of the hospice program and its resources in conformity with the philosophy, goals, and policies established by the board of directors. It is unfortunate that occasionally an adversarial relationship develops between clinical and administrative staff, because a strong positive relationship provides the best medium for the growth and cooperation necessary for good patient care. Care providers sometimes enjoy the role of being "above" petty cost-effectiveness concerns, yet economic concerns are of fundamental importance in securing and managing the money necessary to maintain high quality patient care.

Director of Nursing, Patient Care Coordinator, and Team Nurses

The nursing staff generally comprises inpatient nurses, home-care nurses, a patient care coordinator and perhaps a coordinator of nursing education. Nursing aides and homemaker aides generally work under nursing supervision as well. A director of nursing is sometimes designated instead of, or in addition to, the patient care coordinator. The director makes assignments and supervises work, and it is generally his or her responsibility to implement the policies of the board of directors. In addition to specific nursing skills, she or he provides the primary care supporting the patient's ability to live as fully as possible within the limits imposed by illness. The director is the professional most readily available, and probably the most frequently seen. It is the nurse who most often is brought into close physical contact with the patient and who provides information and assesses and defines problems.

Patient Care Coordination and the direction of managing team meetings may be done by the Director of Nursing or handled by a separate position of patient care. The coordinator of Patient Care serves to match appropriate care and services with patient–family needs. The familiar illustration of the patient-family in the center of a circle of care is accurate in hospice, but frequently those caregivers are orchestrated to the patient's best advantage by a care coordinator who is a "partner in care."

The roles of the hospice program nurse, like those of the home health nurse in cancer care, are many and varied. The hospice program nurse not only delivers skilled care but teaches, counsels, and supports and generally coordinates services for the patient. The nurse may be the only constant in the patient's life of multiple care providers, and she or he must identify the roles of each provider relative to the care that is needed (Baird, 1980). The nurse may interpret instructions and gather needed information for the patient-family. The nurse may also assure all providers of ongoing communication when they are not actually meeting to discuss patient needs (See Table 5-1, p. 79).

Skilled nursing care includes all the functions of asessment; choice of personnel to deliver care; and the inclusion and education of family members. Family involvement is a primary function of the successful at-home care program. The nurse must be able to make accurate judgments about the family's ability to learn and their willingness to participate. This role may lead the nurse into one of patient–family counselor. Providing reassurance, along with training, to the family often guarantees the possibility of the patient staying at home.

A large part of providing care in the home centers on the family's knowledge of available community resources. The home health agency, often through the nurse or social worker, can furnish information about services and equipment, eligibility and costs. The nurse or social worker may be able to pull together a support system of volunteers from a church or social organizaton to augment the hospice team volunteers, due to his or her constant association with the patient and family.

The hospice team nurse, in each of his or her roles, provides for physical, emotional, and spiritual care that is conducive to both relief of distressing symptoms and trust (Baird, 1980). Note that the nurse provides *for,* but does not *provide* all of these kinds of support. In this period of redefinition and expansion of roles, it is important not to burden nurses with unrealistic expectations. Nurses cannot, and indeed should not, provide the care that qualified and available interdisciplinary team members can contribute. A weekly discussion and re-evaluation of any care plan should be held. Professionals from all disciplines, as well as family and volunteers, should have the opportunity to compare and evaluate their observations and to plan the implementation of their various management plans. At the same time, according to Baird (1980), it is the primary nurse who "is responsible for the continuing quantitative and qualitative assessments of needs. This nurse is also accountable for the coordination of the hospice care delivered" (p. 35).

Hospice Clergy

The chaplain is both a facilitator and a provider. If the patient or family has had strong and satisfying ties with a place of worship and a particular minister, priest, or rabbi, then the hospice chaplain's role is to support that relationship; it is extremely important that every possible opportunity be extended to involve the patient and family's own clergy in the team. If the patient or family expresses no desire for spiritual guidance or support, the chaplain should honor that decision. If the patient or family expresses a need for religious, spiritual counseling, however, hospice clergy answers that need. Chaplains should be available throughout both the illness and bereavement, and they may work actively with the bereavement team in the role either of chaplain or of counselor perhaps without a specific denominational mission.

Also important is the role the chaplain plays in educating other religious leaders about the hospice philosophy and program. And the chaplain should be available to counsel staff and volunteers about the effect of the hospice philosophy on their own feelings of personal mortality and about the impact of patients' deaths.

Social Worker

The social worker is trained and experienced in helping patients in a variety of ways. Social workers can aid families with the emotional, social, and financial impact of illness and probable death. They should be able to help patient and family get the optimum benefit from the health care system and from community agencies; they can guide the family as they "negotiate the system." In this capacity, social workers can also serve as a resource to the rest of the hospice team. (See Chapter 11 for a complete discussion of social service needs.)

Volunteers

The volunteer is an excellent position to establish a close and supportive relationship with a family. Volunteers can lessen fear and isolation by keeping the patient and family in touch with the rest of the team and with the community. The volunteer contribution can be as varied as the individual talent, humor, and creativity of those who serve as volunteers. Teams profit from having a core of volunteers who have a wide range of backgrounds, ages, languages, professions, hobbies, and ethnic origins. They can help with almost any activity that a family needs continued, and can be responsive listeners and sympathetic counselors.

Coordination of volunteer selection, training, aptitudes, assignments, and supervision is usually handled by a director of volunteers, or a volunteer coordinator. This person functions as a support to the volunteers by helping them find and use their skills as well as providing education and support to help them understand their reactions to patient–family problems, humor, and grief (Dorang, 1981).

Volunteers must be included in team meetings, for their insights are valuable to the other team members. A patient frequently reveals important truths to the volunteer, who is seen as ever present, more accessible, less professional—one of the family. In addition, volunteers need to be kept informed. For instance, current information about the patient's condition will prevent volunteers from making commitments they cannot keep, such as promise of an outing that is becoming physically impossible. Being informed helps volunteers respond appropriately to family requests.

HOSPICE TEAM RESOURCE MEMBERS

There are many other valuable team members who can be interfaced with the team in an individual patient–family situation. In individual situations they may actually become more important than others in both care and support. In addition to the pharmacologist, psychiatrist, and physical therapist discussed here, these occasional team members include the dietician, music therapist, dentist, speech therapist, psychiatric nurse, genontologist, thanatologist, and attorney.

Pharmacologist–Clinical Pharmacist

Consultation among the primary care physician, the nursing staff, and a pharmacologist can be critical in controlling pain and other distressing symptoms. The pharmacologist has a sophisticated knowledge of drug interactions, dosage, effects, and reactions that is needed for quick and effective symptom management. A similar role in hospice care is being developed by clinical pharmacists, who are becoming highly valuable members of the team. In a recent study, 46% of the hospice directors considered the affiliated pharmacist to be a member of the interdisciplinary team (Berry, 1981).

Psychiatrist

A psychiatrist who is available to team members and families on a consulting basis can be very helpful in the resolution of extreme emotional problems that may result from periods of anxiety, guilt, fear, or grief. A clinical psychologist can also function as part of the team by being available for counseling, either individual or group. Those working with patient–family problems may find that their own lives change and their perspectives shift; counseling can bring new self-awareness.

A group of eminent psychiatrists attending the International Conference on Hospice in London, 1981, issued a statement which addressed the unique contributions their profession could bring to hospice care. They recognized that care of the dying requires an understanding of the "complex interrelationships of the biological psychological and spiritual needs of patients, families and caregivers." (Fergenberg, L. 1981). Since the training of psychiatrists is in both medical and behavioral fields their skills apply to (a) assisting team members in the diagnosis and treatment of organic and functional psychiatric disorders and (b) advising on the use of medications. (Fergenberg, L. 1981).

Their statement was direct and clear in its affirmation that "dying is not a psychiatric illness" (Fergenberg p. 2) and that the skills of the psychiatrist are often directed towards reassurance and support in the normality of the patient and family responses to grief and stress. There was also an offer to assist with staff support and counseling. They also entered a request that if a psychiatrist is available to the team, he or she should be involved as a team member rather than as a "consultant to whom people are passed for treatment." (Fergenberg, L. p. 2).

Physical Therapist

The emphasis in hospice care is on improving the quality of life. The physical therapist working in hospice is not concerned with rehabilitation but with maintaining functions. The dying patient is constantly concerned with his or her deteriorating ability to perform normal daily activities. The physical therapist's training provides him or her with the ability to (1) accurately assess physical potential for movement and activity, (2) work with the patient to enable him or her to function with the greatest possible independence in the face of diminishing resources, (3) help the patient to understand his or her limitations, and (4) advise team members and family regarding positioning, transfers, and various helpful devices for patient comfort and safe functioning (Doutre, 1980).

Such maintenance of daily living activities can provide the patient with release from tension, recreation, and some degree of accomplishment and pride in independence.

Table 5-1. *Roles of the Home Health Nurse*

- Coordinator of services
- Deliverer of skilled care
- Teacher of patients and families
- Counselor and supporter
- Facilitator for community resources

Source: Based on Baird (1980), pp. 30–33.

BUILDING AND MAINTAINING AN EFFECTIVE TEAM

There are ways that an individual can single-handedly improve his or her team's ability to function. Realistically, it takes a coordinated group effort to effect large changes, but substantial and positive things happen when even one more member makes an effort to facilitate team achievement. Ask yourself: Do I—

1. help identify and prioritize tasks
2. keep the group's purpose in mind when suggesting new ideas;
3. help implement what I suggest or support, even assuming a leadership role if necessary;
4. compromise when necessary and remain flexible to suggestions;
5. get and give information freely;
6. evaluate my responsibility and actions;
7. genuinely understand and respect the contributions of other disciplines;
8. accept the proven efficacy of someone else's plan over mine?

Being able to answer 'yes' honestly to each of these questions means that as a team member you will be constructive, not destructive of its purposes.

REFERENCES

Baird, S.B. Nursing roles in continuing care: Home care and hospice. *Seminars in Oncology.* 1980, *7,* 28–37.

Doutre, D., Stillwell, D.M., & Ajemian, I. Physiotherapy in palliative care. In New York: Ajemian, I., & Mount, B. (Eds.), *Royal Victoria Hospital Manual on Palliative/Hospice Care.* Arno Press, 1980.

Epstein, C. *Effective interaction in contemporary nursing.* Englewood, N.J.: Prentice-Hall, 1974.

Hayes-Bautista, D. "Modifying the Treatment: Patient Compliance, Patient Control, & Medical Care," *Social Science of Medicine,* Vol. 10, 1976, pp. 233–38.

Lowe, J.I., Herranen, M. Interdisciplinary team hospice manual. In *Hospice: Education Program for Nurses,* Department of Health & Human Services Publication No. HRA 81-27, 1981, Project Officer Henry, O.M. U.S. Government Printing Office, Washington D.C.
National Hospice Organization,*Standards of a Hospice Program of Care.* 6th Revision, McLean, Va., 1979.
Rubin, J., & Beckhard, R. Factors influencing the effectiveness of health teams. *Milbank Memorial Fund Quarterly,* 1972, *50* (Part I), p. 317–30.

1. F		*6. T*	
2. T		*7. T*	
3. F		*8. F*	
4. F		*9. T*	
5. F		*10. F*	

6

Principles and Standards of Hospice Care

Answer the following questions True (T) or False (F). Answers appear after references in this chapter.

1. *A document developed by the International Work Group on Death, Dying, and Bereavement has articulated the assumptions and principles essential to improving care of the terminally ill.*

2. *The National Hospice Organization's Standards of a Hospice Program of Care have addressed those standards that are intrinsic to all forms of hospice care.*

3. *The NHO standards are reviewed annually by the membership and can be changed through the democratic process.*

4. *The NHO standards support the concepts of interdisciplinary, 24-hour-a-day, patient-centered, appropriate care.*

5. *Any hospice that wishes to join NHO in any category must comply with the NHO Standards.*

6. *The NHO Standards guarantee that all services described must be reimbursible through third-party payers.*

7. *The NHO Standards define the full-service hospice program as offering both inpatient and home care.*

8. *The NHO Standards direct that all medical care must be provided by a physician on the staff of the hospice program*

9. *A standards document may help guarantee a reimbursement system that does not compromise hospice services.*

10. *There is at present no cooperation among professional groups to develop licensing and reimbursement criteria.*

Those whom I have known within this country and within the National Hospice Organization who have functioning programs are generally very interested in seeing that Hospice care takes steps to remain both professionally and humanly appropriate and competent, that it seeks to maintain and improve the quality of care for the terminally ill, that it retains the ability to be responsive to the needs of its patients throughout the final stages of their illness, that it establishes and maintains a dialogue of mutual respect with other elements of the health care system. These concerns are motivated by professional and personal convictions developed both through training and caring for the terminally ill. Hospice cannot avoid the necessity and practicality of assuming responsibility for its actions on the basis of its experience.*

A S THE hospice movement continues to thrive, a great variety of groups with many individual purposes are creating new kinds of hospice programs. In 1975 there were three known United States hospices although such diverse groups as the Frontier Nursing Service in Kentucky and the Benedictine Nursing Center in Oregon have provided hospice-like care for many generations. In 1982 the National Hospice Organization (NHO) had 338 voting, provider members, supported by communities, hospitals, and agencies of various kinds. At this writing, no state is without at least a developing hospice. The movement has advanced primarily as a reform, which, according to Max Weber (1964), "begins with dissatisfaction with an existing system and the subsequent development of ideas for a new approach." In an environment of reform there will be a tension between those maintaining existing systems and those with the new ideas. If the new ideas and approaches are to survive, they must find ways to coexist with the policy makers, licensing agencies, and managers who will institutionalize them.

PRINCIPLES OF THE HOSPICE MOVEMENT

The North American hospice movement is now at that critical point where the position of new ideas within or opposing the existing system is

---

*From Hadlock, D.C. *Letter to Association of Community Cancer Centers,* October 23, 1979. With permission.

becoming highly visible. Some of the challenges are: palliative treatment in a curative system; personal care in an impersonal technological system; family participation in a system that sees the patient as the unit of care; team input in the traditional, medical-model system; warm personal environment in a clinical setting; and holistic care in a specialized, departmentalized service. Also, as Wald, Foster, and Wald (1979) argue, "reformers need credibility, funds and formal permission to carry out their aims. Decision-making inevitably involves compromise, and everyone involved must ask whether the compromise is necessary and, if so, can the ideal survive" (pp. 27–28). A statement of principles that underlie these decisions can often preserve the integrity of the original program.

Decisions, it must be remembered, are often made in reaction to an external event or system. It is often difficult to table such decisions, once they have been made even if there is only partial understanding of the issue. Consultants from the fields of finance, fundraising, and law and experts in legislation are called in and, with their experience, perceptions change and priorities shift. Frequently even the basic caregiver composition of a board of directors may change as individuals are included to help confront the complexities of incorporation, funding, reimbursement, and the like. New areas of decision often result in compromises that endanger the humanistic purpose of the movement (Wald, Foster, & Wald, 1981).

Saunders (1980) has emphasized the principles adhered to at St. Christopher's. She has stated that whether a hospice is a separate unit, part of a hospital, a separate ward or a home care or hospital team," it should establish certain specific principles, some of which are common to any branch of medicine or nursing, others of which are particularly relevant to hospice care. These principles emphasize the importance of interdisciplinary, clinical and emotional-support professional team; open professional communication; home or inpatient care 24 hours every day; research and teaching; bereavement counseling; supportive environment; efficient administration; a community of patients (within some cases, "long-term progressive illnesses, chronic pains... frailty and old age"), and a commitment to a continuous research to improve care (Saunders, 1980). She continues:

It has been important to define the standard of relief that should be achieved so that those in the general field may assess their own practice and recognize the expertise of the special unit or team and when it should be evolved. Only such standards and such integration will ensure that wherever patients are dying, they will receive the best treatment available.*

Although many groups and individuals have adopted specific care principles, the work of three groups has emerged as basic to the hospice

---

*From Saunders, C.M. Hospice care. In I. Ajemian & B. Mount (Eds.), *The Royal Victoria Hospital Manual on Palliative Hospice Care.* New York: Am. Press, 1980, p. 23. With permission.

movement. The discussion in this section utilizes the work of St. Christopher's Hospice (Cicely Saunders, Medical Director), The International Work Group on Death, Dying and Bereavement (Florence S. Wald, Chair of the Standards Committee), and Standards of a Hospice Care Program of the National Hospice Organization (Standards and Accreditation Committee).

St. Christopher's Hospice, London, England

St. Christopher's, the first hospice built specifically with teaching and research purposes set out, with funding from the National Health Service "to establish recognized standards of care which could be interpreted in the home as well as in other settings and cultures and become a part of general medical and nursing teaching" (Saunders, 1980, p. 22).

As the hospice concept of care has spread, a wide variety of innovations and individual interpretations have developed. Although there are almost as many variations as programs, for convenience of discussion they can be grouped loosely into several models including the free-standing hospice, the hospital unit or team; the home-health agency, and the community-coordinated hospice. Some have considerable financial support; others operate within very modest budgets. Their staff may comprise paid or volunteer professionals or both. Some programs are entirely autonomous administratively; others are affiliated with other programs or function as units or departments within a larger entity.

The standards of care that have evolved out of various hospice programs and interest groups are not generally concerned with the manner (model) in which care is provided but emphasize the type, level, and quality of that care and its appropriateness to patient and family needs.

Hospice should never stop evolving and growing; it should retain always the flexibility without which there can be no individualized care or community input. As Mortinson and Hackley urge, we must be willing to share our exclusivity, our market, and our benevolent control over who can care for the terminally ill and in what form they do it as long as it is done well (Mortinson & Hackley, 1979).

The International Work Group on Death, Dying and Bereavement

In November of 1974, the International Work Group on Death, Dying and Bereavement met and formed a standards committee, with Florence S. Wald as chairperson. The membership of the committee includes authorities from the fields of medicine, nursing, religion, social work, psychology, sociology, and anthropology. The task of the committee was to delineate the standards of care essential for dying patients and their families and the support system necessary for caregivers. Although the committee continues to meet every 18 months, committee members recognized the need to publish their work and presented the document titled General Assumptions and Principles in 1978. This document outlines the assumptions, and principles that underlie general standards of care while others have made use of them in developing standards suited to individual institutions.

The International Work Group on Death, Dying, and Bereavement advocates a variety of approaches in providing hospice care as long as the basic principles and assumptions articulated by its standards committee are observed. Thus each community, each institution, has the flexibility to determine its own needs and use its particular resources.

The National Hospice Organization

The National Hospice Organization, working from a variety of sources, including the principles of St. Christopher's and the "Assumptions and Principles" of the International Work Group, has prepared a document, "Standards of a Hospice Program of Care," which the NHO membership has ratified. This work was funded in part through the generosity of the Ittleson Foundation, Inc., New York.

NHO's board of directors gave the organization's Standards and Accreditation Committee (SAC) a mandate "to identify those standards which are intrinsic to all forms of Hospice care....to establish criteria which outline acceptable limits for Hospice care programs....[and] to create and implement mechanisms (Standards and Accreditation Committee, National Hospice Organization, 1979, p. 2). All of these activities were to be carried out under the direction of the NHO's board of directors and in response to input from the membership at large.

It was, and has remained, the intent of the NHO membership to provide a protective document for consumers and care providers as well as a sound program definition for regulatory and reimbursement agencies. The National Hospice Organization's definition of hospice is now generally accepted by most hospice programs. It reads as follows:

A Hospice is a centrally administered program of palliative and supportive services which provides physical, psychological, social, and spiritual care for dying persons and their families. Services are provided by a medically supervised interdisciplinary team of professionals and volunteers. Hospice services are available in both the home and inpatient setting. Home care is provided on a part-time, intermittent, regularly scheduled and around-the-clock on-call basis. Admission to a hospice program of care is on the basis of patient and family need.*

---

*From Standards and Accreditation Committee, National Hospice Organization. *Standards of a hospice care program.* McLean, Va.: National Hospice Organization, 1979, p. 4. With permission.

As can be seen, although a number of services are included in the "total" hospice, there is no attempt to restrict the way in which these services are to be delivered. Communities still have the flexibility within the NHO standards to construct a program according to local needs and resources.

The NHO standards also include a statement of philosophy that parallels the assumptions and principles described earlier.

Hospice affirms life. Hospice exists to provide support and care for persons in the last phases of incurable disease so that they might live as fully and comfortably as possible. Hospice recognizes dying as a normal process whether or not resulting from disease. Hospice neither hastens nor postpones death. Hospice exists in the hope and belief that through appropriate care and the promotion of a caring community sensitive to their needs, patients and families may be free to attain a degree of mental and spiritual preparaton for death that is satisfactory to them" (Standards and Accreditation Committee, National Hospice Organization, 1981, p. 8).

This short definition and the statement of philosophy contain the essence of all that is unique about hospice—the belief in dignity of life, and the preservation of that dignity.

The full text of *Standards of a Hospice Care Program* will be found at Appendix 6-1.* That text includes a statement of each standard and of the principle that underlies it as well as an exclusive interpretation of each standard.

The Standards and Principles of a Hospice Program of Care

The Standards of a Hospice Program are based on certain principles of human behavior and health care. For the purpose of this document the standards have been organized into four categories, which constitute a general framework in which to view Hospice care as a response to the needs of patients and families. The four categories are

      A. Basic Principle Underlying Hospice Care
      B. The Nature of Hospice Care
      C. The Patient and Family
      D. The Hospice Program

A. *Basic Principle Underlying Hospice Care.* One of the tenets of Hospice is the belief and recognition that dying is a normal process whether or not resulting from disease. Every aspect of Hospice care and program development emanates from and is guided by this tenet.

No.	Standard	No.	Principle
1	Appropriate therapy is the goal of Hospice Care	1	Dying is a normal process

*From Standards and Accreditation Committee, National Hospice Organization. *Standards of a hospice care program.* (6th ed.). McLean, Va.: National Hospice Organization, 1981, pp. 1–29. With permission.

B. *The Nature of Hospice Care.*   Appropriate therapy is a goal of Hospice Care; therefore, it is necessary to define that which is appropriate within a given situation. With the recognition that death is inevitable as the final moment of the natural course of human life and that the terminal phase of the disease process is irreversible, it becomes possible to establish goals for caring and interventions to achieve the palliation of the accompanying concerns and distressful symptoms of the process of dying.

No. Standard	No. Principle
2 Palliative care is the most appropriate form of care when cure is no longer possible.	2 When cure is not possible, care is still needed.
3 The goal of palliative care is the prevention of distress from chronic signs and symptoms	3 Pain and other symptoms of incurable disease can be controlled
4 Admission to a Hospice Program of care is dependent on patient and family needs and their expressed request for care.	4 Not all persons need or desire palliative care.
5 Hospice care consists of a blending of professional and nonprofessional services.	5 The amount and type of care provided should be related to patient and family needs.
6 Hospice care considers all aspects of the lives of patients and their families as valid areas of therapeutic concern.	6 When a patient and family are faced with terminal disease, stress and concerns may arise in many asspects of their lives.
7 Hospice care is respectful of all patient and family belief systems, and will employ resources to meet the personal philosophic, moral and religious needs of patients and their families.	7 Personal philosophic, moral, or religious belief systems are important to patients and families who are facing death.
8 Hospice care provides continuity of care.	8 Continuity of care (services and personnel) reduces the patient's and the family's sense of alienation and fragmentation.

C. *The Patient and Family.*   The patient and family are the raison d'etre for Hospice programs. Patient and family participation in the decisions and care giving to the maximum extent possible, should enable the patient and family to live according to their "style" and with the dignity and respect due all human beings until the moment of the patient's death.

No.	Standard	No.	Principle
9	A Hospice care program considers the patient and the family together as the unit of care.	9	Families experience significant stress during the terminal illness of one of their members.
10	The patient's family is considered to be a central part of the Hospice care team.	10	Family participation in care giving is an important part of palliative care.
11	Hospice care programs seek to identify, coordinate, and supervise persons who can give care to patients who do not have a family member available to take on the responsibility of giving care.	11	Not all patients have a family member available to take on the responsibility of giving care.
12	Hospice care for the family continues into the bereavement period.	12	Family needs continue after the death of one of their members.

D. *The Hospice Program.* A Hospice Program is designed to achieve the goals of the patients and families for whom the program exists through the provision of appropriate palliative care. The program has a number of components, each of which makes Hospice care possible and is aimed at ensuring quality care. The components of a Hospice Program are identified in the following standards.

No.	Standard	No.	Principle
13	Hospice care is available 24 hours a day, 7 days a week.	13	Patient and family needs may arise at any time.
14	Hospice care is provided by an interdisciplinary team.	14	No one individual or profession can meet all the needs of terminally ill patients and families all the time.
15	Hospice programs will have structured and informal means of providing support to staff.	15	Persons giving care to others need to be supported and replenished in order to continue to give care.
16	Hospice programs will be in compliance with the Standards of the National Hospice Organization and the applicable laws and regulations governing the organization and delivery of care to patients and families.	16	The need for quality assurance in health care requires the establishment of standards for practice and program operation.

17 The services of the Hospice program are coordinated under a central administration.

17 Optimal utilization of services and resources is an important goal in the administration and coordination of patient care.

18 The optimal control of distressful symptoms is an essential part of a Hospice care program requiring medical, nursing, and other services of the interdisciplinary team.

18 Attention to physical comfort is central to palliative care.

19 The Hospice care team will have: (a) a medical director on staff; (b) physicians on staff; (c) a working relationship with the patient's physician.

19 Medical care is a necessary element of palliative care.

20 Based on patient's needs and preferences as determining factors in the setting and location for care, a Hospice Program provides in-patient care and care in the home setting.

20 The physical environment and setting can influence a patient's response to care.

21 Education, training, and evaluation of Hospice services is an ongoing activity of a Hospice care program.

21 There is a continual need to improve the techniques of palliative care and to disseminate such information.

22 Accurate and current records are kept on all patients.

22 Documentation of services is necessary and desirable in the delivery of quality care.

APPLICABILITY OF STANDARDS

Accreditation, Licensure and Reimbursement

The National Hospice Organization standards have wide applicability in the health care system. In addition to developing the *Standards* document over a period of three years, the NHO's standards and accreditation committee has undertaken the following activities:

• The committee has reviewed the need for hospice accreditation and has engaged in repeated dialogue with major accrediting bodies and has developed pilot accreditation programs.

- The committee has met with leaders of the major, relevant health care and accreditation organizations, explored the possibilities of working in conjunction with the National League for Nursing/American Public Health Association, the Joint Commission on Accreditation of Hospitals, the American Hospital Association, the National Association of Home Health Agencies, Blue Cross, Blue Shield Association, and the Accreditation Association for Ambulatory Health Care, among others.

- The committee has maintained an active dialogue with major medical insurance groups, including the Health Insurance Association of America, regarding NHO input into accreditation as a basis for quality assurance as an integral part of continuing reimbursement.

In a 1980 report to the NHO board, the standards and accreditation committee pointed out the need for these additional areas of activity: "The pressure to develop an accreditation process increases with the rapid increase in the number of Hospice programs and the interest of third party payors to develop reimbursement for Hospice Care" (Standards and Accreditation Committee, National Hospice Organization, 1980, p. 1). The office of Health Care Finance and Accounting (HCFA) began in 1982 to collect data through demonstration projects at 26 sites to determine the feasibility and means for Medicare–Medicaid reimbursement.

The Standards and Accreditation Committee has been sensitive to both the cost and the unnecessary duplication of effort in developing a totally new accrediting agency only for hospice programs. Yet, because hospice programs have developed in a number of settings (e.g., hospitals, home health agencies, nursing homes), no existing accrediting agency is totally experienced in conducting an accreditation visit according to the essentials of hospice care as defined in the *Standards* document. At this writing considerable progress has been made and a cooperative attitude has been displayed by most accrediting organizations in developing a means of insuring Hospice representation to the accrediting process (Standards and Accreditation Committee, National Hospice Organization, 1980).

In addition, other committees of the National Hospice Organization have worked on matters directly related to the developing of a model accreditation process. For example, using a "Basic Data Set," the Research and Evaluation Committee has collected and coded information on the state of the art in hospice care in America.

Evidence from this and subsequent data sets indicates that although these standards are flexible and allow for many individual models or interpretations of ways to deliver care, they are still extremely difficult for a dedicated hospice group to apply. Excellent community-based hospices have begun with some elements of a program such as home care and bereavement counseling but without dedicated inpatient beds. Nursing-directed teams do function with written medical orders but without a paid, full-time hospice medical director. Care must be delivered in the very real world of small rural communities.

Sometimes all the resources just are not there, and yet it cannot be denied that the program functions, and that patients and families receive a higher quality of care because the program exists. But the standards exist to emphasize what hospice can be—should be—at its best. And if a community program lacks some elements, it can continue to strive for maximal resources.

All hospices, particularly recently developed programs, will find real protection in strongly endorsed national standards. Cost-containment will dictate the degree to which some hospices find it possible to keep patient–staff ratios in line with hospice levels of care, to plan and erect environmentally supportive buildings, or to maintain program autonomy. Caution must be maintained, as the less expensive options for overlapping agencies' staffs, buildings, and administrative operations become apparent, so that the resulting compromises of autonomy do not dilute the quality of hospice care.

The process of accreditation will require criteria for assessment standardized enough to be applied nationally. If standards had not existed within the hospice movement, they would have been written by those responsible for licensing. As it is, a cooperative effort among professional groups, using the NHO standards as a central treatise, is progressing. In 1983 a total of 375 hospices nationwide, representative of all administrative types, reviewed a Joint Commission on Accreditation of Hospitals (JCAH) standards manual developed by the JCAH standards and survey procedures committee. Although still to be approved, JCAH has sought hospice provider input and completed extensive field testing prior to beginning their accreditation process.

Reimbursement will have a large impact on the way hospice care evolves. Traditionally, what third party payers select for reimbursement is what survives. Without a clear guide, whole areas of hospice may disappear for lack of funding. More likely, subtle changes will occur as previously volunteered services become reimbursable and staff are hired to provide them. Or requirements for reimbursement will cause shifts in the way medical and nursing orders are written. Care may be restricted to certain settings, and may be provided within only a specific time frame or family support may be decreased. It would be good if vast time were available to develop the accreditation–reimbursement mechanism, but hospices are already experiencing the need for reimbursement for services and pressure from third party payers. For example, segments of American industry have indicated their interest in providing a "hospice benefit" for their employees, provided care is given by an accredited program.

Hospice and Medicare

On August 19, 1982, Congress approved the hospice reimbursement legislation that had been incorporated into the Tax Equity and Fiscal

Responsibility Act of 1982. The legislation authorized coverage under Medicare for hospice care for the terminally ill. Reimbursement levels have not been officially approved.* Table 6-1 presents the defining characteristics of a "hospice program" according to that legislation.

At this writing the legislation provides that "hospice care" includes benefits for nursing care under the supervision of a registered nurse; physical, occupational, and speech–language therapy; medical social services under the direction of a physician; home health services by an aide who has successfully completed an approved training program; homemaker services; medical drugs, biologicals, and appliances; physician services; short-term inpatient care including respite care, pain control and symptom management; and counseling, including bereavement, dietary and nutritional counseling.

National Hospice organization advocacy has concentrated on strengthening the volunteer component of hospice, raising payment levels for inpatient care to correspond to the clinical needs of terminally ill patients, and mechanisms for investigating and preventing fraud. NHO has argued that the government could best contain costs by encouraging the highest quality of

Table 6-1. *Definition of "Hospice Program"*

A "hospice program" is a public agency or private organization (or a subdivision thereof) that—

- provides hospice care and services, as needed, on a 24 hour basis
- provides bereavement counseling to the immediate family of the terminally ill person
- provides hospice care and services in the home, on an outpatient basis, or on a short-term inpatient basis
- assures that care provided an individual on an inpatient basis over a 12-month period does not exceed 20 percent of the aggregate number of days during such period
- employs an interdisciplinary team consisting of at least one physician, one registered nurse, one social worker, and one pastoral or other counselor
- utilizes volunteers and maintains records on volunteer use, cost savings, and expansion of services resulting from volunteer use
- maintains centralized records on all patients and does not discontinue care to an individual because of inability to pay for care
- is licensed according to existing state laws

*As of September, 1983.

hospice care, which would result in a substitution of hospice services for more costly hospitalization.

CHANGE AND THE HEALTH CARE SYSTEM

It is sometimes said, particularly in moments when the "system" seems particularly oppressive, that the high standards of hospice care will never be a reality. It may be true that elements of the health care profession and the institution will continue to exist not in the best interests of the individual patient but for the convenience, expedience, or advantage of the profession or institution itself. Hospice, even in a society where there seems to be a growth of awareness in humane health care values, may not be able to overcome all the limitations on the delivery of health care (Koff, 1980). Implementing the standards of hospice care is difficult; it requires substantial commitment from many powerful professional and community groups.

The aphorism credited to the Duc de La Rochefoucauld, "Plus ça change, plus c'est la même chose" (The more things change, the more they are the same), deserves thought. Even situations changed by revolutionary means have a way of reverting eventually to their original status once they are exposed to the conditions of the bureaucracy (Donovan, 1975).

Etzioni (1972), commenting on change, emphasizes the need to make changes closer to the problem than the person. He points out, through a variety of examples, the limited effect education, even compensatory education, has had on behavior change. The expensive public education effort to decrease driving recklessness and accidents was paralleled by an ever-increasing highway death rate—until the phenomenal decline in 1974, when speed limits were reduced to conserve gasoline. One may speculate whether the health care system also may change more to comply with strictures of regulatory and reimbursement agencies than because people begin to support the change philosophically.

Bringing About Organizational Change

In spite of resistance, change does occur, and frequently it is due to the concerted efforts of just a few very dedicated individuals. The following list outlines suggestions made by Longest (1980) for minimizing the resistance that sometimes results from staff insecurity, misunderstanding, or turf protection.

1. Through education and research, *document the need for change.*
2. *Outline the problem,* clarifying its symptoms and its basic cause.
3. *Identify alternative methods* for improvement. Inherent in the situational approach is the understanding that each organization must adapt in unique ways to its particular strengths and weakness.
4. *Select the approach* in consultation with those who will be affected by the change.
5. *Implement* by
    a. making sure that everyone involved understands and that enough time has elapsed for education
    b. disturbing as little as possible the existing customs and informal relationships
    c. providing information in advance and throughout the process, including the relevance, progress, and impact on the organization and people in it
    d. encouraging constant input from and ownership of the program with *all* involved
    e. providing for a means of releasing tension, doubts, and frustrations as the new program philosophy affects people, departments, or agencies.
6. *Evaluate* the program and thus provide feedback that can lead to corrections and strengthen convictions.

Change is not easy. People resist and become confused by change for many reasons. As Alfred North Whitehead has said, "The art of progress is to preserve order amid change and to preserve change amid order."

What Can One Person Do?

Maybe initially it is not necessary to change or create whole programs. When most patients and families are surveyed regarding the strengths and weakness of the hospice program in which they are cared for, the appreciation they express is usually focused not on some nebulous service or program but on specific people. People who care, who are attentive to needs and quick to respond with appropriate therapies are hospices within themselves. As someone in close contact with the patient, one caregiver can support the dignity of the dying person through total attention and care. One person who can be counted on to "be there" will meet, all alone, the underlying philosophy that staff should "communicate a sense of trust, honesty in their promises, skill in giving care and involvement and concern with the person receiving care" (Koff, 1980, p. 25).

In 1927 Peabody (1927) wrote, "The treatment of disease may be entirely impersonal...but the care of the patient must be entirely personal.... The secret of the care of the patient is in caring for the patient" (p. 877). The patient needs to be shown that she or he is cared for, but how can an individual caregiver do this? Balfour M. Mount has offered a list of some very practical suggestions that are grounded in a profound respect for the individual's unique worth. If an entire hospice program cannot be put in place, perhaps regulations concerning visitation and visitors can be relaxed or areas of privacy can be provided. Multidisciplinary counseling teams can be organized to assist in high-risk situations (surgery, abortion, intensive care, terminal care). Even if departmental changes are slow in coming, the individual caregiver can do a great deal of "hospice-concept care." For example Mount (1980) suggests that as a patient's room is entered, one should take time to look at the patient, address him or her by the name he or she prefers and also acknowledge family and friends present. He recommends, if at all possible, sitting down at the bedside and allowing time for questions and feelings to be expressed. Privacy should be guaranteed for such communications. He advises to be alert to non-verbal communication and willing to share some of our own feelings when appropriate. He also emphasizes the patient/family's need for prompt information. The individual is also paramount in other suggestions he makes regarding the recognition of the adult patient as an adult with physical, emotional and spiritual needs.

In a more general programmatic sense, he encourages goal-oriented team conferences, family conferences with team members and substantial use of volunteers as a way of raising the overall quality of any program. He concludes, quite honestly, with the thought that doing the above requires that you "keep your sense of humor" (Mount, p. 42).

There has never been a time in the history of medical care when attention to the standards of total patient care has been more important. Whether individuals, teams, or comprehensive programs are providing the highly important care of the dying, we should always strive for a broader understanding of dying. "Let us ask how, as individuals, we relate to patients with terminal illness and whether our relationship is near the ideal and, if not, let us take steps now to learn more about the one experience that we have in common with our patients" (Shepherd, 1980, p. 25).

REFERENCES

Donovan, H.M. *Nursing service administration.* St. Louis: C.V. Mosley Company, 1975.
Etzioni, A. Human beings are not very easy to change after all. *Saturday Review,* 1972, *55,* 45–47.
Hadlock, D.C. Letter to Association of Community Cancer Centers, October 23, 1979.
Koff, T.H. *Hospice: A caring community.* Cambridge, Mass.: Winthrop Publishers, Inc., 1980.
Longest, B.B. *Management practices for the health professional,* (2nd ed.). Reston, Va.: Reston Publishing Co., 1980.

Mortinson, L., & Hackley J. There is only one true way. *Cancer Program Bulletin* ACCC, Vol. 5, (3), 1979, p. 2–3.

Mount, B.M. Caring in today's health care system. in *The Royal Victoria Hospital manual on palliative/hospice care,* Ajemian, I., and Mount, B., (Eds.), Arno Press, N.Y., 1980.)

Peabody, F.W. The care of the patient. *Journal of the American Medical Association,* 1927, 88, 877.

Saunders, C.M. Hospice care. In Ajemian, I. & Mount, B. (Eds.), *The Royal Victoria Hospital manual on palliative/hospice care.* New York: Arno Press, 1980.

Shepherd, D.A.E. Terminal care: Toward an ideal. In Ajemian, I. and Mount, B., *The Royal Victoria Hospital manual on palliative/hospice care,* Arno Press, New York, 1980.

Standards and Accreditation Committee, National Hospice Organization. *Standards of a Hospice Care Program.* McLean, Virginia: National Hospice Organization, 1979.

Standards and Accreditation Committee, National Hospice Organization. Statement. July 11, 1980.

Standards and Accreditation Committee, National Hospice Organization. *Standards of a Hospice Care Program* (6th ed.) McLean, Virginia: National Hospice Organization, 1981.

Wald, F., Foster, Z., & Wald, H.J. The hospice movement as a health care reform, in Hospice: Education Program for Nurses, Dept. of Health & Human Services, Public No. HRH 81-77, Project Officer Henry, O.M. U.S. Government Printing Office, Washington, D.C., pp. 25–34.

Weber, M. *Theory of social and economic organization.* (1947; transl. by T. Parsons, New York, The Free Press, 1964).

1. T	6. F
2. T	7. T
3. T	8. F
4. T	9. T
5. F	10. F

Appendix 6-1.   *Standards and Principles of a Hospice Program of Care**

The Standards of a Hospice Care Program are based on certain principles of human behavior and health care. For the purpose of this document the standards have been organized into four categories, which constitute a general framework in which to view hospice care as a response to the needs of patients and families.

Standards of a Hospice Program of Care

Standard: Appropriate therapy is the goal of Hospice Care.

Principle: Dying is a normal process.

Interpretation of Standard.   Appropriate medical care is always a blend of two complementary systems of therapy—curative and palliative. All patients receiving care on a Hospice program are alive and needful of care regardless of the medical care required or of the length of time they are expected to live.

Curative therapies are treatments directed primarily toward eradicating a disease process. Even if they do not produce a cure, they may still be partially successful in establishing disease control. Such therapies are beneficial to the patient to the extent that they successfully remove or control the diseas process causing distressing signs or symptoms. They usually do not directly benefit the patient and may even temporarily increase the patient's distress before their antidisease effect becomes predominant.

Palliative therapies are those therapies directed primarily toward control of signs and symptoms. Their purpose is to control distress that results from a disease process that has not yet responded to curative endeavors, or for which cure is no longer possible. Palliative therapies do not directly affect the disease process itself.

Seldom does a patient receive therapy that is solely curative or palliative in nature. Rather, there is an equilibrium between these two systems of therapy from the time of diagnosis until the time of death.

Appropriate therapy is the blend of curative and palliative therapies that produce the greatest degree of relief from distress caused by disease for the longest period of time with the least number of distressing therapy-related side effects.

Standard: Palliative care is the most appropriate form of care when cure is no longer possible.

Principle: When cure is not possible, care is still needed.

---

*This appendix is excerpted from Standards and Accreditation Committee, National Hospice Organization, *Standards of a hospice care program,* (6th ed.), McLean, Va.: National Hospice Organization, 1981. *The Standards,* which are reviewed annually, are available in their entirety from the national office of the NHO.

The members of the Standards and Accreditation Committee, in 1980, were as follows: Carmian Seifert, Chairperson; Dan Hadlock, Board Liaison; Bill Lamers; Charles Marvil; Clair Tehan; Anne Katterhagen; Mary Kaye Dunn; Peter Keese; Al Sproull; Ruth Kopp; and Jan Williams, Staff Assistant.

Adopted by The Board of Directors of The National Hospice Organization, February 1979. With permission.

Interpretation of Standard. There is a balance to be considered in all medical therapy. The practitioner must weigh the relative values of the likelihood of (a) the benefits from curative therapy, (b) the toxicities of that therapy, and (c) the risks of not treating the disease directly. If it becomes apparent that cure-oriented therapy has a higher risk of causing physical, spiritual, or psychosocial distress than of inducing a state of disease remission or control, the patient deserves the option of palliative care. Palliative care not only enhances the quality of the time left to the patient, even if there is little time, but it may also produce longer survival than expected.

Hospice care is palliative care that is specifically oriented toward meeting the special needs of patients and families who are dealing with an incurable illness with a prognosis of six months or less.

Standard: The goal of palliative care is the prevention of distress from chronic signs and symptoms.

Principle: Pain and other symptoms of incurable disease can be controlled.

Interpretation of Standard. With a balanced perspective regarding the relative indications for, and values of, curative and palliative therapies, the health care practitioner need never say to a patient, "There is nothing more I can do for you." Though there may be little one can do to halt the progress of an incurable disease, there is much that should and can be done to control distressing consequences of that disease.

When signs and symptoms are continuous, palliative therapies should be administered routinely to prevent the re-emergence of symptoms that interfere with comfortable living. The goal of such therapy is not to induce an artificial state of euphoria, but to produce a state of physical and mental relief so the patient can live and relate to others as normally as possible. Such care should neither hasten nor postpone death. Continual and careful monitoring is required to maintain such symptom control. Such monitoring is therefore part of Hospice care.

Hospice care needs to be comprehensive in a twofold sense. First, all signs and symptoms causing distress need to be addressed independently. Second, signs and symptoms secondary to the therapies themselves need to be anticipated and prevented so that such side effects do not overweigh the benefits of controlling the original problems.

Standard: Admission to a Hospice program of care is dependent on patient and family needs and their expressed request for care.

Principle: Not all persons need or desire palliative care.

Interpretation of Standard. The concerns of those seeking assistance in dealing with terminal disease are not only whether they can find appropriate care but also whether they will have any control over the care that is given.

It is important for a Hospice care team to acknowledge a patient's and family's independence by encouraging them to make the initial request for admission to the Hospice program. Others may suggest and refer, but the patient and family need to take the initiative of requesting admission to the program. Thereafter, it is of continued importance for the Hospice program to encourage and respect the patient's and family's central role in the identification of the need for care and in the choice of a care plan.

Hospice care seeks to promote independence among patients and their families in dealing with the distresses and disabilities of terminal disease by encouraging patients and families to do for themselves. Hospice care will support them only when and in the ways in which they desire support. Such actions promote initiative and self-satisfaction and enhance communication between care giver and care receiver. It will avoid imposing therapies without regard to the wishes of the patient and family. For some patients and their families, high-risk, high-technology institutionalized types of therapies are the only forms of treatment they will accept, even when cure is increasingly less likely. For such patients, admission to a Hospice program, with its emphasis on the appropriate use of technology, highly personalized palliative care, and with its acceptance of the inevitability of death, may be stressful, inappropriate, and poorly received. Similarly, patients should not be required to remain on a Hospice care program against their wishes or if aggressive, cure-oriented therapy should again become appropriate.

Standard: Hospice care consists of a blending of professional and nonprofessional services.

Principle: The amount and type of care provided should be related to patient and family needs.

Interpretation of Standard.   For a Hospice care plan, it is the patient who describes the need to be met and the most appropriate kind of care necessary and acceptable to meet that need. It is the responsibility of the Hospice care program to develop the kind of interdisciplinary team that has the capacity to provide comprehensive and appropriate care for the patient. This team should be able to respond on an "as needed" basis to the patient's expressed needs and desires.

To respond fully to these ends, the Hospice patient care team must provide a spectrum of professional and nonprofessional services. The core team is defined as consisting of the patient and the patient's family, the attending physician, and the following Hospice personnel—physician, nurse, social worker, patient care coordinator, volunteer director, and clergy. The significance of each of these professional resources will be considered equal in the functioning of the Hospice team. The team (including volunteers) will work as an interdisciplinary unit with a common commitment to the care of the patient and family. Personnel must be qualified according to standard criteria in their area of practice. Special services will be available on a consultant basis and may consist of such medical, paramedical, legal, financial, religious, and other resources as needed.

The Patient Care Coordinator is that member of the core team whose function is to monitor and coordinate the interrelationships of the various components (both within and outside the Hospice team) of each patient and family's care plan. This individual will also supervise the patient records to ensure that they are current and complete and that they accurately reflect all the components of care being delivered and the effective interaction of those components. This person will also be in charge of regular meetings of the core team to review all aspects of each patient and family's care.

The volunteers are to be carefully selected, trained, and supervised by a member of the core team, the Director of Volunteers. The volunteer staff may consist of professionals and nonprofessionals. It will complement and support the paid professional and nonprofessional staff. The volunteer staff will participate in continuing education programs designed to enhance their effectiveness as part of the Hospice patient care team. These programs are designed to improve and develop specific skills and sensitivities in such areas as individual and group dynamics, supportive counseling, and listening skills.

The volunteer staff provide services under the direction of the Patient Care Coordinator and the Director of Volunteers. The volunteers attend regular supervisory and patient care conferences. They will also contribute to the patient record documenting Hospice intervention.

Standard: Hospice care considers all aspects of the lives of patients and their families as valid areas of therapeutic concern.

Principle: When a patient and family are faced with terminal disease and impending death, stress and concerns may arise in many aspects of their lives.

Interpretation of Standard.   Hospice care recognizes that illness in a person's life can cause disorder and distress in many areas—physical, emotional, intellectual, social, financial, and spiritual. The Hospice care giver considers all of the patient's and family's concerns as important. In attempting to give effective palliative care, the Hospice care giver strives to make available various provisions and resources to meet the patient and family's concerns.

Standard: Hospice care is respectful of all patient and family belief systems, and will employ resources to meet the personal philosophic, moral, and religious needs of patients and their families.

Principle: Personal philosophic, moral, or religious belief systems are important to patients and families who are facing death.

Interpretation of Standard.   Those who are involved with caring for dying persons often have, or develop, strong beliefs about the meaning of life, and their life in particular. Such beliefs sustain them and can allow the care giver to remain sensitive as well as strong in meeting the needs of dying patients and their families.

However, care givers in a Hospice program will not impose any one value system or set of beliefs on patients and their families. Care will be given in such a manner so as not to violate the religious or moral convictions of either care giver or care receiver. Rather those in a Hospice care program shall seek to be sensitive to the values and beliefs of the patients and families and to provide them freedom from distress of any sort so that they have the opportunity to achieve a satisfactory degree of mental and spiritual preparation for death.

Hospice programs will develop resources to meet the moral and religious needs of patients and their families. These resources will include personnel (staff and consultant) and materials sufficiently broad enough to both respect and serve the spiritual needs of those who have no formal religious beliefs. Finally, these resources will be used to educate and inform other staff so that they will be sensitive to the values of patients and their families.

Standard: Hospice care provides continuity of care.

Principle: Continuity of care (services and personnel) reduces the patient's and the family's sense of alienation and fragmentation.

Interpretation of Standard. A Hospice program will provide a continuum of care to the patient and family. Supportive care for the family will be extended through a minimum of the first year of their bereavement.

In respect to the setting where patients receive care, a Hospice program will have the capability of providing *both* home and inpatient care (see Standard 18).

Hospice personnel with whom patients and families develop rapport *should* be encouraged to maintain their involvement with the patient and family for the duration of patient and family admission to Hospice. All Hospice team members will be encouraged to show personal and professional concern for the patients and families with whom they come in contact. All members of the Hospice team will be available to each patient and family. The plan of care for each patient and family will endeavor to provide continuity not only in regard to the plan of care, but also to the setting in which the care is provided, the time during which care is available, and the personnel who have contact with the patient and family. Through such efforts to provide continuity in these areas, it is hoped that the patient and family will not experience stress due to frequent changes of setting, personnel, or fragmentation of services.

Standard: *A Hospice care program considers the patient and the family together as the unit of care.*

Principle: Families experience significant stress during the terminal illness of one of their members.

Interpretation of Standard. It is well recognized that the family in which one member is dying is under significant stress. If not acknowledged and therapeutically addressed, such stress can result in significant physical, emotional, social, and spiritual disorder.

A Hospice care program considers the family along with the patient as the unit of care. The family, and the patient, define the needs to be addressed and provide significant information and assistance in developing an effective plan of care.

A Hospice program develops support systems to spend time, provide information, share insights and reactions, and to assist in referrals as necessary to address family needs—physical, emotional, intellectual, social, financial, and spiritual.

Families have a right to know the specifics of their situation and that of the dying member, so that they may prepare for death and take full advantage of the opportunities of the present. Hospice recognizes that anxiety, fear, depression, and grief are normal in families dealing with dying and death. Hospice recognizes the value of time for patients, families, and staff—time just "to be" in dealing with such reactions, as well as the value of time "to do."

Hospice identifies the patient's family as persons who are legally related and also those persons regarded as significant by the patient.

Standard: The patient's family is considered to be a central part of the Hospice care team.

Principle: Family participation in care giving is an important part of palliative care.

Interpretation of Standard.   The patient's family and friends are to be regarded as an integral and central part of the Hospice care team. By knowing what is happening to the patient (their relative) and by being trained, supervised, and supported in the provision of care to the patient, the family is assisted through a process of preparatory grief which allows them to tolerate bereavement more effectively and satisfactorily.

The involvement of the family in care giving can be therapeutic for the patient as well. The patient belongs to the family primarily, not to the health care team. Patients may more likely accept supportive care from someone they have known and loved, than from strangers.

If a patient's family is unable or finds it difficult to be supportive or to give direct care, the Hospice team will encourage their involvement to the extent that they feel is realistic. It is to be hoped that this encouragement, together with the services of the Hospice team, will enable the patient's needs to be met.

Standard: Hospice care programs seek to identify, coordinate and supervise care for patients without an available family member.

Principle: Not all patients have a family member available in the home to assume the responsibility of giving care.

Interpretation of Standard.   Hospice Home Care requires the presence of a concerned and competent person, other than the patient, in the patient's home. If a patient does not have available a family member or other such person, Hospice will seek to find a person who will be acceptable to the patient and responsible for giving care. Some examples of alternatives to family members are friends, neighbors, social or church group members, and paid companions. The Hospice program will offer teaching, supervision, and support to these persons. The responsibility of these persons will be to attend to the patient's needs.

Standard: Hospice care for the family continues into the bereavement period.
Principle: Family needs continue after the death of one of their members.

Interpretation of Standard.   Family needs do not end when the patient dies. A period of grief and bereavement is to be expected. Hospice encourages the expression of such grief as is consistent with the family's life style. Hospice recognizes the value of social, religious, and ethnic practices in providing emotionally, socially, and ethically acceptable outlets for such emotions. Hospice supports the value of family involvement in the funeral process.

A Hospice program addresses the emotional, social, spiritual, and physical reactions to loss that accompany terminal illness, dying, and bereavement. A Hospice program will develop a bereavement program that provides a continuum of supportive and therapeutic services for the family, including formal and informal individual, family, and group treatment modalities. These will be employed as needed to support the patient's family for at least one year following the death.

Standard: Hospice care is available 24 hours a day, 7 days a week.

Principle: Patient and family needs may arise at any time.

Interpretation of Standard.   Hospice care is intended to be flexible to meet the changing needs of the patient and family. Therefore, a Hospice program of care makes its services available to every patient and family on the program whenever those services are needed.

This standard has a different significance for Hospice home care and Hospice inpatient care. Whereas the delivery of Hospice inpatient care is continuous, the delivery of Hospice home care is intermittent (except as provided by the primary care person) by provision for the delivery of needed services on a regularly scheduled and around-the-clock, on-call basis. Emphasis is placed on the medical and nursing services being available around the clock in the home setting.

Standard: Hospice care is provided by an interdisciplinary team.

Principle: No one individual or profession can meet all the needs of terminally ill patients and families all the time.

Interpretation of Standard. The components of a Hospice care team have been identified in Standard No. 5.

A Hospice team is interdisciplinary. Every member of the Hospice patient care team recognizes the value of his or her own particular level of expertise, in either a professional or personal capacity, for meeting at least one aspect of a patient and family's needs. Each member of the Hospice patient care team should also recognize the limitations of individual capacity in delivering care as well as in meeting all the needs of the patient and family.

The functioning of a Hospice team as an interdisciplinary unit requires that the staff meet regularly to develop and maintain an appropriate plan of care for the patient and family. The development and maintenance of such care plans will be done with the awareness that each discipline relates with other disciplines in the delivery of the overall plan of care to the patient. Each member of the team may thus be involved in delivering aspects of the care plan, resulting in what is often referred to as "role blurring."

Hospice seeks to provide a community of care for patients and families dealing with the distress of terminal illness. The strength of the interdisciplinary team in this regard is that all members of the team have a common commitment to meet the patient and family's needs, and this commitment supersedes the boundaries of their own disciplines. They not only contribute on the basis of their own expertise but also give others insight into their own fields. In this manner a nurse may be involved with developing and delivering social service aspects of care; the physician may perform nursing care; a volunteer may respond to spiritual questionings, etc. The team trains, encourages, and supports itself in the delivery of such a blending of professional and nonprofessional services.

Standard: Hospice programs will have structured and informal means of providing support to staff.

Principle: Persons giving care to others need to be supported and replenished in order to continue to give care.

Interpretation of Standard. An ongoing concern within a Hospice program is to give careful attention to the needs of staff as those needs relate to their personal well-being and ability to continue to give care to patients and their families. Administrative policies and practices, channels for effective communication, individal and group support, as well as personnel practices are means to provide staff the affirmation and necessary resources for continued job performance.

Hospice will provide resources for staff support on a structured and informal basis. For example, the skills of a mental health specialist (or other such person) may be needed when certain individual or group concerns arise. Another example would be the day-to-day support of one care giver to another (e.g. acknowledging a job well done or kindly offering constructive criticism), or providing staff opportunities for quiet and reflection are some ways in which staff support may be given.

In the interpretation of this standard it is not possible to list the many ways in which support can be given to staff. Hospice recognizes that job satisfaction is an important factor in any staff support system. It is through the provision of care of a high quality that care givers are most likely to experience job satisfaction. That "I am my brother's keeper" is a responsibility which Hospice has toward not only patients and families, but to the Hospice staff as well.

Standard: Hospice programs will be in compliance with the Standards of the National Hospice Organization and the applicable laws and regulations governing the organization and delivery of care to patients and families.

Principle: The need for quality assurance in health care requires the establishment of standards for practice and program operation.

Interpretation of Standard. Hospice programs will be in compliance with the Standards of the National Hospice Organization as well as those federal, state, and local regulatory agencies which require licensure and/or certification.

Standard: The services of the Hospice program are coordinated under a central administration.

Principle: Optimal utilization of services and resources is an important goal in the administration and coordination of patient care.

Interpretation of Standard. A governing body (or designated persons so functioning) assumes full legal authority and responsibility for the operation of a Hospice program. The governing body has written by laws and oversees the administration, services, and fiscal management of a Hospice program. A Hospice program will have written and readily available evidence of its organization, services, and channels of authority for responsibility of the care provided to patients and their families.

Hospice care will coordinate the professional and nonprofessional elements of its own care team as discussed under Standard No. 14. In addition, Hospice will seek to coordinate its services with professional and nonprofessional services in the community. Hospice programs will seek to avoid duplication of services and utilize existing resources as needed in the development of care plans. Hospice programs will continually seek to be cost effective. In the interest of quality and efficiency, Hospice programs may contract out for *some* elements of their services. Direct patient service by Hospice personnel (core team) must be maintained with the patient and family. Those elements provided by contract will be primarily and directly responsible to the Hospice program in matters relating to the care of Hospice patients and families.

Hospice will coordinate inpatient and home care. The inpatient component wll be under the direct administration of the Hospice program. Hospice will coordinate its plan of care and services in response to the patient and family's needs and/or requests. The goal of such coordination will be to provide direct and supportive services to enable the patient and family to cope with their situation. Patients and families will frequently be assured of the availability of the home care team on an around the clock basis. At all of these levels of coordination, Hospice will seek to establish a program of care which meets the needs of the care receiver, i.e. the patient and family.

A Hospice program of care will have a central administration whose sole function will be to provide support for the Patient Care Team in the performance of its tasks for the patients and their families. The Hospice administration may be directed by a governing body with broader responsibilities. The main function of the Hospice administrator will be to ensure that the Hospice team will have the necessary support to provide Hospice care. The goal of this administration and coordination is to ensure the integrity of a Hospice program in providing efficient, competent, high quality, loving care for patients and families.

Hospice will not discriminate in its services to patients and their families on the basis of race, creed, sex, national origin, religion or handicap. Likewise, there will be no discrimination on the basis of the above in the personnel policies and practices of a Hospice program.

Standard: The optimal control of distressful symptoms is an essential part of a Hospice care program requiring medical, nursing and other services of the interdisciplinary team.

Principle: Attention to physical comfort is central to palliative care.

Interpretation of Standard. In terminal care there are frequent changes in patient and family needs. Hospice will strive to achieve optimal symptom control of the distressful symptoms of terminal disease. The Hospice care team will be skilled in the management of distressful symptoms. Physicians and nurses skilled in symptom management pursue a course of palliative intervention aimed at enabling the patient to function as optimally as possible. Hospice physicians and nurses, knowledgeable, sensitive, and skilled in diagnosis and treatment of stress, are alert to the physical and nonphysical causes of the signs and symptoms of stress. For these reasons, the Hospice physician and nurse shall have a central role in the development and delivery of a Hospice plan of care, and will need to be available, and involved with every aspect of care at all times. They, together with the skills and services of other disciplines (e.g. social work, pastoral care, physical therapy, etc.) provide skillful intervention for the distressful symptoms according to an established plan of care.

Standard: The Hospice Care program will have:
    a. a medical director on staff.
    b. physician on staff as member of care team.
    c. a working relationship wih the patient's physician (i.e. primary or attending).

Principle: Medical care is a necessary element of palliative care.

Interpretation of Standard. If all components of a plan of care are to be effective there must be medical direction at the level of program administration, clinical services, and professional relationships with other aspects of the medical community and profession.

It is important that the working relationship between the Hospice physician and the patient's own physician (primary or attending) be clearly defined. The Medical Director (Hospice staff) is responsible for the development and maintenance of policies (e.g., medical orders, admission policies) and procedures governing working relationships with physicians as well as for the medical direction of the care plans of patients and families receiving Hospice services.

The Hospice physician on staff is available to make home visits as medically indicated. The Hospice physician will perform those medical services necessary for the diagnostic, prescriptive, therapeutic, and evaluative functions of medical practice.

Hospice medical care interfaces with other aspects of care provided by the Hospice interdisciplinary team. Effective channels of communication and working relationships with other disciplines is required. In particular, there must be effective means for physician-nursing coordination as nursing has a central role in the overall provision of care as well as medical-legal responsibility.

Standard: Based on patient's needs and preferences as determining factors in the setting and location for care, a Hospice Program provides in-patient care and care in the home setting.

Principle: The physical environment and setting can influence a patient's response to care.

Interpretation of Standard. The patient with a limited life expectancy but for whom good symptom control has been achieved, or for whom such symptom control is possible in the home setting may often prefer to be cared for at home rather than in an inpatient setting. In some instances even where such control is not optimally achieved, the patient and family elect to remain at home. Hospice provides patients the option of care at home by meeting the patients' needs and supporting both the patients and their families. Hospice Home Care services are provided on a part-time intermittent basis. When care in the home is not appropriate, Hospice care is available in an in-patient Hospice setting where all the elements of Hospice care remain available. The physical affords a functional, safe, barrier-free, and comfortable setting for patients, family, staff, and the public. Hospice will assist the patient and family to achieve these conditions in the home. In this sense a Hospice program of care will offer the patient with a limited prognosis the freedom to choose the location for care and so increase a sense of personal significance and self worth.

Standard: Education, training, and evaluation of Hospice services is an ongoing activity of a Hospice care program.

Principle: There is a continual need to improve the techniques of palliative care and to disseminate such information.

Interpretation of Standard. Hospice care programs recognize the need for continued education; training, and evaluation of its services and goals. The National

Hospice Organization has as one of its tasks to assist in the accumulation of pertinent data regarding all aspects of Hospice care. It will also establish a national network to disseminate the knowledge acquired within the United States and other countries.

It is to be emphasized that all care provided will comply with regulations relative to the protection of human subjects as are mandated by the United States government.

Standard: Accurate and current records are kept on all patients.

Principle: Documentation of services is necessary and desirable in the delivery of quality care.

Interpretation of Standard.   For each patient/family a Hospice record of care will be maintained in order to ensure compliance with regulatory and quality care standards.

In addition, Hospice considers the record necessary for purposes of education, evaluation, research, and fiscal management.

Appropriate policies and procedures governing the use of the patient/family record are required.

7

Symptom Control

Answer the following questions True (T) or False (F). Answers appear on the last page of this chapter.

1. *The primary focus of palliative nursing is on intensive intervention during crises, with periods of minimal involvement until the next problem occurs.*

2. *Several minutes of whispering "haaah" with each exhalation will slow pulse and respiration.*

3. *Therapeutic touch is a nontraditional massage technique.*

4. *Compazine can cause tremors and jerking movement when used every four hours for relief of nausea.*

5. *Valium can depress respiration and increase pain perception.*

6. *The multiple side effects of steroids are contraindications for their use in terminal symptom relief.*

7. *Vistaril, prednisone, and atropine may all be indicated in the orthopneic lung cancer patient with profuse pulmonary secretions.*

8. *It may be difficult for a good nurse's aide to stop forcing fluids and activity as patient condition declines.*

9. *Intravenous fluids and tube feedings maintain optimum comfort for the dying person.*

Death arises from Life, itself. For every three out of ten born, three out of ten die.—Lao-tzu

W ITH PROGRESSIVE deterioration of body function, many symptoms develop to impair the dying person's quality of life. Too often the attitude of health professionals has been a grim resignation to these symptoms, an assumption that they are to be endured because "nothing more can be done." The thrust of the palliative care and hospice movement is to challenge such assumptions and to continue vigorous efforts to bring syptoms under control. Something more can *always* be tried.

THE ROLE OF THE NURSE

The nurse assists the dying person with physical distress to maintain human functioning at the highest possible level. The physician looks for the underlying causes of symptoms and attempts to control the disease. The nurse focuses on symptom relief and support for the patient's priorities to maintain quality of life (Donovan, 1979). When physicians cannot find a reason for a symptom, they may not take the symptom seriously. For example, a patient suffered for over a year with worsening flatulence, dyspepsia, and vomiting. Whenever the symptoms overwhelmed the patient, he went for more diagnostic tests but these were always "negative." The role of the nurse in this case was to support the need for symptom relief even though the cause of the patient's symptoms could not be pinpointed. Nursing focuses on human experience, not disease analysis.

The nurse's *regular presence* at the patient's side is central to the nursing role. Being with the patient regularly and frequently makes it easier to develop a helping relationship; to observe both distress from symptoms and effects of threapy; to make continual adjustments in palliative measures based on those observations; and to teach patient and family effective ways of controlling symptoms by themselves. The nurse offers independent nursing measures and

109

collaborates with the physician to implement appropriate pharmacological or other medical and surgical measures.

Teaching Symptom Management

Teaching goals are derived from an assessment of the patient's and family's ongoing capacity for caregiving—their knowledge, their motivation for self-help, and their limitations (see Chapter 12). To determine the effectiveness of teaching, the instructor must have or formulate learning objectives that specify how the learner will behave after instruction. *Outcome Standards for Cancer Nursing Practice* (Oncology Nursing Society & American Nurses' Association Divison on Medical–Surgical Nursing Practice, 1979) emphasizes patient–family knowledge, skilled observation, and independent management of symptoms as outcomes of skilled nursing intervention. The *Standards* outline appropriate educational outcome criteria for patient and family managing problems of comfort, nutrition, mobility, elimination, and ventilation.

Anticipatory Guidance

In teaching patient and family to manage the symptoms associated with dying, the nurse *anticipates* those problems most likely to occur and *guides* the patient and family in making plans ahead of time. Anticipatory guidance clearly requires nursing knowledge of the common course of dying and of the likely problems with a particular disease process. Table 7-1 summarizes the kind of information patient and family need to maximize their ability to cope with the physical distresses of a downhill course.

The focus is on what Penny MacElveen-Hoehn (1981) calls *pro-active nursing,* not on *reactive nursing* that waits for a crisis and then attempts to put out the "fire" when symptoms are out of control. Hospice nurses are involved in "fire prevention," albeit at the end of life, and built their practice accordingly. In the following case example, pro-active nursing enabled a family to manage current problems and to prepare for future problems as they cared for a stroke patient who was dying at home.

Case Example: Pro-Active Nursing

Catherine Andrios was a 76-year-old widow living in the home of her 70-year-old sister, Maria. She had three married daughters living nearby who asked for nursing help "to keep Mama at home to die in her own bed." Catherine had suffered a right-sided CVA two years earlier, which left her with expressive aphasia, left hemiplegia, and incontinence managed by an indwelling Foley catheter. She had been up in a wheelchair at the center of family activities in the kitchen and living room, until

Table 7-1.   *Information Needed by Patient-Family*

1. Knowledge of bodily changes and changes in appearance and function that may be expected.

2. Performance of basic nursing measures:
    a. Assistance with nutrition
    b. Assistance with locomotion, other physical activity
    c. Assistance with bowel and bladder function
    d. Giving medication
    e. Care of the bedridden person including hygiene, moving and positioning, skin care

3. Palliative relief measures for common symptoms.

4. Relief measures likely to be needed as condition deteriorates.

5. Use of specific techniques and equipment such as oxygen, dressings, ostomy care, catheters, irrigations.

6. Organizing care, using family and community resources.

7. Determining when to choose hospitalization for symptom control.

8. Determining whether to choose death at home and making special preparations:
    a. Capable caregivers at the bedside
    b. Palliative drugs and equipment available
    c. Knowledge of what to expect and when to call for professional help.

---

a recent second CVA left her bedridden and dysphagic. Physical examination revealed her to be somnolent, but able to respond to commands if repeated several times. The patient's tongue was shiny red and caked with yellow exudate; lungs were clear, with diminished breath sounds throughout; hands were cool and grey; blood pressure was 86/34; abdomen was soft, with bowel sounds present; perineum was reddened and odoriferous; feet were cool with bilateral 2+ edema to the knee and nonpalpable pedal pulses; Foley was draining amber urine with large amounts of mucopurulent material. She was unable to take fluids without choking, and the family had been giving her ice cream and gelatin.

Nursing guidance involved explaining the patient's symptoms to the family and advising them of the likely causes of death. The nurse saw signs of cardiac decompensation and ascertained that the patient was also prone to developing pneumonia or pyelonephritis. Because the family did not want these to be actively treated but wanted Catherine to be comfortable, the nurse secured an order for injectable hydroxyzine (Vistaril) 25–100 mg, to be stored in the kitchen cupboard and used for restlessness or shortness of breath. Arrangements were also made with the physician to obtain other palliative measures, such as oxygen or morphine, if needed. The family was taught basic nursing measures to take care of the patient in bed and, because the nurse anticipated that the patient would soon go into coma, she began teaching the family methods of caring for the comatose patient. Teaching focused also on palliative measures to relieve Catherine's existing stomatitis, poor perineal hygiene, cystitis, and dysphagia. In addition, the nurse *thought ahead* to anticipate problems that might well arise with the catheter and / or when the patient stopped taking food or fluids altogether. The family was taught how to irrigate the Foley catheter should it become obstructed, and an extra catheter and insertion kit were left in the home. The nurse also began discussions with the family about the meaning of food and the difficulty of watching Catherine stop eating because that meant that "the end is near."

Nursing Goals

The process of contracting joint patient, family, and professional team goals is described in detail in Chapter 4. The nurse's plan for symptom relief is always determined by negotiation; the patient-family choose what they believe will be of most help. The nurse serves as an advocate for their choices as she or he works toward ongoing clarification of values and goal re-evaluation.

Case Example: Symptom Management Goals

A man in his 70s was suffering from advanced metastatic lung cancer. Though his progressive weakness, diminished energy level, and accumulating edema from toe into the groin, refractory to treatment, all indicated that he was approaching death, he requested a feeding tube to improve his nutrition. Although he was aware that he was dying, no manner of counseling had been able to relieve his fear of starvation. He had been a chef all his life, and food held great symbolic meaning for him. His wife was slow mentally and wanted him to "get better." Occasionally she would acknowledge that he was dying, but she lamented, "I can't get on without him." The nurse believed that a feeding tube would prolong a life that held no quality, but she supported the patient's choice while she honestly pointed out the drawbacks she saw. The patient believed that both the nurse and the social worker were listening to him and respecting his decision. Both nurse and social worker continued to provide "sounding boards" for husband and wife as the latter faced home management of the husband's many physical symptoms. Not imposing one's own values subconsciously can become difficult for many nurses when patient choice and sound symptom management collide.

Training Nonprofessional Paid Caregivers

The greater portion of bedside terminal care for pay continues to be provided by nurse aides and practical nurses in nursing homes and hospitals, and by nurse aides, practical nurses, and "self-made" caregivers at home. These paid caregivers in the home are provided by home health agencies or private duty agencies, or they are self-employed. The first concern of the professional working with the nonprofessional is to train and supervise the latter regarding integrity and competence in basic nursing skills. In the home, the patient and family are the ones to hire and fire, and the nurse can only report her concerns and make recommendations. If the family will permit, the nurse should advise regarding criteria for hiring and retention. It is best to consult private-duty agencies with high standards, but economics may force many families to hire the "cheapest" available person who claims nursing competence.

Nonprofessionals with strong basic nursing skills need significant support and education to adapt those skills most effectively to caring for the terminally ill. They need help to understand the switch from restorative goals to palliative goals. Refraining from pushing fluids and not coercing the person to get out of bed may be quite difficult for those who took pride in how well "their" patients drank and in the fact that no one was left in bed during "their" shift! These nonprofessionals may also need help in learning to accept and effectively administer many "strong" drugs in which they may not at first believe. Finally, they will need encouragement to sit at the bedside and "do nothing" except *listen,* a behavior not likely to have been rewarded in the past on a task-oriented job! And, just like the rest of us, they need emotional support in dealing with dying people.

INDEPENDENT NURSING MEASURES

Symptoms are often alleviated by the use of nursing measures that are chosen and implemented independent of "orders" from other professionals. These measures are a facet of the collaborative plan developed by the interdisciplinary caregiving team, and nurses teach their use to other professional and nonprofessional caregivers.

Creative Basic Nursing

A significant portion of effectively helping the dying person involves the creative application of such familiar fundamentals of nursing as assistance with nutritional modifications; modification of activities of daily living; bowel and bladder training; medication systems that work for the individual and family; easy ways of caring for the bedridden person; creative use of equipment available in the home; re-orientation techniques; ways of saving energy, promoting sleep, and treating bedsores; and the management of countless other physical problems and related medical equipment. The nurse's familiarity with a wide range of problems and his or her attitude of "we will overcome" as new problems arise are of invaluable assistance to patient and family. The nurse who can think of countless alternative approaches is the one to be at the side of the dying patient, not the nurse who needs to follow a "cookbook" when trouble occurs.

Stress Reduction Techniques

Several mind–body techniques can be used to elicit the *relaxation response* (sense of calm, reduced pulse, reduced respirations, decreased metabolic rate, decreased emotional and mental activity) in patients whose stress is contributing to physical symptoms. Because of their low energy, terminally ill patients are best led through the exercises by caregivers, family members, or tapes; one cannot expect them to do the exercises themselves. The setting should be quiet and comfortable. In leading the exercises one's voice should be slow-paced and restful, tuning into the patient's own breathing and images. The exercises should be modified so as to find what is most useful to the patient; use images that the patient can relate to his or her own life style. These exercises, of course, can also help family members and caregivers relax. The information in this section is adapted from guidelines prepared by Lynne Talley (1981).

Slowing one's *breathing* and paying attention to it is calming by itself, and this exercise is used as a prelude to other techniques. When the patient is in a comfortable, supine position, have him or her rest one hand on the chest and one on the abdomen. Have the patient practice abdominal breathing so that the hand on the chest barely moves at all. After some practice, have the patient breathe in through the nose and out through the mouth, whispering "haah" with each exhalation as the jaw and tongue are relaxed open without tension. Ask the patient to pay attention to the sounds and feeling of the long abdominal breaths for between five and ten minutes.

Progressive relaxation involves the tensing and relaxing of whole muscle groups. Following instructions should be adapted to the individual and repated slowly on tape or in person. Families can be trained to use these instructions with the sick person or for themselves. When patients have muscle or bone pathology or severe weakness, and ask them to become aware of the tension in each part of the body but not to increase the muscle tension.

Get in a comfortable position and relax. Now clench your right fist, tighter and tighter, studying the tension as you do. Keep it clenched and notice the tension in your fist, hand, and forearm. Now relax. Feel the looseness in your right hand, and notice the contrast with the tension. Repeat this procedure with your right fist again, always noticing as you relax that this is the opposite of tension. Relax and feel the difference. Repeat the entire procedure with your left fist, then both fists at once.

Now bend your elbows and tense your biceps. Tense them as hard as you can and observe the feeling of tautness. Relax, straighten out your arms. Let the relaxation develop and feel that difference. Repeat this, and all succeeding procedures at least once.

Turning attention to your head, wrinkle your forehead as tight as you can. Now relax and smooth it out. Let yourself imagine your entire forehead and scalp becoming smooth and at rest. Now frown and notice the strain spreading throughout your forehead. Let go. Allow your brow to become smooth again. Close your eyes now, squint them tighter. Look for the tension. Relax your eyes. Let them remain closed gently and comfortably. Now clench your jaw, bite hard, notice the tension throughout your jaw. Relax your jaw. When the jaw is relaxed, your lips will be slightly parted. Let yourself really appreciate the contrast between tension and relaxation. Now press your tongue against the roof of your mouth. Feel the ache in the back of your mouth. Relax. Press your lips now, purse them into an "O". Relax your lips. Notice that your forehead, scalp, eyes, jaw, tongue, and lips are all relaxed.

Press your head back as far as it can comfortably go and observe the tension in your neck. Roll it to the right and feel the changing focus of stress; roll it to the left. Straighten your head and bring it forward, press your chin against your chest. Feel the tension in your throat, the back of your neck. Relax, allowing your head to return to a comfortable position. Let the relaxation deepen. Now shrug your shoulders. Keep the tension as you hunch your head down between your shoulders. Relax your shoulders. Drop them back and feel the relaxation spreading through your neck, throat and shoulders, pure relaxation, deeper, and deeper.

Give your entire body a chance to relax. Feel the comfort and the heaviness. Now breathe in and fill your lungs completely. Hold your breath. Notice the tension. Now exhale, let your chest become loose, let the air hiss out. Continue relaxing, letting your breath come freely and gently. Repeat this several times, noticing the tension draining from your body as you exhale. Next, tighten your stomach and hold. Note the tension, then relax. Now place your hand on your stomach. Breathe deeply into your stomach, pushing your hand up. Hold,and relax. Feel the contrast of relaxation as the air rushes out. Now arch your back, without straining. Keep the rest of your body as relaxed as possible. Focus on the tension in your lower back. Now relax deeper and deeper.

Tighten your buttocks and thighs. Flex your thighs by pressing down your heels as hard as you can. Relax and feel the difference. Now curl your toes downward, making your calves tense. Study the tension. Relax. Now bend your toes toward your face, creating tension in your shins. Relax again.

Feel the heaviness throughout your lower body as the relaxation deepens. Relax your feet, ankles, calves, shins, knees, thighs and buttocks. Now let the relaxation spread to your stomach, lower back, and chest. Let go more and more. Experience the relaxation deepening in your shoulders, arms, and hands. Deeper and deeper. Notice the feeling of looseness and relaxation in your neck, jaws and all your facial muscles*

Autogenic training achieves the relaxation response by imaging the sensations of warmth and heaviness throughout the body. The following sentences are repeated slowly with pauses between each:

I am calm and quiet, calm and quiet. Nothing around me is of any importance. My thoughts pass like clouds in the summer sky. My right hand is heavy and warm, heavy and warm. My right hand and my right arm are heavy and warm. My left hand is heavy and warm, heavy and warm. My left hand and my left arm are heavy and warm, heavy and warm. My right foot and my right leg are heavy and warm, heavy and warm. My

---

*From Talley, L. *Noninvasive techniques: Symptom management in terminal illness.* Seattle: Hospice of Seattle, 1981. Adapted from Martha Davis (see references).

left foot and my left leg are heavy and warm, heavy and warm. My body is heavy and warm. My forehead is light and cool, light and cool. My eyes are calm and quiet; there is nothing to see. My breathing is calm and regular; it breathes me. I'm going deeper and deeper into my relaxation; deeper and deeper.*

The person is then instructed, slowly and at his or her own pace, to stretch, open his or her eyes, and come back to the room.

Meditation is the discipline of blocking out the business and distractions of the everyday world to focus attention on single aspects of being. For example, one can focus on one's breathing, as described earlier; one can fix one's attention on an external object, become mindful of bodily functioning, attend to a particular image, or repeat a word or concept that brings positive associations. The consequence of this focused attention, with the accompanying elimination of worldly distractions is the relaxation response and an enhanced sense of calm and peace. "When a man can *still his senses* I call him illumined" (Bhagavad-Gita). Two excellent books, by LeShan (1975) and Benson (1976), can aid in the development of the meditative discipline. For patients whose illness leave them with little energy for concentration, it may be most useful to recommend counting breaths or repeating a comforting word like *one* or *peace* or, for those with spiritual grounding, a short prayer. Meditation should be practiced for several minutes periodically during the day.

Imagery or visualization involves vivid imagining of pleasant sensations and experiences, and typically leads to a change in bodily state. At the simplest level, this can happen simply by encouraging the patient to remember certain experiences, perhaps to "walk through" them again with you. One imagery exercise format is as follows:

Begin by breathing in a comfortable position. Imagine inhaling light and exhaling darkness. Imagine inhaling warmth and exhaling cold. Create a door over the area of tension or pain, and watch yourself exhale through the door, blowing the tension or pain out. Close the door and slowly come back to the room.

Describe how the symptom feels (like a big knot, a red-hot poker, etc.) and then imagine reversing the image (untie the knot, cool the poker in water, etc.)*

Find images that are pleasurable for patients, and help them go there in their imaginings. Consult *Seeing with the Mind's Eye* (Samuels & Samuels, 1975) for more discussion and illustration.

Therapeutic touch is a meditative healing technique adapted from the laying-on of hands and developed by Dolores Krieger, professor of nursing at New York University. Using this technique, healers place their hands over

---

*From Talley, L. *Noninvasive techniques: Symptom management in terminal illness.* Seattle: Hospice at Seattle, 1981, adapted from the teaching of Heida Grenneke. With permission.

areas of tension in the patient's body and, while in a meditative state, center their minds on the transmission of healing energy. The technique is clearly described in Krieger's book, *Therapeutic Touch* (1979). The result of the technique is the relaxation response and, often, specific symptom relief for the patient.

PHARMACOLOGICAL SYMPTOM RELIEF

The nurse works collaboratively with the physician in the recommendation of palliative drugs, the ongoing assessment of patient response to medication, the titration of drugs to relieve symptoms with the smallest number of side effects, and the active instruction of the patient-family in the effective use of drugs for symptom management. The nurse needs to establish his or her expertise in critically observing patient response to the drugs used. The goal is to get the physician to provide flexible, sliding-scale drug orders for the nurse who has demonstrated knowledge of pharmacology, expertise in patient assessment, and communication skills both with the physician and with the patient. Flexible orders are particularly essential when the patient's status is continually changing or when a symptom is out of control. Four types of drugs are used frequently in the relief of terminal symptoms: antianxiety agents, antidepressants, antiemetics, and corticosteroids.

Antianxiety Agents

Tranquilizers are carefully adjusted to diminish anxiety without impairing mental clarity. The *antihistamine sedatives,* hydroxyzine, (Vistaril, Atarax) and diphenhydramamine (Benadryl) are drugs of choice for the relief of anxiety, insomnia, dyspnea, and nausea. These drugs also enhance the effects of narcotics. They cause minimum circulatory and respiratory depression. At high doses, anticholinergic actions can cause a range of problems including drying of mucous membrane, urinary retention, constipation, tachycardia, and excitability. Daily doses of 400 mg for hydroxyzine and 200–300 mg for diphenhydramamine can cause convulsions (Halpern, 1982). Benadryl and Vistaril are given at doses of 12.5–50 mg every 4–6 hours, or one hour before meals if vomiting is a problem. *Stat* intramuscular doses of 50–100 mg are given for agitation or acute respiratory distress. Bedtime sedative doses range from 25 to 100 mg. Promethazine (Phenergan) is another antihistamine with antiemetic and calming effects, but it is reported to increase pain perception in those for whom pain control is a problem. (McCaffery, 1979).

Phenothiazines are often chosen to control nausea and/or anxiety. Adverse reactions can occur with long term administration, high doses, or an incompetent liver. Mental sluggishness and postural hypotension are frequent problems. A primary concern is extrapyramidal effects due to increased cholinergic activity: parkinsonism, dyskinesias, and dystonias (coordinated rhythmic movement or uncoordinated jerking), or feelings of restlessness and agitation. These effects can be blocked by the adjunctive use of diphenhydramamine (Benadryl) for its anti-cholinergic effects. Phenothiazines also cause some anti-cholinergic reactions such as dry mouth, constipation, and urinary retention. They lower the seizure threshold, possibly requiring increased anticonvulsant dose. Blood dyscrasias and jaundice are other notable adverse reactions. Prochlorperazine (Compazine) is given at doses of 5–10 mg orally, 25 mg by suppository, or 10 mg intramuscularly around the clock or one hour before meals if nausea is the problem. Chlorpromazine (Thorazine) is chosen if more sedation or narcotic enhancement is the goal. Haloperidol (Haldol) is very similar pharmacologically to the phenothiazines and is effective in the control of nausea and anxiety. It is chosen particularly for its effectiveness in controlling restlessness and disorientation; it has less sedating hypotensive effect than Thorazine. Haldol 2 mg is approximately equal to 100 mg Thorazine. For an extensive discussion of phenothiazine-type drugs, see Elizabeth Harris (1981).

The *benzodiazepines* are tranquilizers often chosen for their quieting effect. Diazepam (Valium) and chlordiazepoxide (Librium) are effective daytime anti-anxiety agents, and flurazepam (Dalmane), triazolam (Halcion), or tamazepam (Restoril) is used for sleep. Most common side effects include daytime sedation and paradoxical excitement, particularly in the elderly. Disadvantages of the use of these drugs with the terminally ill include the mental side effects just mentioned as well as respiratory depression, lack of antiemetic effect, antianalgesic action, and withdrawal symptoms when discontinued abruptly (Harris, 1981).

The *barbiturates* and non-benzodiazepine tranquilizers are generally not drugs of choice for the terminally ill. Barbiturate "sleeping pills" have a narrow range of safety (the effective dose is close to the toxic dose), frequently cause a "hangover" effect, produce sleep for no more than 14 days, and cause rebound restlessness after the drug is withdrawn. Non-benzodiazepines like meprobamate or chloral hydrate have a narrow range of safety and cause withdrawal when discontinued. Chloral hydrate causes gastric irritation (Harris, 1981).

Antiemetics

Drugs that control vomiting act on the vomiting center and the nerve pathways to or from the vomiting center, the chemoreceptor trigger zone, or the gastrointestinal tract itself. The antihistamines (Vistaril, Benadryl) act on the vomiting center, on the nerve pathways to the vomiting center from the chemoreceptor trigger zone, and directly on the gastrointestinal tract to slow motility. The phenothiazines (Compazine, Torecan, Thorazine) act on the chemoreceptor trigger zone.

Trimethobenzamides (Tigan) is less effective than the phenothiazines and has little use in terminal care. Antihistamines and phenothiazines have been described under "Antianxiety agents." Metoclopramide (Reglan) acts on the chemoreceptor trigger zone and directly on the stomach to increase emptying, on the small bowel to increase motility, and on the gastroesophageal sphincter to increase tone and diminish regurgitation (Weis & Weintraub, 1982). Intravenous Reglan has significantly more antiemetic effect than Compazine, with the primary side effect being sedation. (Gralla, 1981) Extrapyramidal effects and diarrhea are occasionally associated with Reglan administration. The lower serum levels obtained by oral administration of Reglan appear to explain the lesser effectiveness of the oral route in contrast to the highly effective intravenous route. (Strum, 1982, p. 2685)

Marijuana derivatives and scoplomamine are also being used as antiemetics in hospice care. Delta-9-tetrahydrocannabinol (THC) and nabilone and homemade marijuana concoctions (teas, suppositories, cigarettes, baked goods) often will diminish nausea and increase appetite, but the effects are unpredictable. Side effects commonly include ataxia, sedation, and dysphoria. (Gralla, 1981) Some hospices are using scopolamine administered by the Transdermal Therapeutic System (Transderm—V). The drug is slowly absorbed over a three day period from a small pad that is applied to the skin behind the ear. The effect is anticholinergic with side effects including dryness of the mouth, drowsiness, and sometimes disorientation and confusion.

Antidepressants

The *tricyclic antidepressants* have calming, antidepressant, and analgesic effects. Commonly used are imipramine (Tofranil), amitriptyline (Elavil), and doxepin (Sinequan). Side effects include those that are anticholinergic (dry mouth, blurred vision, urinary retention, constipation, excitability), cardiovascular effects (tachycardia, orthostatic hypotension, arrhythmias), paradoxical excitement, daytime sedation, and tremors. The threshold for seizure activity may be lowered (DeGennaro, 1981). Maximum daily dose is 300 mg; dosages begin at 50–75 mg before bedtime, and can be gradually titrated upward as tolerated. The sedative effect occurs immediately. The analgesic effect takes a few days, and it may take up to two weeks for a mood-elevating effect to occur. Amoxapine (Ascendin) is a new antidepressant claimed to have reduced cardiotoxicity and anticholinergic side effects with more rapid 4–7 day onset of antidepressant effect. (Smith, 1982) See Table 7-2 for a quick review of the adverse reactions most common with the antianxiety and antidepressant drugs, particularly with the adjunctive use of several agents at once.

Table 7-2. *Adverse Effects of Some Psychoactive Drugs*

Problem	Representative Drugs That Can Cause Problem
Daytime sedation	Valium, Librium, Thorazine, Elavil, Vistaril
Slowed thought processes	Librium, Thorazine, Elavil, Vistaril
Paradoxical excitement	Valium, Librium, Elavil, Vistaril
Postural Hypotension	Valium, Librium, Thorazine, Elavil, Vistaril
Dry mouth, constipation, urinary retention, blurred vision, excitability	Thorazine, Elavil, Vistaril, Atropine

Note: A patient receiving several of these drugs is at high risk.

Corticosteroids

The physiological effects of steroids are outlined in Table 7-3. Prednisone and dexamethasone (Decadron) are used widely in the management of symptoms of terminal illness. Dexamethasone, which has high anti-inflammatory potency and does not promote salt retention, is often the agent of choice for increased intracranial pressure and spinal cord and nerve root compression. Prednisone is used for most other purposes; it is a potent anti-inflammatory agent, it has minimal salt-retentive properties, and it is inexpensive. Prednisolone is prescribed if the liver is incompetent to convert oral prednisone to prednisolone, the substance that is pharmacologically active (Newton, 1977). Because prednisone will reduce the edema layer around a tumor, it can be used effectively to suppress symptoms from the pressure of tumors in lung cancer. Sometimes, at least for a while, it will help relieve the obstructive symptoms with superior vena cava syndrome or partial tracheal obstruction (Stolinsky, 1978). Prednisone is also used to manage hypercalcemia because it increases the renal excretion of calcium. The drug's generalized effect on the central nervous system may improve mood and appetite, but it can also cause behavior changes and depression. Corticosteroids may be used to reduce symptoms in the patient dying with fulminant hepatitis, and injectable or inhalable corticosteroids (like Vanceril) will often be used for brochospasm in advanced lung disease.

It is argued that the relief afforded by corticosteroids for those close to death far outweighs their multiple side effects. However, the nurse needs to be totally familiar with adverse effects lest they cause more problems than they relieve. Acute adrenal insufficiency (fatigue and weakness, nausea, orthostatic hypotension progressing to shock) is a great risk when a patient is on multiple drugs at home and, by accident, steroid dose is abruptly stopped. Patient and

Table 7-3. *Physiology of Corticosteroids*

Type of Effect	Processes Involved
Glucocorticoid	
Antiinflammatory	Stabilization of lysosomes to reduce release of irritating chemicals
Immunosuppression	Reduced lymphocyte production
Reduced edema layer around tumor	Reduced capillary permeability
Increased serum glucose	Gluconeogenesis by liver
	Reduced cellular use of glucose
Protein depletion throughout body	Reduced protein synthesis and increased protein catabolism in all cells except liver
muscle wasting	
osteoporosis	
"tissue paper" skin	
fragile capillaries	
Mineralcorticoid	
edema	Increased sodium retention at kidney tubule
hypertension if predisposed	
hypokalemia	Increased potassium excretion at kidney tubule

family need very careful instruction to maintain safe dosage regimens (Gotch, 1981). When your terminal patient suddenly develops symptoms that appear to indicate adrenal insufficiency, check first to be sure the steroid prescription has been refilled ("Oh *that!* We stopped it 5 days ago. He didn't think he needed it anymore.") Patients are also at risk for gastric irritation; they should *always* take oral steroids with food and/or cimetidine (Tagamet) and/or antacid, and they should be taught to observe for hematemesis and melena. If patients live to use steroids for a prolonged period of time, other effects that may become of concern include hyperglycemia, hypokalemia, hypertension, muscle wasting, osteoporosis, and increased susceptibility to infection. "Moon face" will develop over time and may cause distress with body image.

COMMON NURSING DIAGNOSES
AND EFFECTIVE PALLIATIVE MEASURES

People who are dying obviously can suffer from an endless list of possible symptoms, and, as a consequence, many nursing problems and most nursing diagnoses. Appendix 7-1 identifies some of the most common nursing diagnoses, as well as the problems that typically accompany them, their underlying dynamics, and the most effective palliative measures. The diagnoses that are identified and explored are: ineffective *airway* clearance or *breathing* pattern; alteration in *bowel* elimination; ineffective individual *coping;* impaired physical *mobility; nutrition* less than body requirements; *fluid* volume deficit; impaired *skin* integrity; *sleep* disturbance; and alterations in *thought* processes and/or consciousness. (See Chapters 3, 8, and 9 for explorations of psychological disturbances, pain, decreased cardiac output and tissue perfusion, respectively.) These categories are adapted from the list of nursing diagnoses developed at the Fourth National Conference of the National Group for Classification of Nursing Diagnoses, held in 1980 (Kim, 1982). The reader is referred to Baines (1978), Ajemian (1980), and Geltman (1983) for their summaries of common symptoms and hospice palliation.

Examine Appendix 7-1, "Ineffective Airway Clearance," before considering the following case discussion:

Case Example: Terminal Respiratory Distress

Ada Josephson was a 43-year-old, single mother with a "mind of her own." She had been a union organizer most of her life. As her metastatic lung cancer reduced her endurance and physical mobility, she called her two young-adult children home to live with her. She resisted nursing referrals made by her physician and relied on her own common sense and that of her children until one morning she desperately "dispatched" a friend for nursing help. She was found trembling and in a panic, with respirations 32, bibasilar rales, frequent cough productive of white sputum, and desperate "air hunger." She was alternately resting on her side, with multiple pillows, or shakily sitting up cross legged in her double bed. If you were the nurse, what drug might you carry legally in your bag at all times to inject immediately after phone orders from the doctor? What equipment would help? What do the children need to be taught? What else would be involved in anticipatory guidance for this patient and family?

WHAT ABOUT EMERGENCIES?

The management of successively appearing problems in the terminally ill person is guided by an understanding of patient–family goals, the course of the illness, and the closeness of death. The person with a terminal prognosis who is considered to have months of quality life remaining will usually be treated aggressively to reverse a new problem (see Stolinsky, 1978, on palliative measures in oncological emergencies). For example, a 48-year-old carpenter with slowly progressing brain tumor suddenly developed "crushing" chest pain. He wanted to live and to continue to be with his children. The hospice nurse was called first. Because of the possible implications of the patient's symptoms, the nurse chose not to make a home visit. Instead, with family concurrence, she called an "aide car" and had the patient admitted first to an emergency room and then to a critical care unit for pulmonary embolism. In two weeks, he was back home on anticoagulants and enjoying his extended family.

In a similar case, a terminally ill breast carcinoma patient with extensive bony metastasis who was still ambulating and working in her kitchen with good pain control from several drugs, suddenly developed numbness and tingling in her lower extremities, coupled with lumbosacral pain extending into the groin. She was admitted immediately for high-dose radiation to the vertebral metastasis that was compressing her spinal cord. Paraplegia was thus avoided.

When illness is considered extensive and endstage and the patient has no desire for prolongation, the goal of care is anticipatory guidance to ensure that resources will be on hand to manage symptoms as they emerge and before they can really become an "emergency" (see Chapter 9 for a discussion of the management of commonly expected problems during the last few days of life). When the 48-year-old carpenter with the brain tumor became bedridden, aphasic, and incontinent and could swallow only ice cream or sherbet, the nurse had planned ahead for two likely "emergent" problems—pneumonia and increased restlessness. The family no longer desired acute medical care and instead learned to use injectable Vistaril and morphine, to administer oxygen, and to provide capable nursing care for a comatose and dying person. Another family would be more comfortable choosing hospitalization, where the palliative goals at the end of life would be the same.

CARE OF THE DYING CHILD

The child who is dying touches us profoundly, for a life is passing that has barely begun. Too often such children never experience the comforts and little delights provided by palliative, family-focused care because the adult authorities in their lives focus on death-denying technologies, at great cost to the little persons who must endure them to the end. Ida Martinson describes a contrasting goal for a child's last days: "Extracting maximum pleasure from life while critically ill" (Martinson, 1979, p. 471) Let us look first at the experience of the dying child.

The Child

Bluebond-Langner (1978) notes that children as young as three come to understand that they are dying. However, children will often not express what they fear will upset their parents and caregivers. Children's response to life-threatening illness can be understood only in the context of their developmental demands. Children under five cannot understand death as permanent. They fear separation and bodily hurt. Children of school age come to understand the finality of death and of themselves as separate people. The adolescent who is dying is caught in the developmental task of struggling for identity and independence while facing the reality that she or he will die before achieving these goals. It is important to review in detail the specific developmental tasks for each age and to consider the impact of dying in the light of those tasks. Remember also that children, when threatened, are likely to regress to earlier developmental levels.

A child who is dying requires comprehensive pediatric nursing assessment (see a standard pediatric text). Such an assessment explores areas unique to children such as developmental accomplishments; eating, toileting, and sleeping behavior; play; school involvement; socialization with peers; and family interaction. (See also Chapters 4 and 12 for discussions of family assessment and dynamics.)

Psychosocial care of dying children recognizes their need for concrete information; for a role in decision making as appropriate to their age level; for security of love and consistent discipline and structure; for the ability to continue with their developmental tasks, with special effort on everyday pleasures; and for channels to express feeling. The child relieves his or her emotional burden primarily through acting it out. The preschool and young school-age child is helped best to express feelings through the use of therapeutic play. Dolls or clay models can be used to work out dramas within the family or the health care team. Older school-age children or adolescents are often helped by the third-person approach to articulate feelings which they cannot express directly. For instance, the nurse might say, "Many kids like you begin to wonder whether they will ever get better. What do you think?" (Rothenberg, 1979).

Dying children typically have remarkable maturity and a capacity for making decisions that is beyond their years. The Center for Attitudinal Healing, in San Francisco, and other centers have brought children together to help each other, and to discover joyful purpose in their time remaining (Center for Attitudinal Healing, 1978). Group sessions for parents and children can also be highly effective in increasing self-help skills in an atmosphere of mutual support (Craft, 1982). Moldow and Martinson (1979) note that children over 5 can be involved in decisions to stop treatment and organize their final days.

The Parents

The emotional, spiritual, marital, physical, and economic burden on the parents of a dying child is extreme. Moldow and Martinson (1979) point out that years of aggressive therapy for such illnesses as congenital heart disease, cystic fibrosis, and cancer often exhaust parents, and then they must still cope with the culminating stress of the child's dying. If the child is hospitalized, parents often incur the problems of travel, hotels, restaurants, loss in wages, and costs of babysitting for other children. If the child is dying at home, the primary pressure of responsibility and care is on the mother (Martinson, 1978), for most fathers are compelled to work full time. Keeping the child at home makes it possible for the father to be more involved than he could if the child were institutionalized (Lauer & Camitta, 1980).

Nursing and counseling professionals need to work closely with these parents to support their coping skills, both for the parents' own sakes and because the parents are important to their children's physical and emotional well being. The parents need instruction and counseling in order to understand their own feelings and those of their child. They need to be encouraged to express their feelings rather than experience the hidden, unshared anger and despair that tears individuals and families apart and to make realistic plans for day-to-day living as the child is dying. They are highly vulnerable to marital difficulties and emotional decompensation following the child's death and thus need sensitive bereavement follow-up and referral. Moldow and Martinson (1979) note that home care enables parents to feel more needed and in control. The family is reunited and less at risk during the bereavement period.

The Siblings

Life is rough for other children in the family when a child is dying. Their own relationships with their parents are disrupted, they experience the physical deterioration of their sibling, their own routine is disturbed and they often come home to an empty house while the sick child is hospitalized (Iles, 1979). The sister or brother experiences sadness, anger at being neglected, fear of his or her own dying, jealousy at the attention the sick child is getting, and guilt because of his or her own good health (Moldow & Martinson, 1979). The challenge for the professional and the parent is to help siblings express their feelings through play and verbalization. Iles (1979) notes that siblings' experience can be positive and growth-producing if they are given the opportunity to contribute actively to the care of the dying child. They can develop empathy for their parents; increased cognitive understanding, respect, and compassion for the brother or sister who is dying; and a strengthened self-concept. Martinson (1978 b) notes that children who have been involved in home care as a sibling dies have a healthier bereavement course. The psychiatric literature abounds with descriptions of possible sibling grief reactions such as depression, anxiety, and problems at school, as well as somatic symptoms such as bedwetting, headaches, and stomach aches. It is useful for family and child to see that such reactions are normal and expected and self-limiting over time and not to label a child "abnormal" because of them. The most useful intervention is encouraging acceptable ways of expressing feeling while helping the family to recreate a secure, predictable living situation.

Dying at Home

The fact that a child is dying is often never faced. Hospital treatment is continued until the last breath. The decision to stop treatment should be made when treatment no longer offers life that includes some comfort and quality. Family and health team need to confer. Ambivalence must be worked through because it is very painful to abandon the struggle for the life of a young person.

Most communities have few resources to encourage and support bringing a child home to be with comforting family, friends, surroundings, toys, food, and activities. Both Martinson and Lauer and Camitta report the effectiveness of making 24-hour, 7-day home nursing care available in the community for dying children (Lauer & Camitta, 1980; Martinson, 1978). The programs described by Martinson and by Laver and Camitta strongly emphasize extensive family teaching and anticipatory guidance. They demonstrate outcomes of patient comfort, cost effectiveness, and healthy bereavement reactions.

Marty Keyser (1973) describes the experience of bringing her two-year-old son home to die. She contrasts hospital restrictions with the special features of having her son Sammy at home "nestled between his Dada and me on a double bed with comforters, 'getting' lip smacking squirts of coffee with extra milk and extra sugar," and "held for the final hours in our dear, old, easy chair."*

Physical Care

Daily caring for the child near death focuses on touch and holding, tempting the child with favorite food and fluids, bathing and keeping the child warm and dry, and toileting. Parents can be reminded that these are familiar activities that they used to perform when the child was very young. In Martinson's (1978) (b) study of 32 children dying at home, 17 required no specialized equipment. In a few cases, parents were taught to manage oxygen therapy, intravenous fluids, suctioning, or urinary drainage. Of these children, 18 needed analgesics.

Pain and symptom management for the child follow the same principles discussed in this chapter and in Chapter 8, with drug dosages reduced. All drugs should be carefully titrated to symptoms, which may require doses

---

*From Keyser, M. At home with death: A natural child death. *Journal of Pediatrics*, 1973, *90*, p. 487.

higher than usually recommended for pediatric user. Parents need thorough instruction to administer and adjust drugs for comfort at home. Bleeding and seizures are greatly feared by parents, requiring thoughtful anticipatory guidance if considered likely (Moldow, Martinson, 1979). Keyser (1973) writes about the dying symptoms of her baby son, "I was afraid of the physical agony of dying. Sam's death was amazingly similar to his own birth. He looked as if he were in labor. He seemed to know that he had a difficult and important job and he worked hard to accomplish it" (p. 487).

REFERENCES

Ahmed, M.C. Op-Site for Decubitus Care. *American Journal of Nursing,* 1982, 82, 61–64.

Ajemian, I. General principles of symptomatic management. In I. Ajemian & B. Mount, (Eds.). *The Royal Victoria Hospital manual on palliative/hospice care.* New York: Arno Press, 1980.

Baines, M.J. Control of other symptoms. In C. Saunders (Ed.), *The management of terminal illness.* London: Edward Arnold, 1978.

Baines, M.J. Symptom control in the dying patient. In C. Saunders (Ed.), *Hospice: The living idea.* London: Edward Arnold, 1981.

Benson, H. *The relaxation response.* New York: Avon, 1976.

Bluebond-Langner, M. *The private worlds of dying children.* Princeton, N.J.: Princeton University Press, 1978.

Center for Attitudinal Healing. *There is a rainbow behind every dark cloud.* San Francisco: Celestial Arts, 1978.

Craft, M. *et al.:* Nursing care in childhood cancer—coping. *American Journal of Nursing,* 1982, 82, 440–442.

Daeffler, R. Oral hygiene measures for patients with cancer. I, II, III. *Cancer Nursing,* 1980, 2, 347–355, 423–432; 1981, 3, 29–34.

Davis, M. *The relaxation and stress reduction workbook.* Richmond, Calif.: New Harbinger, 1980.

DeGennaro, M. Antidepressant drug therapy. *American Journal of Nursing,* 1981, 81, 1304–1309.

Donovan, M. Relaxation with guided imagery. *Cancer Nursing,* 1980, 2, 27–32.

Donovan, M. *Symptom management: The nurse is the key.* Seattle, Washington: Fred Hutchinson Cancer Research Center, 1979.

Foltz, A. Nursing care of ulcerating metastatic lesions. Oncology Nursing Forum, 1980, 7, 8–13.

Geltman, R.L. Symptom Management in Hospice Care. *American Journal of Nursing,* 1983, 83, 78–85.

Gotch, P.M. Teaching patients about adrenal corticosteroids. *American Journal of Nursing,* 1981, 81, 78–81.

Gralla, R.J. Antiemetic Efficacy of High Dose Metoclopramide. *New England Journal of Medicine* 1981, 305, 905–909.

Groer, M., & Pierce, M. Anorexia-cachexia. *Nursing,* 1981, 81, 39–43.

Guyton, A. *Human physiology and mechanisms of disease.* Philadelphia: Saunders, 1982.

Halpern, L. Conference with Hospice of Seattle staff, May 19, 1982.

Harris, E. Sedative–hypnotic drugs. *American Journal of Nursing,* July, 1981, 81, 1328–1334.

Hushen, S. Questioning TPN as the answer. *American Journal of Nursing,* 1982, 82, 852–854.

Iles, J.P. Children with cancer: Health siblings' perceptions during the illness experience. *Cancer Nursing* 1979, 2, 371–377.

Keyser, M. At home with death: A natural child death. *Journal of Pediatrics*, 1973, *90*, 486–487.

Kim, M.J., & Moritz, D.A. *Classification of nursing diagnoses*. Philadelphia: Saunders, 1982.

Krieger, D. *Therapeutic touch*. Englewood Cliffs, New Jersey: Prentice Hall, 1979.

Lauer, M.E., & Camitta, B.M. Home care for dying children: A nursing model. *Journal of Pediatrics*, 1980, *97*, 1032–1035.

LeShan, L. *How to meditate*. New York: Bantam, 1975.

McCaffery, M. *Nursing management of the patient with pain*. Philadelphia: Lippincott, 1979.

Martinson, I.M. Caring for the dying child. *Nursing Clinics of North America*, 1979, *14*, 467–474.

Martinson, I.M. *Home care: A manual for implementation of home care for children dying of cancer*. Minneapolis: University of Minnesota, 1978. (a)

Martinson, I.M. Home care for children dying of cancer. *Pediatrics*, 1978, *62*, 106–113. (b)

Moldow, D.G., & Martinson, I.M. *Home care for dying children: A manual for parents*. Minneapolis: University of Minnesota, 1979.

Newton, D. You can minimize the hazards of corticosteroids. *Nursing*, 1977, *77*, 26–33.

Oncology Nursing Society, American Nurses' Association Division on Medical-Surgical Nursing Practice. *Outcome standards for cancer nursing practice*. Kansas City: American Nurses' Association, 1979.

Plum, F., & Posner, J. *Diagnosis of stupor and coma*. Philadelphia: F.D. Davis, 1969.

Rothenberg, M.B. The dying child. In J. Noshpitz (Ed.), *Basic handbook of child psychiatry*, (Vol. 1). New York: Basic Books, 1979.

Samuels, M., & Samuels, N. *Seeing with the mind's eye*. New York: Random House, 1975.

Smith, R.S. A Critical Appraisal of Amoxapine. *Journal of Clinical Psychiatry*, 1981, *42*, 238–242.

Stolinsky, D. Emergencies in oncology. *Western Journal of Medicine*, 1978, *129*, 169–176.

Strum, S.B. Intravenous Metoclopramide: An Effective Antiemetic in Cancer Chemotherapy. *Journal of the American Medical Association*, 1982, *247*, 2683–2686.

Talley, L. *Non-invasive techniques: Symptom management in terminal illness*. Seattle: Hospice of Seattle, 1981.

Weis, O., & Weintraub, M. New developments in the treatment of nausea and vomiting. Drug Therapy; Hospital, 1982, *12*, 66–72.

Welch, L.B. Simple new remedy for the odor of open lesions. *RN*, 1981, *44*, 42–43.

Zerwekh, J. The dehydration question. *Nursing 83*, 1983, *13:* 47–51.

THE DYING CHILD—RECOMMENDED READING

Baker, L. *You and leukemia: A day at a time*. Philadelphia: W.B. Saunders, 1978.

Benoliel, J.Q. The terminally ill child. In G. Sciplen (Ed.), *Comprehensive pediatric nursing*. New York: McGraw-Hill, 1975.

Benoliel, J.Q., & McCorkle, R. A holistic approach to terminal illness. *Cancer Nursing*, 1978, *1*, 145–149.

Gaddy, D.S. Nursing care in childhood cancer—Update. *American Journal of Nursing*, 1982, *82*, 416–421.

Grollman, E. *Talking about death: A dialogue between parent and child*. Boston: Beacon Press, 1976.

Gyulay, J.E. *The dying child*, New York: McGraw-Hill, 1978.

Jackson, E. *Telling a child about death*. New York: Channel Press, 1965.

Martinson, I.M. et al.: Nursing care in childhood cancer—methadone. *American Journal of Nursing*, 1982, *82*, 432–435.

Mills, G. Books to help children understand death. *American Journal of Nursing,* 1979, *79,* 291–295.

Nilsen, J.D. Nursing care in childhood cancer—adolescence. *American Journal of Nursing,* 1973, *82,* 436–439.

Rudolph, M. *Should the children know? Encounters with death in the lives of children.* New York: Schocken Books, 1978.

Sahler, O.J.Z. *The child and death.* St. Louis: C.V. Mosby, 1978.

Schiff, M. *The bereaved parent.* New York: Crown Publishers, 1977.

Stephens, S. *Death comes home.* New York: Monehouse-Barlow, 1973.

1. F	*6. F*
2. T	*7. T*
3. F	*8. T*
4. T	*9. F*
5. T	

Appendix 7-1. *Common Nursing Diagnoses*

Ineffective Airway Clearance or Breathing Pattern

Related Problems	Underlying Dynamics	Psychosocial Impact	Palliative Measures
1. *Dyspnea/hypoxia—signs:*	Pneumonia	Patients with chronic lung disease may not identify this as a problem, because they are so accustomed to shortness of breath.	Position in semi-Fowler's or support upright.
Dropping pO_2	Pulmonary edema		Patient may be able to sleep only in chair or hospital bed with headrest elevated.
Rising pCO_2	Pulmonary embolism	Acute air hunger is terrifying.	Don't leave patient alone.
Breathing with mouth open or pursed lips	Atelectasis	Fear of suffocation as cause of death is common.	Use oxygen.
Using accessory muscles	Pleural effusion		Use humidity.
Complaining of shortness of breath	Invasive tumor		Try hydroxyzine (Vistaril) or diphenhydramine (Benadryl) every 4–6 hours and/or *stat* 50–100 mg IM for respiratory crises.
Interference with talking	Obstruction		Glucocorticosteroids can be used (prednisone 5–10 mg TID) for advanced lung cancer.
Respiratory rate over 24 and/or irregular	Emphysema, bronchitis		Bronchodilators and/or steroids are used for bronchospasm.
Tachycardia and/or cardiac arrhythmias	Adult respiratory distress syndrome		Pleural tap is considered for effusions if patient chooses.
Cyanosis	Fever, anemia		Try morphine for unrelieved severe respiratory distress.
Apprehension			
Restlessness			
Reduced mentation			
Possible progression to increased neuromuscular irritability, agitation, coma			
Possible progression to increased neuromuscular irritability, agitation, coma			

| 2. Cough/excessive respiratory secretions | Presence of inflammation or excessive secretions or pressure of tumor against bronchi or trachea will set off impulses that are transmitted to the medulla to initiate the cough reflex. | Interferes with talking and resting. Increased anxiety as cough and/or secretions are not controlled. Panic. | Increase fluids as tolerated. Avoid milk products. Try humidifier or vaporizer. Try O.T.C. syrups with dextromethorphan. Use codeine 30–60 mg po q4–6h. Add other narcotics if cough still not suppressed. Expectorants or antihistamines are of questionable effectiveness. Use postural drainage, and clapping, if patient tolerates it and finds it effective. Treat pulmonary edema with digitalis and diuretics. Treat pneumonia if patient wants prolonged life. Try atropine .4 mg BID for excess secretions. For severe attack, use *stat* atropine .4 mg and narcotic IM. Consult with speech therapist, physical therapist for help with stimulating swallowing. |

131

Ineffective Airway Clearance or Breathing Pattern (cont.)

	Related Problems	Underlying Dynamics	Psychosocial Impact	Palliative Measures
3.	*Dysphagia/choking*	Esophageal obstruction	Panic	When swallowing is no longer possible, begin atropine .4 mg and narcotic IM to reduce distress from accumulating pharyngeal secretions.
		Increased salivary production with pressure on walls of esophagus		
		Reduced strength & coordination of tongue; depressed pharyngeal swallowing reflex		Values clarification instruction and advocacy when patient being considered for feeding intubation.
4.	*"Death rattle"*	Air bubbling through accumulation of pharyngeal secretions due to inability to swallow. Accumulation of pulmonary secretions due to end-stage lung pathology	Sound is distressing to those in attendance at bedside, but not usually to patient whose level of consciousness is depressed.	Give atropine or scopolamine .4 mg–.6 mg q4–6h IM or more frequently prn. Trauma of nasopharyngeal suctioning is rarely justified.

Alteration in Bowel Elimination

	Related Problems	Underlying Dynamics	Psychosocial Impact	Palliative Measures
1.	*Constipation—signs:*	Reduced peristalsis due to immobility, narcotic use, anticholinergic drugs	Increased preoccupation with bowels reduces quality of life.	Determine history of elimination, normal patterns, and aids.
	Hard stools			
	Less-frequent-than-usual stools	Reduced intake of fluids and fiber		Increase water and dietary fiber as tolerated.
	Straining at stool			
	Feeling of rectal pressure	Reduced abdominal muscle strength		Maintain normal position and timing.
	Liquid stool leaking around palpable impaction	Reduced awareness of urge to defecate		Encourage activity if possible.
				Psyllium (Metamucil) 1 tsp.–several Tbsp. will work well if patient can drink it fast before it turns into unpalatable gel.

2. *Bowel obstruction (inoperable)—signs:*

Rushes of loud, high-pitched bowel tones with cramping pain *or* bowel tones absent

Vomiting of intestinal contents

Abdominal distention

Malignant invasion and block of small or large intestine

Ascites, massive

Mesenteric vascular occlusion

Frightening until symptoms controlled.

Diagnosis of inoperable total obstruction heralds the end of life.

Use stool softeners: diocytyl sodium (or calcium) sulfosuccinate **BID** to **QID** to prevent constipation.

Titrate dose to softness and frequency of stool. Add bisacodyl (Dulcolax) tablets or daily suppositories to stimulate large bowel contraction.

When obstruction is complete:

1. Minimize fluid intake to minimize amount of gastrointestinal fluid.

2. Use narcotic to slow peristalsis. Diphenoxylate with atropine (Lomotil) 2.5–5 mg q4–6h will have least effect on mentation. Other narcotics can also be increased.

3. Try antiemetics that act on vomiting center (antihistamines).

When obstruction is incomplete:

1. Since metoclopromadide (Reglan) promotes emptying of stomach and peristalsis of small bowel, use with incomplete obstruction, paralytic ileus. Stop with complete obstruction.

2. Try antihistamine antiemetics.

3. Try stool softeners.

133

Ineffective Individual Coping

Related Problems	Underlying Dynamics	Psychosocial Impact	Palliative Measures
1. *Anxiety/fear—signs:* Expressed apprehension Preoccupation with self Diminished problem solving Increased muscle tension GI distress Sweating Headache Trembling	Fear of loss of identity, roles and relationships; changed body image and function; loss of power Fear of the unknown Fear of uncontrolled suffering Fear of death	Discussed in Chapters 3 and 10	Attentive listening, presence at the person's side. Encouragement of ventilation of feelings and identifiable fears. Teaching and advocacy to increase knowledge and power. Meditative and relaxation techniques. Spiritual counseling.
2. *Depression—signs* Sad affect, posture Slowed movements Expressions of hopelessness Disturbances in appetite, sleep, sexuality Intense preoccupation with self	Normal grief response but can be disabling	Discussed in Chapters 3 and 10	Challenge hopelessness with realistic hope. Teach normal grief process. Facilitate expression of angry feelings. Teach healthy coping strategies. Try positive imagery techniques. Use of antidepressants. Though conscientious psychiatric practice generally considers antidepressant drugs to be contraindicated for "exogenous depression," (sadness that is a

natural response to circumstances), use of those drugs in the terminally ill will "lighten the burden" enough to make possible some quality of living and some movement in the grief process.

Spiritual counseling.

Impaired Physical Mobility

Related Problems	Underlying Dynamics	Psychosocial Impact	Palliative Measures
Impaired ambulation	Underlying disease affecting bones, joints, muscles, and peripheral or central nervous system.	Losses of ability to perform normal activities are visible indicators to the patient of diminishing health and independence.	Assist to conserve energy, identify priorities, maximize capacity as patient chooses.
Impaired use of upper extremities			Teach to use supportive appliances (walkers, wheelchairs, transfer belts, etc.)
Reduced endurance	Underlying disease reducing oxygen, hemoglobin, circulation, glucose availability	Ability to communicate and ventilate feelings is impaired.	Teach safe transfer, ambulation techniques.
Reduced capacity to maintain role performance (job, household, family, community)	Depression		Occupational and physical therapy consults to maximize function if patient chooses.
Eventually reduced ability to manage basic self-care			When chair-bound or bedridden, teach methods to prevent skin breakdown.

Impaired Physical Mobility (cont.)

| | Other methods usually used to prevent complications of immobility are not relevant when the goal is comfort for a person near death.

Therefore, eliminate *forcing* of fluids, deep breathing, and range-of-motion exercises; do not insist on transfer or ambulation. |

Nutrition Less Than Body Requirements

Related Problems	Underlying Dynamics	Psychosocial Impact	Palliative Measures
1. *Anorexia/starvation—signs* Weight loss Emaciation Reduced skin fold thickness Anemia Low serum protein Inadequate intake of calories and protein	Diminishing energy for eating Nausea/diarrhea Altered taste Dysphagia Malabsorption Increased catabolism in cancer Depression Emotional withdrawal	Everyone equates food with life. Family, patient, and caregivers often interpret diminishing food intake as "giving in" to dying. Eating becomes a burden, a "chore."	Perform diet history to determine food enjoyed that is nourishing, usual meals, meaning of food, cost factors. Consult dietitian. Plan rest before meals. Avoid food aversions (commonly red meat). Power pack foods to concentrate protein & calories (add an egg, cream, butter, commercial supplements). Encourage small, frequent meals.

Encourage nutritional fluids and fluids generally as tolerated.

Create pleasant setting for meals.

Use alcohol as appetite stimulant.

Consider THC as appetite stimulant.

Treat nausea and vomiting.

Try glucocorticosteroids: prednisone 5 mg TID as appetite stimulant.

Use values clarification, teaching, and advocacy for patient when tube feeding or hyperalimentation is being considered.

2. *Nausea and vomiting*

Stimulation of integrative vomiting center by—
a. Effects on chemoreceptor trigger zone of biochemical changes (uremia, hepatic failure, hypercalcemia, narcotics, chemotherapy drugs).
b. Gastrointestinal distention or irritation, which occur with esophageal obstruction, intestinal obstruction, ascites, stomach cancer or ulcer

Unpredictable vomiting is socially isolating. Meal time is lost as a social event.

Assess for *reversible* causes: metabolism, electrolyte balance, drug effect, obstruction, ulcer, intracranial pressure, stress. Treat underlying cause.

Antiemetics (use 1 hour before meals or every 4 hours with severe vomiting):

Phenothiazines

Antihistamines

Metoclopramide (Reglan)

Droperidol (Inapsine)

Tetrahydrocannibinal (THC, or marijuana)

137

Nutrition Less Than Body Requirements (cont.)

    c. Increased intracranial pressure

        Combine several agents when vomiting uncontrolled.

    d. Anxiety

        Try relaxation and imagery (imagine immersing face in cold water while breathing slowly).

        Counsel to reduce anxiety.

3. *Stomatitis (mucositis)—signs:*
Oral mucosa red, shiny, edematous, bleeding easily
Ulcerations
White or brown coating

Radiotherapy or chemotherapy causing direct damage to mucosa.

Dehydration.

Inadequate protein intake.

Reduction in saliva secondary to radiation (xerostomia).

Defective immune response.

Poor oral hygiene.

Mouth breathing.

Continuous O_2

Local trauma

Discomfort of eating.

Impaired social interaction due to altered appearance of mouth.

Symptoms of stomatitis are sometimes ignored because person is preoccupied with other problems.

Stimulate saliva: use sugarless gum, sour candies, ice chips, and popsicles.

Encourage high fluid and protein intake if acceptable to patient.

Clean routinely every 2–4 hours; saline mouthwash; avoid the drying and irritation caused by commercial products or dilute such products.

Avoid the drying and irritation caused by lemon and glycerine.

Remove debris: use soft toothbrush and floss if there is a bleeding problem. Try sodium bicarbonate or hydrogen peroxide diluted to tolerance. Rinse afterward.

Relieve pain: Dyclone .5% spray lasts about an hour, while viscous xylocaine lasts a few minutes. Diphanhydramamine (Benadryl) has local anti-inflammatory effect. The alcohol based elixir can be irritating. Powder from capsules can be placed in Maalox or cream to coat mouth. Chloraseptic spray has phenol which may irritate.

Treat infections: Use frequent cleansing, culture, mycostatin suspension and suppositories for monilia.

Fluid Volume Deficit

Related Problems	Underlying Dynamics	Psychosocial Impact	Palliative Measures
1. *Fluid depletion—signs:* Reduced intake Disproportionate output Oliguria, concentrated urine Postural hypotension Dry skin and mucous membranes	Weakness and withdrawal, causing person to drink less. Gastrointestinal losses. Dysphagia. Reduced extracellular fluid volume, causing diminished level of fluids throughout body.	People equate fluid with life. Dehydration naturally occurs at the end of life, but many find this difficult to accept and so force fluids or start IVs.	Special mouth care with rinses, favorite beverages, brushing, ice chips, lubricant to lips. Encourage fluids that the patient can enjoy, but do not force fluids against the patient's wish. When intravenous feeding is being considered, assist patient-family to clarify goals and expectations.

Fluid Volume Deficit (cont.)

		A patient near death who is hydrated can experience the unpleasant consequences of increased edema and ascites, increased discomfort from tumor swelling, increased pharyngeal and respiratory secretions, increased GI secretions to cause vomiting, increased urine output that may require catheterization.
		Evaluate risks and benefits of intravenous therapy as discussed above.
2. Electrolyte imbalance— signs:	Hypernatremia secondary to serum concentration with reduced water intake.	Manage hypercalcemia with diuretics, corticosteroids, indomethacin (Indocin).
Clouded mentation	Acidosis secondary to kidney failure, lactic acid accumulation, ketosis, CO_2 retention.	
Neuromuscular irritability		
Cardiac irritability	Hyperkalemia secondary to kidney failure, tissue catabolism, acidosis.	
Nausea and vomiting	Hypercalcemia secondary to serum concentration; immobility; cancer of bone.	

Impaired Skin Integrity

Related Problems	Underlying Dynamics	Psychosocial Impact	Palliative Measures
1. *Fungating ulcerating metastatic lesion—signs:* Malignant skin lesion Purulent drainage Frequently foul odor	Local extension into epithelium and the supporting lymph and blood vessels. Resulting necrosis, rupture of capillaries, infection.	Social stigma causes withdrawal. Odor may increase isolation.	Nursing to minimize infection, bleeding, odor: 1. Cleansing with soap or detergents. 2. Debridement by enzymes (Elase, Trypsin) or oxidizers (H_2O_2, Dakin's solution) 3. Bacteriostatic agents like silver sulfadiazine (silvadene) or provodine iodine (Betadine). 4. Odor control by baking soda between bandage layers or using odor antagonist (like Banish or Hexon) on bandages. Room temperature yogurt or buttermilk used to irrigate wound, followed by saline rinse. Lactobacillus capsules opened, and powder sprinkled on wound. 5. Clean dressing covering at all times. Medical Management: 1. Excision 2. Radiation 3. Chemotherapy

141

Impaired Skin Integrity (cont.)

2. *Decubiti*	Pressure over bony prominences, poor circulation, poor nutrition.	Caregivers may judge quality of care provided by self or others based on *preventing* pressure sores. When they appear in someone near death, it may *not* be a sign of poor care.	Methods of management include that basic *necessity* or turning, positioning, cleanliness plus that *vast array* of alternative "potions and powders" and dressings that are always being tried. See a recent Basic Nursing text. It may be impossible to avoid pressure on some areas in the dying person. The orthopneic patient may develop coccygeal or ischial breakdown. Some patients may be comfortable in only one position, and complain bitterly when turned. When near death, they can be left in a position of comfort. Caregivers should not be criticized if breakdown occurs. Dressings should cover the sore and analgesic used as needed. "Op-Site" is useful in these cases.
3. *Ostomies, fistulas*	Cancer surgery to divert stool or urine. Extension of infection or malignancy.	Impaired body image, social stigma of being "unclean."	Management does not differ from standard approaches. Consult enterostomal nurse therapist for problems.

Sleep Disturbance

Related Problems	Underlying Dynamics	Psychosocial Impact	Palliative Measures
1. *Insomnia—signs:*	Increased state of arousal due to anxiety, worry.	Vicious cycle of inability to relax.	Review history to determine normal pattern and conditions that usually promote sleep.
Reports of inadequate sleep each night	Occasionally night sweats	Sleep deprivation affects ability to concentrate, solve problems, and maintain equilibrium.	Encourage daytime activity, avoidance of naps.
Reports of inability to fall asleep, waking early, periods of wakefulness during night.			Try relaxing evening activities including relaxation techniques.
Signs of sleep deprivation in daytime: fatigue, poor concentration, irritability.			Modify environment.
			Try warm milk at bedtime.
			Try sedative drugs at bedtime:

			Hydroxyzine (Vistaril)
			    Diphenhydramamine (Benadryl)
			    Flurazepam (Dalmane)

			Avoid barbiturates, except for occasional use to block disturbing vivid dreams.
2. *Increased sleeping-fatigue-lethargy.*	Reduced circulating oxygen and hemoglobin.	Requires withdrawal from usual activities of life.	Help prioritize activities to choose where to place energy.

143

Sleep Disturbance (cont.)

Sedative effects of altered body chemistry due to organ failure, electrolyte imbalance.	Encourage alteration of rest and activity.
Sedative effects of medication.	Assist with energy conserving modifications of activities of daily living.
Depression.	Try iron supplement and increased iron in diet.
Emotional withdrawal.	Those with ongoing blood loss or inadequate production of RBC's often receive regular transfusions until they feel quality of life makes it no longer "worth it."
Reduced nuritional intake.	As death nears, explain increasing sleeping as a natural process.

Alterations in Thought Processes and/or Consciousness

Related Problems	Underlying Dynamics	Psychosocial Impact	Palliative Measures
1. *Reduced concentration and problem solving*	Fever	Dramatic reduction in role performance.	Work up to reverse causes if possible.
	Expanding cerebral mass.	Increased dependency very distressing.	Carefully titrate drugs.
	Reduced cerebral circulation.	Loss of "mind".	Teach patient-family to anticipate this problem as death draws near.
	Cerebral hypoxia, hypercapnia.		
	Metabolic changes (renal, hepatic), electrolyte imbalance.		
	Drug effects.		
	Anxiety, depression.		
2. *Confusion, disorientation*	As above	Increasing dependency on others. Loss of mind very distressing to self and others. Safety hazards with increasing confusion, lack of judgment.	Haloperidol (Haldol) for acute disorientation.
			Dexamethasone may be prescribed for cerebral edema.
			Oxygen can diminish hypoxia.
			Create a calm, structured environment.
			Teach re-orientation techniques.
			Look for safety hazards.
			Patient cannot be left alone.

Alterations in Thought Processes and/or Consciousness (cont.)

3. *Declining level of consciousness—signs:* Downward progression from dull indifference with slow responses, to *coma* with no response or only reflex response to stimulus. Metabolic coma is distinguished by the presence of resting tremor, asterixis ("liver flap") and multifocal myoclonus (gross twitching of muscle groups).	Caused by expanding lesions of the brain and metabolic encephalopathy (hypoxia, ischemia, CO_2 narcosis, sedative drugs, acid-base and electrolyte imbalance).* Sign heralding approaching death.	Implement excellent care of comatose patient; family involvement and teaching as they desire. Prepare to manage possible problems with neuroexcitability, "death rattle."

Sources: Ahmed (1982), Baines (1981), Daeffler (1980), Foltz (1980), Groer (1981), Hushen (1982), Plum and Posner (1969), Welch (1981), Zerwekh (1983).
*See Plum and Posner (1969) for full discussion of dynamics underlying coma.

8

Control of Pain

Answer the following questions True (T) or False (F). Answers appear on the last page of this chapter.

1. *Narcotics should be prescribed sparingly because they are not effective at high doses.*

2. *The best way to control pain is to ask the patient to take medicine whenever she or he becomes uncomfortable.*

3. *Aspirin relieves metastatic bone pain.*

4. *Respiratory depression is a major complication with scheduled use of narcotics in the advanced cancer patient.*

5. *A stool softener should usually be prescribed whenever round-the-clock narcotics are taken.*

6. *Aspirin Grains X is equivalent to a Demerol 50 mg tablet.*

7. *Methadone 10 mg p.o. (2 tablets) is approximately equal to one 10 mg morphine shot IM.*

8. *Intravenous narcotics should be scheduled regularly every four hours.*

9. *The patient on high doses of methadone will sleep most of the time.*

10. *Prednisone can reduce metastatic cancer pain by minimizing the fluid layer around tumors.*

The beginning of healing is in the solidarity with the pain. In our solution-oriented society it is more important than ever to realize that wanting to alleviate pain without sharing it is like wanting to save a child from a burning house without the risk of being hurt. *

I N CONTRAST to our most deep-seated fears and expectations, severe pain need not be a common problem for the dying person. About 50 percent of terminal cancer patients experience pain that requires use of palliative measures (Twycross, 1978); the proportion of those dying from cerebrovascular, cardiovascular, and respiratory diseases who suffer severe pain is even lower. The physical, emotional, and spiritual distress engendered by this kind of pain has been a focal point of palliative and hospice care. This chapter explores the dynamics underlying terminal pain, defines the nursing role in the assessment of pain, and describes the use of palliative measures.

UNDERLYING DYNAMICS

Pathophysiology

The sensation of pain arises from a variety of underlying mechanisms. Some of the processes involved in the spread of cancer include infiltration into and inflammation of pain-sensitive structures (fascia, periosteum, mucous membranes); compression or infiltration of nerves; ischemia from obstruction of blood vessels; and spasm from obstruction of hollow organs or their ducts (Bonica, 1980). Myocardial ischemia is the most common cause of severe pain in cardio-respiratory pathologies. Peripheral arterial ischemia and/or venous engorgement are common problems with vascular disease processes. Inflammation and muscle spasm may complicate many terminal courses. As terminal illness progresses, with multiple organ involvement, often several

---

*Nouwen, H. *Reaching Out,* Garden City, N.Y.: Doubleday, 1975, p. 43.

underlying mechanisms trigger pain at once. Some degree of reflex muscle spasm is usually present.

The sensation of pain is transmitted to the brain through multiple pathways. The endings of the fibers that transmit the pain impulse are stimulated by chemicals such as histamine and bradykinin. Smaller, myelinated fibers carry sharp, pricking sensations and larger, nonmyelinated fibers transmit burning, aching pain. Both enter the cord at the dorsal roots, cross over to the opposite side, and pass upward in the lateral and ventral spinothalamic tracts. These divide at the brainstem into multiple collaterals that are relayed through the reticular regions to the thalamus, with some reaching the cortex.

It is known that the sensation of pain can be blocked or diminished in the presence of other neural impulses. This is the basis of the gate control theory, which states that there is a gating mechanism located in the dorsal horns of the spinal cord. The gate may be closed by sensory input that triggers inhibitory impulses from the brain stem. Heat, cold, pressure, acupuncture, and electrical stimulation are some therapies that provide this kind of sensory input. The gate can also be closed by inhibitory impulses from the cerebral cortex. Techniques such as biofeedback, distraction, and counseling affect this gate (Melzack, 1980).

Transmission of pain is also blocked naturally by the endorphin compounds, which inhibit transmission of pain impulses along the central nervous system. Endorphins, which are found throughout the central nervous system, are similar in action to morphine; they have effects on pain perception, mood, and respiratory rate (Wilson, 1981). It is hypothesized that the effectiveness of some pain-relief measures may be based on their ability to stimulate the release of these naturally occurring pain relievers. Significant research is now being directed at examining how endorphins are released and how this release could be stimulated for the person in pain.

Psychosocial Dynamics

The pain of organic illness is never an isolated phenomenon. All dimensions of the human experience are interwoven. Therefore, pain impairs the mental, emotional, social, and spiritual well-being of the individual. Likewise, diminished mental, emotional, social, and spiritial health will often aggravate the experience of physical pain. As a result, there can be a vicious circle of suffering at all levels.

The terminally ill person coping with a long-term pain experience manifests a familiar pattern of psychosocial responses. Depression is common. Chronic anxiety may be manifested in irritable behavior, hostility, and changes in eating and sleeping. It is common for people to withdraw and isolate themselves. Coping with their suffering becomes the exhausting, consuming center of their existence. Relief permits a return to less burdened human experience, an opportunity for choices and fullness of life in the time remaining. Unrelieved terminal pain hastens death, as the individual exhausts physiological, psychosocial, and spiritual resources for coping.

NURSING ROLE

The nurse assists the dying person who is in pain to maintain human functioning at the highest possible level. When the person is incapable of choice, the nurse provides independent nursing measures and collaborates with the physician to implement appropriate pharmacological or other medical–surgical therapies. When patient and/or family are more autonomous, the goal of nursing is to *empower the patient-family to control the pain effectively by themselves* and to ask for help early whenever the pain is no longer controlled. The nurse assures that relief measures are multi-faceted and individualized. He or she is frequently present at the patient's side to assess comfort level, adjust appropriate relief measures, and teach the family.

A Therapeutic Relationship

Pain can be dreadfully isolating and emotionally very debilitating; the person often feels powerless. There is little energy to reach out to others. The relationship offered by the nurse needs to be one of genuine encounter; the nurse's nonverbal and verbal behavior should communicate attention and receptivity to the sufferer as an individual. Persistence is essential; trust may develop very slowly, appearing only after the nurse has "proven" his or her reliability by persistently but unobtrusively being present and by implementing pain-relief techniques that work. A therapeutic relationship develops as nurses share their understanding of the patient's experience and as patients validate and clarify what they are actually experiencing; patients' experience is affirmed and isolation diminishes. Spiritual and emotional pain are thus eased through the experiencing of another's presence.

This relationship with the nurse can help sustain a patient through the pain experience, and it can motivate people to take back power in their own lives by learning methods to effectively control their pain.

A Teaching Relationship

Effective teaching is central to achieving the goal of empowering the patient-family to learn to manage pain by themselves. A teaching relationship begins with a therapeutic relationship, wherein the person's concerns, knowledge, and both motivation and ability for self-care are assessed. It is also essential to assess where family and friends interested in assisting with pain relief are "coming from," as they approach learning about pain control. What knowledge have they? What are their capabilities and limitations in learning?

The nurse must then determine learning objectives based on his or her own knowledge of pain relief and on the assessment of what information the particular patient-family needs to manage self-care. Because there are so many behaviors that must be learned in order to manage pain effectively, the teaching relationship needs to be extended over time whenever possible.

A behavioral objective on first meeting a patient with uncontrolled pain might be stated as follows: "The patient takes prescribed narcotic plus two aspirin tablets every four hours as demonstrated by his or her recording the times." Once pain is under control, the nurse proceeds in later contacts to identify behavioral objectives based on the patient-family absorbing increasingly complex information about pain relief. Two examples of such objectives might include the following: "The patient-family can state how to adjust narcotic dose based on the patient's mental state and respiratory rate." and "The patient-family demonstrate a progressive relaxation exercise to the nurse." The objectives are not stated in terms of what the nurse teaches, but rather *in terms of how the learner behaves following teaching.* Thus the outcomes of the teaching relationship are measurable.

Assessing the Pain Experience

Assessment of the pain experience has three components: analysis of the characteristics of the physical pain, exploration of its impact on quality of life, and identification of the patient's wishes regarding pain relief.

The following questions should provide strong descriptive data to characterize a patient's physical pain:

1. Where exactly is the pain in your body? (It may be helpful to have the patient mark painful areas on drawings of the human body; see Figure 8-1 for a sample response.) Commonly, a patient suffers from several different kinds of pain. Origins should be differentiated (such as muscle spasm, dyspepsia, infection, bony metastasis) to determine different forms of palliation.
2. When did the pain start? What makes it worse and what provides relief? Does it change over time?
3. How severe is your pain?
4. Describe how your pain feels.

The McGill Pain Questionnaire (Melzack, 1975) provides multiple tools for clearly eliciting descriptive information from a person in pain. This assessment tool, which is still in the developmental stage, has been adapted for use by many hospice and palliative care programs around the country. The three parts of Figure 8-2, which is based on that questionnaire, are particularly helpful to patients in describing their experience and in answering questions 2 to 5 above.

Assessing the impact of pain on quality of life can be far ranging. Areas to consider include mental health as reflected in verbal and nonverbal expression; changes in eating, sleeping, activities of daily living; changes in interpersonal relationships; and effects on quality of life as reported directly by the patient as well as by family and friends. Cultural variations in the way people respond to pain and express discomfort must be considered.

It is not always easy to identify the patient's wishes regarding pain relief. Patients' wishes are influenced by their knowledge of the cause of pain and of the nature of relief measures available, the meaning and value of the pain experience as useful or destructive, and motivation to take charge of the pain. Most patients seek to avoid pain, but some patients choose, either overtly or covertly, not to have their pain relieved. One patient, an alcoholic "on the wagon," chose to experience pain rather than accept relief from any drugs that he considered potentially addictive. Another patient gained significant emotional support from his family when he sabotaged regular scheduling of medicine ("I can remember to take my pills without a schedule.") and faced pain crisis after crisis. One patient believed that he could control his life best if he were not interrupted by a variety of pain-relief techniques initiated one after the other as oral narcotics failed. He rejected such techniques as not worth the effort. In order to determine joint goals for pain relief, it is vital to keep working to make explicit what the patient wishes and resists. Patient

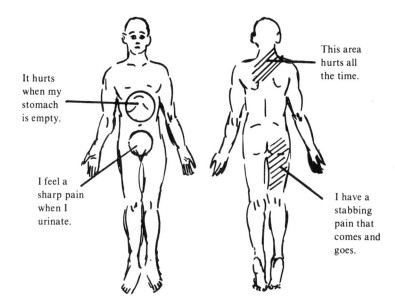

Figure 8-1. Body drawings, with sample marking of pain areas.

Figure 8-2. Pain assessment tools.*

A. **Pattern of Pain**

Which word or words would you use to describe the *pattern* of your pain?

1	2	3
Continuous	Rhythmic	Brief
Steady	Periodic	Momentary
Constant	Intermittent	Transient

B. **Severity of Pain**

Which of the following describes the intensity of your pain?

1	2	3	4	5
Mild	Discomforting	Distressing	Horrible	Excruciating

To answer each question below, write the number of the most appropriate word in the space beside the question.

1. Which word describes your pain right now? _____
2. Which word describes it at its worst? _____
3. Which word describes it when it is least? _____
4. Which word describes the worst toothache you ever had? _____
5. Which word describes the worst headache you ever had? _____
6. Which word describes the worst stomachache you ever had? _____

C. **How the Pain Feels**

Circle *only* those words that best describe your present pain. Leave out any category that is not suitable. Use only a single word in each appropriate category.

1	2	3	4
Flickering	Jumping	Pricking	Sharp
Quivering	Flashing	Boring	Cutting
Pulsing	Shooting	Drilling	Lacerating
Throbbing		Stabbing	
Beating		Piercing	
Pounding			

5	6	7	8
Pinching	Tugging	Hot	Tingling
Pressing	Pulling	Burning	Itchy
Gnawing	Wrenching	Scalding	Smarting
Cramping		Searing	Stinging
Crushing			

9	10	11	12
Dull	Tender	Tiring	Sickening
Sore	Taut	Exhausting	Suffering
Hurting	Rasping		
Aching	Splitting		
Heavy			

13	14	15	16
Fearsome	Punishing	Wretched	Annoying
Frightful	Grueling	Blinding	Troublesome
Terrifying	Cruel		Miserable
	Vicious		Intense
	Killing		

17	18	19	20
Spreading	Tight	Cool	Nagging
Radiating	Numb	Cold	Nauseating
Penetrating	Drawing	Freezing	Agonizing
Piercing	Squeezing		Dreadful
	Tearing		Torturing

*Adapted from Melzack, R. The McGill pain questionnaire. Major properties and scoring methods. *Pain,* 1975, *1,* pp. 277–299.

wishes may change, and they must be continually validated, as there are changes in the pain experience, in trust, and in patient understanding.

Nursing Goals for Pain Relief

As discussed in Chapter 4, the goals of care are determined by negotiation. In the present context, the patient-family choose the pain relief tools and outcomes they believe will be of most help. As the nursing relationship expands, goals are continually re-evaluated and expanded.

INDEPENDENT NURSING MEASURES

Though the plan of care is determined by interdisciplinary consultation, there are a number of pain-relief tools that can be chosen and implemented by nurses independent of "orders" from other professionals. The therapeutic and teaching relationships are instrumental in the use of all these "tools of the trade." The use of "noninvasive pain-relief methods," as they are called by Margo McCaffery, is thoroughly discussed in her excellent text, *Nursing Management of the Patient with Pain* (1979).

Environmental Modification

The nurse can create a physical environment in which the *patient* feels comfortable, avoids boredom and monotony, and experiences specific distraction strategies as indicated. The nurse may begin by assisting with the choice of mattress, pillows, cushions, chair, location of room at home, familiar objects, pleasing colors. Cleanliness and order contribute to comfort for many people but may be distressing to those unaccustomed to these qualities. One patient allowed herself to be hospitalized only after she was assured that ward staff would not force her to bathe or give up her own blankets.

To prevent monotony and the increased pain perception that commonly accompanies it, the nurse assesses the patient's interests and previous everyday life activities. Given the limitations of the patient's energy, the nurse can help patient and family to plan a day that schedules regular, pleasant activities such as visiting with people, exercising as much as possible, reading or being read to, watching favorite television programs, eating special foods, performing household and job-related tasks as able, and pursuing crafts and hobbies. Occupational therapy can assist in generating useful activity and in modifying former activities so that they are still possible. Immersion in activities, for those who can tolerate it, enhances pain relief.

Distraction strategies are used to focus attention away from the pain experience on to *alternative sensory input.* Distraction techniques vary, from simply talking to a patient to asking personal questions during a painful procedure to specific distraction exercises that provide relief for brief periods of time. Techniques used include rhythmic breathing that accelerates and decelerates and rhythmic massage, used in ways that have become familiar in childbirth preparation. Listening to music and other forms of entertainment are also effective distractors. Norman Cousins has popularized the analgesic effects of laughter: "I made the joyous discovery that 10 minutes of genuine belly laughter had an anesthetic effect and would give me at least two hours of pain-free sleep" (Cousins, 1976).

Imagery

As indicated in Chapter 7, the imagination may be used to alter one's bodily state. Inducing relaxation facilitates the development of sensory images that reduce the intensity of the pain experience or substitute pleasing images. *Images should be identified that are appropriate to the patient's experience.* McCaffery's version of the "ball of healing energy," for example, which is described next, may be adapted to make it comfortable and meaningful for yourself and for each patient:

You may close your eyes now. Take a slow, deep breath, breathing slowly and deeply. Feel yourself relax as you breathe out slowly. Concentrate on your breathing, breathing slowly and deeply from your abdomen. Breathe as deeply as is comfortable for you. Feel the air going in your lungs, out of your lungs. To help you concentrate on your breathing you may say silently to yourself as you inhale "in, 1, 2" and as you exhale, "out, 1, 2".... I am going to pause now and let you concentrate on breathing slowly and deeply, feeling the air going in and out of your lungs, feeling yourself more relaxed each time you exhale, counting for yourself, if you wish, to help you concentrate on breathing slowly and comfortably. (Pause for approximately 15 to 30 seconds depending upon the response of the group or the individual). Now, if you wish, you may begin to imagine a ball of white light and healing energy forming on your chest or in your lungs. This ball of white light and healing energy need not be terribly clear or vivid. Anything you wish to imagine is suitable. It may be dim or abstract. Anything will be effective as long as you understand it as a mass of healing energy. (Pause for a few seconds). When you are ready you may circulate this ball of white light and healing energy in the area that hurts. The next time you inhale you may use that air to send the ball of healing energy to the area that hurts. When you breathe out you may use that air to send the ball away from your body, letting it take with it the discomfort and hurt, accumulated toxins, dysfunctional cells, bacteria, tension (these particular causes of pain may be omitted and the focus may be only on healing), leaving behind improved blood supply, feelings of relaxation, comfort, and healthy tissue. You may, if you wish, continue to circulate the ball of healing energy with every breath you take. The ball of healing energy enters your body again purified and as you breathe in you may send the ball of healing energy to the area that hurts. As you breathe out you may send the ball of healing energy away from your body letting it leave behind comfort, relaxation, and health. Each time the ball of healing energy leaves your body, it may take away twice as much of the hurt and leave behind twice as much relaxation, comfort and health. The ball may get larger and larger as it performs this function. I will pause now to allow you time to circulate the ball of healing energy and white light. (Pause 15 seconds or longer, depending upon the response of the group or individual). You may end the guided imagery for yourself when you are ready. Count silently to yourself from one to three. At the count of three inhale sharply and deeply, open your eyes, and say to yourself, "I feel relaxed and alert."*

Physical Methods

The traditional nursing art and science of *positioning*—of helping a patient in pain find a comfortable position must never be overlooked. Fundamentals like maintaining body alignment and proper support for head and extremities must be considered. Skillful use of pillows, knee gatch, and head rest to support and avoid pressure on a painful body part is an essential element of care.

Of great comfort to many patients may be *touching*. Caring and human presence can be expressed meaningfully through touching the hand, the shoulder, the forehead of the suffering person. Remember, though, that many people—in our culture and in others—are uncomfortable with this way of expressing a human bond. It is important for such people to maintain their territoriality; your touch might be perceived as a violation. Touch with the intention to comfort or help those in pain can also have a healing effect that is becoming increasingly well understood by those who are studying and applying "therapeutic touch" techniques (see also Chapter 7).

Techniques that involve *stimulation of the skin* include many such counterirritation or counterstimulation methods which block or oppose the pain stimulus. McCaffery (1979) presents an excellent summary of those commonly used in nursing practice.

Heat for example, improves blood supply and causes muscle relaxation. Unfortunately, it also increases inflammation, edema, and bleeding and should not be applied to areas where it would aggravate those problems. *Cold* reduces inflammation, edema, and bleeding and may cause muscle relaxation. Cold, however, sometimes causes spasm. Moreover, it reduces circulation and is thus contraindicated where circulation is poor. Hot baths, electric heating pads, and light bulbs in goose neck lamps are most frequently used to apply

---

From McCaffery, M. *Nursing management of the patient with pain.* Philadelphia: Lippincott, 1979, p. 177. With permission.

heat. Cold packs may be applied using icy wet, wrung-out towels or a cold plastic gel pack (McCaffery, 1979). When heat or cold are being considered as major adjuncts to pain relief, it is wise to consult with physical therapists, who have expertise in choosing modalities best suited to a patient's type of pain.

Massage and *pressure* can relax muscles, provide a counter stimulus to the pain stimulus, and also provide a way for the patient to receive touch and comforting. People who reject being touched as an expression of caring, may respond enthusiastically to the suggestion of "a good back rub." To use massage and pressure effectively at a level of expertise beyond the back rub, the nurse should consult closely with the physical therapist to determine the best plan and perhaps to implement some of the treatment. A licensed massage therapist can be a very helpful member of the caregiving team, but must be briefed and carefully supervised by the nurse regarding limitations and hazards of pressure and massage because of the underlying pathology. For instance, therapeutic touch techniques and massage are contraindicated directly over metastatic sites.

Acupuncturists, trained in an art developed by Eastern healers and physicians, insert needles into specified points of the body, plotted to correspond to areas of imbalance. Because western medicine has been reluctant to adopt what it cannot fully explain, acupuncture has not yet gained wide acceptance in the medical professions. However, acupressure techniques have been integrated into the practice of some nurses, physical therapists and massage therapists.

COLLABORATIVE PALLIATIVE MEASURES

In the case of many palliative measures, although physicians choose the specific procedures, nurses have significant responsibility for managing their implementation. This is true, for example, in the use of palliative analgesics and, sometimes, palliative cancer chemotherapy. In addition, transcutaneous electric nerve stimulation (TENS) units are ordered by physicians and implemented by physical therapy and nursing. On the other hand, palliative radiotherapy, surgery, and nerve blocks are implemented primarily by physicians, whereas nurses are responsible for skilled care following these procedures.

Palliative Chemotherapy

Oncology nurse specialists are assuming increasingly independent roles in the assessment and management of the cancer chemotherapy patient (see oncology nursing texts and journals for detailed discussion of this topic). It should be noted, however, that chemotherapeutic drugs and hormones are usually not indicated in the terminal cancer patient when there is no sign of tumor response. Sometimes oral drugs are continued, at low dose and thus with minimal side effects, to reduce discomfort from tumor spread. Palliative chemotherapy is much more worthwhile in cancers in which tumor response is reasonably good. At St. Christopher's Hospice, for example, oral cyclophosphamide (Cytoxan) at an average dose of 100 mg daily causes a significant response in one third of their terminal breast cancers; this regimen is often combined with palliative use of tamoxifen, 20 mg bid (Bates & Vanier, 1978).

Palliative Radiotherapy

Radiation therapy is commonly used to manage pain in the patient with metastatic cancer. Its use is determined by the expected radiosensitivity of the tumor, the ability of surrounding tissues to tolerate radiation, and the amount of prior radiation dose to the site. Because bony metastatic sites respond well to palliative radiotherapy, the underlying source of pain can often be completely eliminated in a person who has been suffering severe skeletal pain. If the nurse is caring for a patient in pain with known or probable new bony spread, it is his or her responsibility to inquire about the person's past history of radiotherapy and to consider the possibility of using radiation for pain relief. The probable benefits must always be balanced against the disadvantages, which are primarily weakness and tiredness. The dosage should minimize side effects, and it should be administered in as few treatments as possible, to avoid the exhaustion and trouble of daily travel over time.

Palliative Surgery

The nurse's role in respect to the terminal patient being considered for surgery is that of an advocate within the decision-making team. The nurse should be concerned that the patient not undergo a surgical procedure that might lead to more suffering than if surgery were avoided and palliative analgesia and/or sedation chosen instead. Michael Williams offers a guideline:

It may be possible, however, to provide relief by surgery at the cost of a lesser morbidity, in which case it is essential to count the cost. Apart from minor procedures such as draining abscesses which are justifiable in the last days, my own rule of thumb is that one week spent in a surgical ward is justifiable if there is a prospect of three months' useful life at home, two weeks for six months' respite, while three weeks in hospital is justified for a year of worthwhile survival.*

---

*From Williams, M. The place of surgery in terminal care. In C. Saunders (Ed.), *The management of terminal disease.* London: Edward Arnold, 1978, p. 134. With permission.

The difficulty of such a formula is that each decision must be in accord with the values and individual situation of each patient-family.

Nerve Blocks and Neurosurgery

Nerve blocks are chosen in selected pathologies, usually when pharmacological measures are not working well. Blocks involve the injection of a chemical agent, such as alcohol or phenol, which causes local nerve destruction and thus blocks transmission of pain impulses. Anesthetic agents may also be injected to provide short-term relief. *Intrathecal* blocks involve a lumbar puncture, with injection into the interspace in the middle of the painful area; the goal is to block those posterior nerve roots that transmit pain of bony or nerve involvement in the pelvis or lower extremity. Side effects can include impaired bladder and rectal function; the lower extremities may also be impaired but usually only temporarily. *Brachial plexus nerve blocks* are used to curtail the hand and arm pain of brachial plexus invasion (Pancoast's syndrome). Undesirable side effects include sensory and motor impairment in the arm. *Celiac plexus blocks,* introduced in front of the first lumbar vertebrae, can be chosen for pain in the upper abdomen (stomach, liver, pancreas) or retroperitoneum. Postural hypotension is a problem at first because of local vasodilatation. *Intercostal nerve blocks* are sometimes chosen to relieve rib pain.

A *chordotomy* involves the transection of the spinothalamic tracts in the spinal cord. The procedure can be performed through percutaneous needle into the cervical cord. Pain sensation below and on the opposite side is no longer transmitted. The risk is impairment of nearby motor and sensory fibers in the cord. Many patents choose drug palliation rather than the possibility of paralysis and loss of bowel and bladder control.

Hypophysectomy, destruction of the pituitary, through transnasal injection of alcohol or freezing is occasionally chosen for "uncontrollable" pain. The risk of complications and claim of effectiveness varies according to surgeon. The physiological rationale for this procedure remains uncertain. The patient undergoing this procedure needs extensive discussion with the surgeon regarding expected risks and benefits; he/she will require corticosteroid and thyroid hormone maintenance therapy following surgery.

Use of TENS Units

Transcutaneous electric nerve stimulation (TENS) units are small, battery-powered generators that produce a tingling sensation that can block pain sensation. Electrodes are placed over or near the site of pain. These electrodes, the amount of electrical output, and the particular TENS unit often require repeated adjustments until relief is achieved. Refer to Meyer 1982 to understand management of a TENS unit. Many physical therapists have special training in this procedure. An adequate trial should be allowed this low-risk, noninvasive tool, which is best tried with prolonged pain that is not coming under good control with more conventional methods.

PHARMACOLOGICAL PAIN RELIEF

Nurses have traditionally taken a "back seat" when decisions about pain drugs are being made by the physician. Most of us have absorbed the unspoken maxim that "the best pain medication is the least pain medication." We have worried about addiction, depressing respiration, and the "complaining" patient who wasn't satisfied with his or her Demerol tablet. We have learned a great deal since becoming hospice and palliative care nurses, and we now assume joint responsibility with the physician to *assure* that analgesic medications are used effectively to relieve pain.

Principles of Analgesic Use in the Terminally Ill

Prevention of Symptoms

Symptoms are prevented through regular use of medication. The lowest dose of an analgesic is administered at the widest interval possible to achieve constant control of pain. Medications are scheduled at appropriate regular intervals, not prn. If medicine is taken only when pain reappears, the person will experience an "up and down" quality of life with peaks of relief and valleys of suffering. Instead, the goal is a steady level of medicine in the bloodstream and a steady predictable level of pain relief. The diabetic does not wait until symptoms of hyperglycemia reappear, but rather takes a carefully titrated dose of insulin each day. Likewise, the cardiac patient takes digoxin regularly rather than wait for symptoms of decompensation to appear. The foregoing analogies often help patients and professional colleagues grasp the advantage of preventive analgesic scheduling rather than waiting for painful decompensation before using a drug.

Effective scheduling of analgesics to prevent pain recurrence requires an understanding of the expected duration of drugs used. Table 8-1 provides information on the likely duration of commonly used narcotics, based on the second author's experience at Hospice of Seattle. The literature provides conflicting information on drug duration; more research is needed. One reason for these contradictions is the fact that the pharmacological dynamics of narcotics change with long-term use. Halpern (1982[a]) says, for example, that the necessary interval between narcotics doses can lengthen after five days of regular administration. *The primary nursing implication is the need to watch individual response so that drug dosage can be scheduled just before*

Table 8-1. *Likely Duration of Effects of Common Narcotics*

Drug	Hours of Effectiveness per Method of Administration		
	Oral	IM	IV
Morphine sulfate	4	4	2
Methadone	6–8	4–6	4–6
Levorphanol (Levo-Dromoran)	6–8	4–6	?
Meperidine (Demerol)	3–4	3–4	2
Dyhydromorphone Dilaudid	3–4	3–4	2

pain would reoccur. The intervals never should be determined in cookbook fashion; schedules are always individualized.

No Fear of Drug Dependency

Drug dependency is not to be feared with regularly scheduled use of narcotics. *Physiological* dependence does occur, as demonstrated by the need to gradually reduce narcotics if the source of pain is diminished. With sudden discontinuation of narcotics, symptoms of physiological withdrawal will occur. People do not become *psychologically* dependent, however, when narcotics are used for pain control in the terminally ill. Psychological dependence occurs when an individual experiences an overwhelming craving for the psychic intoxicating effects of narcotic. These intoxicating effects do not occur with appropriate use for pain relief.

Tolerance need not be feared. To relieve a constant level of pain, terminal patients do not require higher and higher levels of narcotics. Rather, the amount of narcotic required to control pain often levels off. Twycross (1978) reports that many British hospice patients experience a drop in narcotic need once their pain is under good control. International hospice experience has shown that there is no ceiling of effectiveness with drugs such as morphine and methadone; patients can receive hundreds of milligrams of these drugs daily, if they are carefully titrated.

The central issue around drug dependency continues to be a deep-seated cultural prohibition against the palliative use of drugs that also happen to be drugs of abuse. Attitudes change slowly. In our experience, those who are most resistant to new knowledge about appropriate medical use of narcotics are patients themselves. At the end of their lives, their self-concepts are assaulted by fears of becoming addicts. Their fears need to be heard over and over again, and the choice to "try and get by with as little medicine as possible" must be respected. The nurse listens and teaches and assists with coping in crises that are a result of noncompliant drug-taking secondary to fear. Most patients come to knowledgeable acceptance of the quality of life they achieve with regular narcotic schedules.

Balancing Pain Control and Side Effects

Narcotics are titrated carefully to minimize effects on respiration and mentation. Just the right amount of narcotic is used to cut out pain perception without depression of respiration and mentation. When the proper balance is achieved, the patient is comfortable, mentation is clear, and respiration is within normal limits. When the dosage is too high, the patient is comfortable but feels sedated, mentation is clouded, and respiration may be suppressed. To achieve a proper balance requires ongoing monitoring of pain, mental status, and breathing. The nurse is regularly at the patient's side when new drugs are started, and the patient-family are taught the basics of systematic assessment in these areas. *A common error in the use of narcotics for terminal pain is starting a patient on an effective analgesic and then considering the problem solved.* The nurse provides regular follow-up, checking back with patient and family from wherever she or he is based, be it the physician's office, the home health agency, or the hospital–nursing home unit. Terminal pain may not be constant day to day. Effective pain control requires that the patient-family be taught the indications for increasing or decreasing dosage.

The goal in titrating narcotic dose to respirations is to control pain while keeping the respiratory rate above 10. A lower rate predisposes to cerebral hypoxia. Respirations stabilize with prolonged narcotic use at a constant level, even if the necessary narcotic dosage is very high. Respiratory rate must be monitored whenever a new narcotic is started, dosage is increased, or the amount of pain is diminished (such as following radiation or nerve block). *When death is imminent and cardiorespiratory failure is causing slow, irregular breathing, narcotics may be administered to avoid suffering even in the presence of very low respiratory rates.* It is a challenge to nursing to assess critically all those factors that may be slowing breathing as death approaches and not to deprive a patient of pain relief at the end of life. When death is not near, however, and pain is not controlled by narcotic levels that *appear* to be depressing breaths below 10, drug titration is best performed by admission to the hospital, where narcotic antagonists and nonnarcotic pain-relief strategies are available.

Narcotic dose can usually be adjusted to avoid significant clouding of thought. When a new narcotic is started at levels expected to control pain completely, the pain often experiences several days of sedation and clouded mentation. If this effect does not clear in three days, the dosage is gradually reduced to a level that controls pain and permits mental clarity. For some patients, the slight mental effects that remain may be a source of irritation and

Figure 8-3. Hospice pain control

Use of medication: A self-help guide for family and patient.*
Pain may be a problem with progressing illness, but it can be well-controlled to permit quality living. The goal of this guide is to help people learn the basic principles of pain control in order to apply them to their own situation.

Pain is an intensely unpleasant feeling that only the person experiencing it can know. The causes of pain include bodily change from the physical effects of disease, pressure on sensitive structures, swelling from inflamation, and irritating chemicals produced. Pain almost always causes anxiety or fear at first; when it lasts for a long time, many people become depressed and have sleeping difficulties. As a vicious cycle, pain is accelerated by anxiety and tension, depression, and sleeplessness. A comprehensive plan for pain relief always should include methods to relieve emotional distress and promote relaxation. Pain can also be reduced by specific techniques using distraction, creative imagery, and stimulation to the skin over the painful area. The hospice team can provide guidance on the use of these approaches. This guide focuses on your understanding the use of medication to control pain.

Drug control of pain is effective when applying the following principles:

1. When pain is constant, drugs need to be taken around the clock *at regular intervals.* This keeps enough medication in the blood *at all times* so that pain is *always* controlled. If a person waits until the pain comes back before taking the drug she or he will need a larger dose to quiet the pain. Just as the diabetic does not wait until signs of coma before taking insulin, so the hospice patient does not wait for pain to take drugs to control it. In both situations, the purpose is *prevention of symptoms* by keeping a constant level of drug active in the blood.

   Some medicines last longer than others. For example, methadone may be taken as infrequently as every 6 hours, whereas morphine by mouth is usually taken every 4 hours. Moreover, each individual responds differently.

2. The amount of narcotic needs to be carefully *adjusted and patiently readjusted* in order to prevent suffering.

amount of drug	Balanced Use of One Drug	amount of pain
☐ ☐ ☐		☐ ☐ ☐

The amount of narcotic should be just enough to quiet the pain, but not so much as to cloud the mind.

a. When people first start taking a narcotic regularly, they may become sleepy or feel their thinking is foggy. If the drug dose is right to control the level of pain, the mind will clear in 2 or 3 days. Waiting for the fog to clear is difficult but worthwhile.

b. Sometimes a person will be comfortable on narcotic drugs for a long time and then start feeling confused. Confusion may be due to chemical or physical changes in the body, but drugs should also be reviewed. Too much drug may be in the body, or the pain itself may be less. Drug dosage can be dropped back for a few days to see if the mind clears.

c. When pain reappears after a period of comfort, the amount of narcotic can be increased or other medicines or approaches can be added to balance with the increasing pain.

*Adapted from Hospice of Seattle.

163

may be experienced as a significant loss of self. Such patients may choose to experience some pain rather than lose their mental sharpness. Some persons experience disorientation and hallucinations with one narcotic and need to be switched to another. Some will have these effects after prolonged successful use of a narcotic, particularly those with long action such as methadone, and will stabilize with downward adjustment of the dose.

Figure 8-3 offers a portion of a guide used by Hospice of Seattle to teach patients how to titrate analgesics.

Use of Oral Drugs

Oral drugs are the first choice for terminal pain. One of the most exciting early revelations from St. Christopher's and the British hospice experience has been the evidence that terminally ill patients can achieve excellent pain relief from the use of oral narcotics. This has freed patients from the discomfort and tissue destruction of multiple injections, and it has increased patients' options as to mode of life because repeated injections are not necessary. Oral narcotics are effective for most terminally ill people with pain until they are no longer able to swallow. Occasionally a patient on a scheduled oral regimen may require an injection for acute, "breakthrough" pain, but usually oral dosage can simply be increased or the patient can take extra oral doses of medicine between the regularly scheduled doses.

Combined Drug Regimens

Drugs should be used in combination to treat several dimensions at once. Table 8-2 presents two combined regimens. A narcotic can be used alone and carefully adjusted to the level of pain, but a narcotic dose can be minimized and pain control maximized by the addition of other drugs to the pain control regimen. To this end, acetaminophen (Tylenol) or aspirin may be added for

Table 8-2. *Two Sample Combination Oral Drug Regimens for Pain Relief.*

Regimen 1

Levo-Dromoran 2 mg every 6 hours
Vistaril 25 mg every 6 hours
Aspirin 650 mg every 6 hours
Elavil 75 mg at H.S.
Surfak 50 mg BID
(stool softener)

Regimen 2

Tylenol #3 every 4 hours
Thorazine 25 mg TID
Colace 50 mg BID

peripheral analgesic effect. An antianxiety agent, such as hydroxyzine (Vistaril) or diphenhydramamine (Benadryl), may be added to tackle the anxiety component of the pain experience. Tricyclic antidepressants are also very effective adjuncts to the pain relief regimen, utilized to allay the depressive dimension of pain and also for their bedtime sedative and direct analgesic effects. Sometimes stimulants, such as cocaine or dextroamphetamine, are added to counter the sedative effect of narcotics. Their use is appropriate for only a few days, because tolerance develops rapidly. Stimulants may be used to counter the depressive effects that almost invariably occur during the first days of a narcotic schedule, or to improve mental alertness as requested by a terminal patient close to death (McCaffery, 1979).

The "Pain Cocktail"

Liquid pain medication, "pain cocktail," can be useful in the control of terminal pain. Pain cocktails, which contain a combination of pain-relief drugs, have several advantages in the control of pain. They make it easy for patients in that they need take only one preparation instead of many pills and capsules. Pain cocktails are easy to swallow, and they are easy to titrate by increasing or decreasing teaspoonfuls rather than multiplying or breaking tablets and capsules.

Pain cocktails, however, have several disadvantages that may lead the nurse to recommend other vehicles for some patients. Some patients have problems with the taste of the syrup, whatever the flavor. Some have difficulties with nausea that are diminished with the use of capsules. At Hospice of Seattle, a significant clinical problem with the use of cocktails has been titrating the dose upward as the patient's pain accelerates. If three or four ingredients are present in a syrup, there is a danger of toxic effects when dosages of all drugs are gradually increased. For instance, a patient may start with a cocktail that contains 5 mg methadone, 25 mg hydroxyzine (Vistaril), and 325 mg acetaminophen (Tylenol) in 5 cc cherry syrup; the patient is to take 10 cc (2 teaspoonfuls) every 6 hours. If the pain increases, it will be necessary to increase the teaspoonfuls of this cocktail. The methadone can be safely increased, but the other drugs have toxic limits. When pain is increasing, it is safer to titrate the dosage of each drug individually, rather than to increase all in combination. Therefore we might choose, for instance, to quadruple the methadone dose, double the hydroxyzine, and keep the acetaminophen dose constant.

A major problem with effective use of pain cocktails is the tendency of many institutions to fail to label contents of the bottles that go home. It is impossible to safely titrate a drug unless you know what it is. Nurses should check with the pharmacy or physician immediately upon encountering an unlabeled bottle so that the contents are known. Pharmacies and physicians need to understand the necessity for nurse, patient, and family to know the drugs and dosages that they are adjusting to level of pain.

Common Adjunctive Drugs

Drugs that *diminish peripheral pain sensation and perception* include the steroidal and nonsteroidal anti-inflammatory drugs and acetaminophen. Corticosteroids, paricularly prednisone 5–10 mg tid, are commonly prescribed for the terminally ill person in pain to reduce inflammatory processes, to diminish edema around tumors causing pressure on pain-sensitive structures, and to increase the general feeling of well-being. Dexamethasone (Decadron) is prescribed to reduce intracranial pressure and consequent headache. Aspirin is the first choice in the nonsteroidal anti-inflammatory analgesic class of drugs; it interrupts peripheral nervous system transmission of the pain impulse, it reduces inflammation, and it is also a prostaglandin synthesase inhibitor. Prostaglandin sensitizes nerve endings at bony metastatic sites. The pain of bony metastasis will often be significantly relieved by 650 mg aspirin every 4 hours (Twycross, 1978). To minimize danger of gastric bleeding, aspirin should never be taken on an empty stomach. Since aspirin prolongs bleeding time by inhibiting clumping of platelets, it should be used with caution for patients with known coagulation disorders, such as thrombocytopenia secondary to chemotherapy. The growing class of other anti-inflammatory drugs, much more costly and with many side effects, should be tried as adjuncts for terminal pain only if aspirin has been given a fair trial. This includes drugs like indomethacine (Indocin), ibuprofen (Motrin), and zomepirac (Zomax). Acetaminophen has a peripheral analgesic effect equal to aspirin without the anti-inflammatory action. It is chosen when there is concern over the gastric irritation or lengthened bleeding time with aspirin use.

The *antianxiety agents* of choice are the antihistamine sedatives, hydroxyzine (Vistaril, Atarax) and diphenhydramine (Benadryl). Dosages are commonly effective at 25 mg every 4 to 6 hours, given with each narcotic dose. These drugs possess narcotic-enhancing, antianxiety, antiemetic effects with minimum side effects (see also Chaper 7). Promethazine (Phenergan) is not a drug of choice when the patient is in pain. It is also an antihistamine with calming and antiemetic properties, but it has been observed to increase perception of pain and produce more sedation, hypotension, and respiratory suppression (McCaffery, 1979).

Phenothiazines are often chosen as adjunctive antianxiety, antiemetic agents. Prochlorperazine (Compazine) is popularly used at doses of 5–10 mg orally or 25 mg by suppository every 4–8 hours, administered with analgesics. Chlorpromazine (Thorazine) is often prescribed at doses of 10–25 mg with each narcotic dose; it enhances relief of pain, but oversedation can be a problem (see also Chapter 7).

The minor tranquilizers, diazepam (Valium) and chlordiazepoxide (Librium) are not first choice as adjuncts for terminal pain control. They are often antianalgesic (Halpern, 1982[a]), depress respiration, have no antiemetic effect, and cause withdrawal symptoms when discontinued abruptly.

The *stimulant drugs*—amphetamines or cocaine—are sometimes used as adjunctive drugs to increase analgesia and brighten mentation. However, tolerance develops quickly. They are perhaps best used for brief periods when the patient wants to be particularly clear and functional.

The *tricyclic antidepressants* should be used as adjuncts to pain relief when ever depression is significantly contributing to discomfort, as is commonly the case with chronic pain. Amitriptylene (Elavil), doxepin (Sinequan), and imipramine (Tofranil) are often chosen for their ability to provide immediate bedtime sedation. After a few days, they have a direct analgesic effect. It may take up to two weeks to recognize a mood-elevating effect. To take advantage of the sedative effect, the entire dose is best given at bedtime. Dosages begin at 50–75 mg daily at H.S., and can be gradually titrated upward as tolerated (see also discussion of multiple side effects in Chapter 7).

The *anticonvulsants,* particularly carbamazepine (Tegretol) may be useful to control the pain of progressive nerve invasion that is causing neural hyperexcitability with "seizures of pain" that are not controlled with narcotics (Halpern, 1982[b]).

Using Specific Narcotics

Narcotics bind with the opiate receptor sites, located throughout the central nervous system, to reduce the central perception of pain. The possible adverse effects of the narcotic class of drugs are summarized in Table 8-3. Many narcotic-class drugs are useful for the control of moderate pain in the

Table 8-3. *Some Possible Adverse Narcotic Effects*

Physiological Effect	Observable Problems
Central nervous system depression	Sedation, disturbed mentation, respiratory center depression, depressed cough reflex
Chemoreceptor trigger-zone stimulation	Nausea and vomiting
Increased smooth muscle tone	Increased gastrointestinal tone with reduced motility resulting in constipation, Bronchospasm in asthmatics
Reduced arterial resistance, venous tone	Peripheral vasodilation causing postural hypotension

Table 8-4. *Narcotics Commonly Used for Terminal Pain*

Drug	Oral Dosage (in milligrams)	Effectiveness	Limitations
Dosage Equivalent to 650 mg Aspirin			
Codeine	30	Relief for moderate pain. Enhanced by combination with acetaminophen or aspirin	Dosages over 60 mg may provide no significantly increased analgesia
Meperidine (Demerol)	50	Relief for severe acute pain in IM form only	Poor oral absorption (400 mg p.o. = 100 mg IM) Short acting. Possible drug ceiling of 150 mg (convulsant)
Pentazocine (Talwin)	30	Relief for moderate acute pain in IM form only	Disorientation extremely common side effect Narcotic antagonist: Patient switched from another narcotic to Talwin can have withdrawal symptoms. Short acting
Proproxyphene hydrochloride (Darvon)	65	Relief for mild acute pain Aspirin probably just as effective	Much more toxic than aspirin
Dosage equivalent to 10 mg morphine 1M			
Dyhydromorphone (Dilaudid)	7.5	Relief for severe acute pain in IM form Minimum local irritation with IM and subcutaneous injection; 3–6 mg suppository may relieve moderate pain	Poor oral absorption (7.5 mg p.o. = 1.5 mg IM) Short acting

Drug	Dose (mg)	Comments	
Drugs with oxycodone 5 mg: Percodan (Oxycodone, ASA, homatropine, phenacetin, caffeine) Percoset (actaminophen, oycodone) Tylox (acetaminophen, oxycodone)	30	Relief for moderate pain, long action indicated in some patients.	Percodan's mixture of homatropine, phenacetin, and caffeine is irrational and may be contra-indicated in some patients.
Levorphanol (Levo-Dromoran)	3	Long acting May be given subcutaneously Good oral absorption (3 mg p.o. = 2 mg IM)	Unclear whether less effective than methadone Needs more trials in management of terminal pain
Morphine	15–55	See text	
Methadone (Dolophine)	10–20	See text	

Source: Portions adapted from Halpern (1980), McCaffery (1979).
Note: This table is based on the sources cited as well as on the second author's experience at Hospice of Seattle. The reader should note that there is great variance among "experts" on equal analgesic dosages.

terminally ill, but only a few are desirable drugs in managing severe terminal pain. Table 8-4 charts the effects of commonly used narcotics and identifies their strengths and limitations in managing severe terminal pain. Buprenorphine (Temgesic), a new narcotic antagonist, promises to be an effective, long-acting (8–12 hours) analgesic; it has been quite useful in British hospice care.

British experience with the legal use of heroin for terminal pain has been highly successful. Large doses can be dissolved in smaller amounts of water than can morphine, which is advantageous for high-dose parenteral administration. There is some movement to legalize heroin for this purpose in the United States. In the authors' opinion, however, our patients do not suffer any significant disadvantage from the unavailability of heroin, for high doses of morphine and other drugs can accomplish the same level of pain control.

Morphine sulfate in water is currently the agent of choice in treating severe terminal pain in the British hospices. For a long time, American palliative medicine was hesitant to use oral morphine because the pharmacology literature stated that morphine was largely inactive when taken by mouth. Research by Robert Twycross, pharmacologist at St. Christopher's Hospice, has demonstrated the clinical effectiveness of oral morphine preparations. Twycross (1978[b]) concludes that two-thirds of any given morphine dose is absorbed by the gastrointestinal tract. Other studies show a much smaller fraction absorbed. Morphine liquid is now available in the United States, and more and more pharmacies are preparing morphine in solution. Morphine must be given about every 4 hours by mouth or intramuscularly, and every 2 hours intravenously. Oral morphine 55–60 mg is usually considered equivalent to morphine 10 mg given intramuscularly. However, after prolonged regular use, Arthur Lipman (1980), pharmacologist at the University of Utah and formerly of St. Christopher's, says that 15 mg of oral morphine can be equivalent to 10 mg by injection. The average dose at St. Christopher's is under 30 mg (Twycross, 1978[a]). It is wise to begin with 15–20 mg p.o. and then titrate upward according to need.

Methadone is becoming the oral analgesic of choice in the United States in treating terminal pain. It is long lasting (half-life of about 22 hours), easily absorbed by the gastrointestinal tract, capable of relieving severe pain, and gives only minimal sedation after the first few days. Usually an oral dosage interval of 6–8 hours is effective. Dosage may be started a bit higher than the estimated need, and may be required at 4-hour intervals initially. Sedation is normal at first. As the drug level accumulates and stabilizes, the dosage can generally be reduced and the intervals stretched to 6–8 hours. Halpern (1982[a]) notes that methadone can have a duration of 24–36 hours in a patient who has been taking any opiate regularly for a month. This means that it will have a short duration just like morphine when it is the first narcotic to be used regularly, and the intervals can be stretched out in those with prolonged narcotic use. Intramuscular methadone is very irritating to tissue, which is an argument for switching to morphine when shots are required. Intravenous methadone is extremely useful because of its prolonged duration of action, in contrast to the brief IV durations of most other narcotics. Start with three-quarters of the oral dose, and individualize the intervals by staying with the patient to titrate to pain, respiration, and mentation.

All narcotics, including morphine and methadone, can have troublesome side effects that require switching to alternate drugs. Methadone seldom causes nausea; morphine frequently does and may be relieved by an antiemetic or by discontinuing the drug. In the Hospice of Seattle experience, mental aberrations—hallucinations, agitation, disorientation—can be a critical problem that require ongoing assessment. All factors that are affecting a patient's mental status, such as hypoxia, hypercalcemia, and high anxiety, should be considered before rejecting a drug without adequate clinical trial. The elderly have particular difficulty with unpleasant mental changes from methadone.

The most predictable problem with long-term regular narcotic use is constipation. Immobility, dehydration, lack of roughage in the diet, and reduced muscle strength all predispose the patient to this difficulty. The only answer is a vigorous bowel regimen, initiated when regular narcotics are initiated. Start with psyllium (Metamucil) and other natural sources of fiber, if the patient can tolerate these. We begin our patients immediately on a stool softener (dioctyl sodium sulfosuccinate or dioctyl calcium sulfosuccinate) two or three times daily. A bowel stimulant (bisacodyl) may be added initially or as needed. Milk of Magnesia or bisacodyl (Dulcolax) suppositories daily may be needed. It is essential to prevent impaction.

Parenteral Narcotics

Oral narcotics should be the rule unless a patient cannot or will not swallow. When other routes are indicated, oxymorphine (Numorphan) suppositories 5–10 mg or hydromorphine (Dilaudid) suppositories 3–6 mg can be tried for moderate pain; absorption from the rectum is quite unpredictable. For intramuscular administration, morphine is generally the first choice because its use is very familiar to practitioners. It works very well every four hours and is nonirritating to tissues. Methadone is more irritating but, in the patient who has been receiving narcotics regularly for awhile, has the advantage of longer intervals between shots. In the terminal patient close to death the subcutaneous route is undesirable because of poor absorption. Parenteral drug dosages are determined by calculating the 24-hour total for the patient's oral narcotic dosage, converting that to the equivalent dosage for the parenteral drug, and then dividing by the number of doses in a 24 hour period (see Table 8-4 for drug equivalencies). For example, consider how you would switch to intramuscular morphine when a patient has been receiving 30 mg oral methadone every 4 hours. First calculate the 24 hour total oral methadone dose: $30 \times 6 = 180$ mg. Examine the equivalency chart (10–20 mg oral methadone equals 10 mg IM morphine) and calculate (conservatively) the

24 hour equivalent morphine dose: 180 ÷ 20 = 90 mg. Since morphine is given about every 4 hours IM (6 times daily), determine the amount of each dose: 90 ÷ 6 = *15 mg*. Each patient will respond differently. Effective titration depends on adjustment of dosage and interval to patient response.

The intravenous route is sometimes chosen for severe pain, or to avoid the pain of intramuscular injections. With the growing popular practice of inserting a Hickman line into the superior vena cava to expedite blood drawing, giving drugs, and fluid administration, many patients now enter the terminal phase with a Hickman line in place. Even if this route is available, intravenous bolus narcotics should not be started unless oral administration is no longer possible or unless there is acute pain "breakthrough." This restriction is owing to the typical up-and-down pain-relief pattern obtained from injecting most intravenous narcotics every two hours. This is an immensely burdensome life rhythm to maintain day and night. As intravenous methadone becomes more commonly prescribed, its longer duration of action may allay this problem.

Intravenous narcotics should be diluted in 10 cc normal saline, and administered slowly over 5 min. Rapid administration can cause nausea and dizziness, marked circulatory and respiratory depression.

Continuous morphine drip, managed by an infusion pump, has become a tool to maintain a much more constant blood level, rather than the up-and-down pattern seen with "IV push." It should be chosen for those temporary periods when pain is "out of control" until oral drugs can be properly titrated again. An occasional patient, usually with extensive carcinomatosis and often nerve infiltration, may require continuous morphine infusion to remain comfortable during the last days of life. Dosages involved can often be as high as 10–100 mg morphine hourly. Patients can be maintained on such high-dose infusions for days to months with good pain control and still be "reasonably coherent and alert" (Holmes, 1978). Miser and Clark (1980) describe eight children, 3 to 16 years old, who received .8–80 mg of morphine hourly to provide stable effective pain control for one to sixteen days. Constipation and drowsiness were the most frequent side effects, but mentation was not so suppressed that the children could not communicate with their families.

The elements of a morphine infusion protocol are summarized in Figure 8-4. Because of restrictions on movement, cost, and need for 24-hour skilled

Figure 8-4. Determining a morphine infusion protocol

1. Morphine solutions, prepared by the pharmacist, can be varied in concentration from 50 mg to 500 mg morphine sulfate in 500 ml D₅W.

2. The milligrams of morphine per cc are calculated. If 100 mg morphine sulfate are added to 500 ml D₅W, there will be 1 mg morphone sulfate for each 5 cc infused. If 200 mg morphine sulfate are added, there will be 2 mg for each 5 cc infused. 500 mg in 500 cc should be used for high hourly doses.

3. Prepare a dosing chart to be attached to the pump:

Figure 8-4 (continued)

For instance, for 200 mg MS in 500 cc, 2 mg MS = 5 cc/hr, 4 mg MS = 10 cc/hr.

4. Many different methods are being used to determine dosage. A common strategy is to convert the patient's past 24-hour narcotic dose to an equivalent dose of parenteral morphine, and divide by 24 to obtain a beginning hourly dose by infusion. Many protocols start with a loading dose that involves slow IV push until the patient experiences pain relief.* ·

5. A consistent system for monitoring patient response to infusion must be established. Observations are made every 15 minutes, extended to one hour and then to every 4 hours as response stabilizes.

6. Drug orders are best written for a dosage range after the physician has determined the initial dose, such as "morphine sulfate 20–30 mg/hr. Increase or decrease at 1 mg increments until pain controlled and respirations over 10." If the patient is dying, the need for morphine may diminish somewhat and respirations certainly may be under 10.

Continuous Infusion Morphine: Flow Sheet†

Time
Bolus (mg)
Infusion rate mg/hr
Vital signs: respiration
pulse
blood pressure
pupil size*
Level of consciousness (LOC)**
Pain Assessment (0–3)***
Additional medications: List any pain medications along with infusion

Pupil size*: pinpoint, 1–2 mm; normal, 3–5 mm; dilated, 6 mm or greater.

LOC**: 4+, Normal requires no arousal; 3+, Rouses to alertness with minimal stimulation; 2+ Needs greater stimulation and/or does not reach full alertness; 1+ Deep coma or reflex activity only

PAIN ASSESSMENT***

0 *Absent:* No symptoms to cause physical distress
1 *Relieved:* Treatment resulted in symptoms ceasing to distress patient.
2 *Unrelieved and inconstant:* In spite of treatment physical discomfort.
3 *Unrelieved and constant:* Physical distress persists.

*Cohen, M.A.: Morphine infusion protocol. *Hospital Pharmacy,* 1981, *16,* 296–297.
Boyer, M.W.: Continuous drip morphine. *Amer. Journal of Nursing,* 1982, *82,* 602–604.
† Adapted from Virginia Mason Medical Center, Seattle, Washington. John Horn, Pharm. D. and Meredith Bolt, R.N.

nursing care, this tool should not be chosen for a prolonged period of weeks if there is any alternative that effectively controls pain.

Intrathecal Morphine

Recent experience indicates that the intrathecal injection of morphine into the lumbar region or lateral ventricle provides significant pain relief with minimal side effects. Leavens, Mill, and Lech (1982) describe six patients who received *once daily* injections for 3 to 7 months of 1–7 mg into an implanted Ommaya reservoir.

UNCONTROLLED PAIN

It is difficult to evaluate how frequently pain would be considered "out of control" in a caring system that systematically implements those pain-relief strategies described in this chapter. Twycross (1978[a]) described great success at St. Christopher's in managing pain that before hospice admission had been out of control. Inpatient care at St. Christopher's permits a well-organized continuity-of-care program that facilitates management of the multiple dimensions of pain. Many illness-care systems are more fragmented, with lack of continuity between clinic, hospital departments, and home; and little joint planning between professionals and with the patient and family. In the author's opinion, most pain that appears out of control despite knowledge of palliative measures among the caregivers is a result of an illness-care system that is "out of control" and thus impeding effective continuity of palliative care. Examples of patients caught in such out-of-control systems include those whose history of treatment is fragmented and difficult for the nurse to obtain; who have received trials of drugs without documentation of their effects or any attempt to titrate to need; who have not been taught or able to learn basic principles of pain relief and given control over their own drugs; who have no knowledge of nonpharmacological methods of pain control; who have professional caregivers who seldom confer and are unavailable to one another; and whose caregivers have given in to hopelessness.

Sometimes pain that is "out of control" despite the most appropriate palliative management techniques for the organic cause has an intense emotional–spiritual component. People who suffer in this way need much attention and counseling if they are to move through their agony; sometimes they will refuse this help.

Occasionally patients may present with organic processes that will submit to pain relief techniques only when drugs are frequently adjusted and several adjunctive measures are used. For instance, the pain of nerve infiltration can be difficult to control with narcotics and may require the use of a nerve block and/or imagery and/or acupressure and/or a TENS unit. Sometimes the patient and/or family will exert their control by resisting the learning of new measures for pain relief. Some will choose to experience pain rather than side effects which they find unacceptable. Energy to try new approaches can be very limited at the end of life. Given these limitations, the nurse will sometimes be at the side of a terminally ill person whose pain is poorly controlled, despite "all efforts." These interludes should be marked by ongoing assessment and a willingness to *remain present at the side of the suffering individual.*

Following is a description of the course of pain of a dying woman. Use the knowledge from this chapter to develop ongoing plans for pain control as her condition changes.

Case Example: Ongoing Control of Pain

June 14.   Marian Jorgensen, age 41, has metastatic breast cancer with metastasis to left clavicle, 2nd right anterior rib, right femur, and liver. She transfers with difficulty due to back pain and is afraid to move. She has refused further chemotherapy secondary to weakness, and the physician does not believe there is significant chance of improvement anyway. The patient is about to be discharged on "Percodan tab 1 q3–4h prn." Her doctor is discouraged by her poor response to chemotherapy and asks you, "What more do you think we can do for her?" What specific suggestions would you have?

August 6.   Another bony metastasis is found. Oral morphine 20 mg p.o. q4h is ordered for Ms. Jorgensen. She becomes progressively more confused the following day. What are the possible causes? What would you recommend?

August 23.   Marian is stabilized on 1 tsp pain cocktail with morphine sulfate 15 mg and Vistaril 25 mg every 4 hours. But her chest pain exacerbates and is controlled only with 4 tsp of the cocktail every 3 hours. What would you recommend?

November 1.   Marian is switched to methadone 30 mg p.o. with Vistaril 50 mg q6h. Since her last hospitalization, she has had a Hickmann line to draw blood and give infusions. Her level of consciousness has fallen and she cannot swallow. What would you consider as you prepare to switch her to IV meds and to teach the family to administer them?

REFERENCES

Bates, T., & Vanier, T. Palliation by cytotoxic chemotherapy and hormone therapy. In C. Saunders (Ed.), *The management of terminal disease.* London: Edward Arnold, 1978.

Bonica, J. Cancer pain. In I. Ajemian & B. Mount (Eds.), *The Royal Victorial Hospital manual on palliative/hospice care.* New York: Arno Press, 1980.

Cousins, N. Anatomy of an Illness (as Perceived by the Patient). *New England Journal of Medicine,* 1976, *295,* 1458–1463.

Halpern, L. *Advances in pharmacological control of terminal pain: Current state of the art.*

Address given at Advanced Symposium on Care of the Terminally Ill, Seattle, Washington, February 26, 1982a.

Halpern, L. Dialogue with Hospice of Seattle Team. May, 1982b.

Halpern, L., & Bonica, J. Analgesics. In W. Modell (Ed.), *Drugs of Choice 1980–1981*. St. Louis: C.V. Mosby, 1980.

Holmes, A.H. Morphine IV infusion for chronic pain. *Drug Intelligence and Clinical Pharmacy*, 1978, *12*, 556–557.

Leavens, M.E., Hill, C.S., & Lech, D.A. Intrathecal and intraventricular morphine for pain in cancer patients: Initial study. *Journal of Neurosurgery*, 1982, *56*, 241–245.

Lipman, A. Drug therapy in cancer pain. *Cancer Nursing*, 1980, *13*, 39–46.

McCaffery, M. *Nursing management of the patient with pain*. Philadephia: Lippincott, 1979.

Melzack, R. Current concepts of pain. In I. Ajemian & B. Mount (Eds.), *The Royal Victoria Hospital manual on palliative/hospice care*. New York: Arno Press, 1980.

Melzack, R. The McGill Pain Questionnaire: Major properties and scoring methods. *Pain*, 1975, *1*, 277–299.

Meyer, T.M. TENS relieving pain through electricity. *Nursing*, 1982, *82*, 57–59.

Miser, A.W., Miser, J.S., & Clark, B.S. Continuous intravenous infusion of morphine sulfate for control of severe pain in children with terminal malignancy. *Journal of Pediatrics*, 1980, *96*, 930–932.

Oncology Nursing Society & American Nurses' Association Division on Medical–Surgical Nursing Practice: *Outcome standards for cancer nursing practice*. Kansas City, Missouri: American Nurses' Association, 1979.

Twycross, R. Bone pain in advanced cancer patients. *Topics in Therapeutics*, 1978, *4*, 94–110. (a)

Twycross, R. Relief of pain. In C. Saunders (Ed.), *The management of terminal disease*. London: Edward Arnold, 1978. (b)

Williams, M. The place of surgery in terminal care. In C. Saunders (Ed.), *The management of terminal disease*. London: Edward Arnold, 1978.

Wilson, R.W. Endorphins. *American Journal of Nursing*, 1981, *81*, 722–725.

1. F	*6. T*
2. F	*7. T*
3. T	*8. F*
4. F	*9. F*
5. T	*10. T*

9

The Last Few Days

Answer the following questions True (T) or False (F). Answers appear on the last page of this chapter.

1. A person can have extensive endstage disease but will not actually die until heart or lungs or nervous system fail.

2. Hypoxia and reduced tissue perfusion cause cyanosis in the extremities and impaired mental function.

3. "Death rattle" is best managed by pharyngeal suctioning and Valium.

4. Fluids should be forced in those near death to avoid the discomforts of dehydration.

5. Determining vital signs is essential to identify the course of dying in the last days.

6. Pain is usually a problem at the end of life.

7. The patient who is lingering may have unfinished business remaining.

8. The great religious traditions share some common teaching regarding the spiritual tasks at the end of a lifetime.

9. The family who has received guidance in anticipation of the expected course of dying can often manage the vigil and death effectively without the presence of a professional.

0. It is less traumatic for family and friends to have the deceased body removed as soon as possible.

No ship can outsail death.... When I seem to be dying, I don't want to be stimulated back to life. I want to be made comfortable to go.*

T
HE LAST FEW DAYS and hours of life comprise a vital time of partnership between the dying person and those, including helping professionals, who would provide vigil and comfort at his or her side. The nurse needs to know what to expect physically, physiologically, and emotionally so that she or he will be equipped to provide anticipatory guidance for the patient-family.

CAUSES OF DEATH

Trauma and disease cause death. The incidence of different problems varies according to age group. In school age children, accidents, leukemia, brain tumors, birth defects, and pneumonia are predominant causes of death. In adults over 60 years of age, cardiovascular disorders, cerebrovascular disease, cancer, obstructive lung disease, and pneumonia are the most frequent cause of death. A study at the M.D. Anderson Hospital in Houston revealed the following underlying causes of cancer death, listed in order of frequency: infections (septicemia, pneumonia, peritonitis, pyelonephritis); organ failure (lungs, heart, liver, central nervous system, kidney); infarction (lungs, heart); hemorrhage (gastrointestinal, brain, rupture of major blood vessel, lungs); or the presence of extensive carcinomatosis (Inagaki, Rodriguez, & Bodey, 1974).

Death draws closer as there is irreversible failure of normal integrated bodily functions. Whatever the underlying pathology with multiple systems failing, it is *cardiopulmonary failure* that is the final cause of death. The heart or lungs must fail for death to ensue. Therefore the best indicators of imminent death are cardiac and respiratory signs.

---

*Mark Twain, in Donaldson, N., and Donaldson, B. *How Did They Die?* New York, St. Martins, 1980, p. 373.

Circulatory failure may be sudden due to myocardial infarction, arrhythmias, or blood loss. Gradual decompensation and hypovolemia are common dynamics preceding death. Failing circulation causes reduced tissue perfusion, of which common indicators are dropping blood pressure, tachycardia and irregular pulse, reduced mentation (less blood to the brain), cooling and cyanosis of extremities (slowing of blood flow in periphery), reduced urine output (diminished circulation to kidney), possible chest pain (reduced coronary artery blood), and possible pulmonary and peripheral edema (back-up of venous blood).

Pulmonary failure can have multiple causes including pneumonia, thromboembolism, pleural effusion, pulmonary edema, pulmonary or tracheal obstruction, obstructive lung disease, and depression of the medullary respiratory centers secondary to central nervous system failure. Signs of pulmonary failure include the effects of hypoxia and eventually hypercapnia (slowed mentation, confusion, restlessness, apprehension, coma) as well as orthopnea and air hunger, irregular or rapid breathing, tachycardia, and use of accessory muscles to breath. Excessive accumulating secretions can cause frequent productive cough and a fear of choking or drowning.

Cardiopulmonary failure associated with an imminently terminal status can be well managed palliatively by the use of oxygen if it provides subjective relief, injectable hydroxyzine (Vistaril) or diphenhydramamine (Benadryl) to allay dyspnea and restlessness, and morphine for the pain of infarction or when additional palliation is needed for air hunger. Atropine can reduce excessive secretions in the hours before death. All these measures and their use in the time just before death will be explored further in the next section.

PREDICTABLE CHANGES
AS DEATH APPROACHES

Signs and symptoms in the final days and hours of life frequently follow a pattern that can be anticipated. They are accelerated in a rapid downhill course and slowed in a lingering death, when a person remains "on the brink" for days. These symptoms are not so well known to those of us who practice in a context of contemporary technological medical care because we have so often seen the natural course interrupted by technical intervention with multiple life support systems. Traditionally, the face of imminent death has been only too familiar to physician and nurse, who recall Hippocrates' description of "a sharp nose, hollow eyes, collapsed temples, cold contracted ears with the lobes turned out, forehead skin rough, distended, and parched, and a green, black, livid, or lead coloring of the face" (Hippocrates quoted in Martinson, 1981, p. 344). Though the face and dying course of each person is highly individual, there are some recognizable landmarks and preparations that can be made to assure comfort at the end of life.

No More Food or Drink

The second author once had a patient who consumed pancakes and pizza right up to the morning of the day of his death, but this is most unusual. Stopping eating is a predictable sign that life is drawing to a close; dying requires no nutrition. People stop eating when their disease prevents swallowing or digesting food, or when they have no energy or desire to force themselves to eat. Usually the intake of fluids also deteriorates to perhaps a few sips of water or a favorite beverage. It is unkind and useless to force food or fluid on a person considered to be within a few days of death. Dryness of the mouth is relieved by sips of fluid, small ice chips, frequent cleansing of the mouth, and oil to the lips.

The family and dying person should discuss choices about using intravenous fluids. It may be desirable to consider hospitalizing for hydration a person who is not drinking, or even to consider intravenous fluids in the home. An intravenous line should be inserted only after careful consideration of goals to be accomplished for the dying person. Intravenous hydration increases the level of fluids throughout the body, and the dying body may not be able to handle the load. Thus nasogastric intubation and Foley catherization may be needed to handle increased gastrointestinal and urinary fluids; increased respiratory secretions may require suctioning. Symptoms from accumulating ascites and edema, including edema surrounding tumors, may present problems. Two to three liters of intravenous fluids daily are much more likely to cause problems for the dying person than one liter daily.

Dehyration as a natural course of events may be preferred. The technological problem of safely keeping an IV running is avoided. There may be symptom relief with less edema, less pressure from tumors, less vomiting, less need to void, less rattling secretions as the person "dries out." The resulting effects on level of consciousness may be considered to be a "natural anesthesia." The greatest problem with dehydration is usually dry mouth. (Zerwekh, 1983)

The choice between administering intravenous fluids or allowing dehydration to occur should always be individualized. The benefits of the former choice are sometimes prolongation of life, better control of nausea, the confidence that "everything is being done." The risks are sometimes prolongation of suffering, aggravation of symptoms as detailed above, and a focus on technological rather than human needs. The nursing role is to clarify options and listen carefully to the patient and family, support patient–family choice, and encourage deliberative health team decisions that are consistent with patient–family wishes.

In the hospital, the nurse has the responsibility for maintaining a prescribed intravenous line, often difficult in the dying person whose veins are either scarred from repeated venipunctures or collapsing in the presence of circulatory failure. The nurse assesses and documents the patient's response to intravenous hydration. In the home, the nurse occasionally trains a family who wants to keep intravenous fluids running. It is easiest at home to use a heparin lock and run the actual infusion over a 6–8 hour period, during which it is watched carefully. Infiltrations should be expected and a plan made to realistically cope with the problem of finding a professional with a high level of venipuncture skill to reinsert. A Hickmann line is most reliable to maintain. Private-duty nursing coverage is highly desirable, and most insurance companies will pay for this level of skilled care.

Oliguria and Incontinence

The urine of a person who is dehydrating gradually diminishes in volume and increases in concentration. Circulatory failure also precipitates prerenal failure and oliguria. Progressive fatigue and weakening of muscles often affect ability to control urination; incontinence is not unusual. When the person is just not drinking, the volume of urine may be so small that she or he may need to urinate only once or twice daily, possibly less. Therefore, incontinence may occur only a few times, or not at all, before death.

Caregivers should prepare for the possibility of loss of urinary control by protecting the bed with a plastic cover. Bedclothes will need to be changed, and the lower part of the body bathed immediately after incontinence is discovered. It is easiest to place soft towels or incontinence pads over the bottom sheet. For the person at home, the latter are commercially available through hospital supply houses.

A person who has continued to drink well or receive IV fluids may be expected to urinate several times in large volume during a day. If incontinence becomes a problem, it may be desirable to insert a retention catheter into the bladder to prevent repeated wetness and skin irritation. In Lamerton's (1979) study of 600 patients dying at home, 22 percent required catheterization before death. At home, equipment is obtained through a hospital supply company, hospital central supply room, or, if a visiting nurse is involved, a home health agency.

Changes in Breath

Some difficulty breathing is commonly seen at the end of life. Pneumonia, tumors, and fluid in the lung due to sluggish circulation from organ failure (heart, liver, kidneys) all cause problems with increased lung congestion. Other disease processes block movement of air in the lung or upper respiratory passages. Thromboembolism blocks pulmonary circulation. In the final days of life, the resulting difficulties may include an intense hunger for air, frequent productive cough, rattling sounds with each breath. The first rule with respiratory distress is to achieve a sitting, upright position to allow full expansion of the chest. Try a chair with high back and arm rests (recliners are excellent) or bolsters in bed. Mountains of pillows are a problem over time, for they keep collapsing as a person tosses and turns. Breathing problems are greatly eased by a hospital bed with a backrest that cranks up, but many people at home prefer to modify their own beds. Narcotics suppress cough and ease breathing and apprehension. Sedatives like Benadryl or Vistaril also ease breathing and fear. Any person dying at home who has had progressing lung disease as a primary problem should have these drugs at home in readiness. Pills can be used until the person can no longer swallow. Injections are necessary with severe distress. Begin with Vistaril or Benadryl 25 mg by injection every 2–6 hours; you may have to increase dosage to around 100 mg for great trouble breathing. Combine with narcotic.

Oxygen therapy may ease breathing by making more oxygen available for exchange. Often the lungs are so filled with fluid or tumor that little gas can travel across that barrier to reach the blood. Nevertheless, oxygen blowing into the nostrils is comforting to a dying person who feels desperate for air. At home, oxygen is available only with a doctor's order from medical supply companies and specialized firms. Employees of such firms are trained to teach the safe use of equipment.

Once, a special friend of one of the authors died with extensive pulmonary metastases. She was a very bright and independent sort who had pretty much run the show and had not asked for any help. About a week before her death, she had preferred to discuss politics and flowers and common friends. One morning at 6 A.M. I received word that she was overwhelmed with terror at her inability to breathe. I received the physician's permission to begin injections of morphine and Vistaril every 4 hours, and her vast community of willing friends was mobilized to continue the shots. A hospital bed was ordered. By evening, she was sitting up cross-legged, breathing easily with her oxygen prongs and admitting her astonishment: "I really do feel all right now. I didn't think it was possible."

Caregivers should understand that the only stimulus for breathing in people with chronic advanced lung problems is the low oxygen level in their blood. If the oxygen is turned up higher than prescribed, the person's oxygen level may rise significantly and she or he may stop breathing.

Change in breathing pattern is another useful yardstick of death approaching. Often breaths are very shallow or noisy. The periods of apnea may lengthen, and the number and depth of breaths is reduced until the last breath comes.

The Death Rattle

This sound is heard with the breath passing through the accumulation of pharyngeal and pulmonary sections. This occurs when the person is neither able to completely cough up sputum or to swallow the saliva that gathers in the back of the throat. The sound is an unmistakable, loud, coarse bubbling. Generally, the person experiencing this has a reduced level of consciousness and is not bothered. If she or he is aware, Vistaril or Benadryl, as described in the last section, will relieve apprehension. Atropine .6 mg subcutaneously or intramuscularly can be used to dry up the secretions. Usually only a few injections are needed every 4 hours before death occurs. Often, the family suffers more than the patient, as they must listen to the rattle. It is perfectly acceptable to administer drugs to make the family's vigil easier.

Patients with a death rattle should be turned on their sides, unless this is uncomfortable. A side-lying position allows the secretions to run out of the mouth. Though commonly used, a suction machine has little purpose at the bedside of a dying person. It often gags the patient and traumatizes the mouth and throat. In addition, the noise can be as disturbing to the family as the rattle itself. Dying hospice patients generally do not need this. If they are dehydrated, there is very little fluid to cause rattling in the air passages. Likewise, morphine and the antihistamine action of Benadryl and Vistaril cause drying of secretions. If rattle occurs nevertheless, atropine injections are preferable to suctioning. An exception exists with those who already have tracheotomies in which routine suction is usually needed for comfort. The use of IV fluids in the last days increases the chance that a death rattle will occur.

Slowing Circulation

As the heart puts out less and less blood, the peripheral part of the body begins to cool down. The skin becomes cyanotic when slowed circulation results in greater extraction of oxygen and thus the presence of more reduced hemoglobin. A typical pattern begins with the observation of a blue discoloration in the feet; the purple-blue mottled appearance and cold temperature change often proceed gradually up the legs while the hands also become cold and increasingly dark. This process progresses in step-wise fashion, but in many people there are times when skin color and warmth return briefly to normal. Then the progressive cooling in the extremities spreads. *The color and temperature of extremities is one of the most useful indicators that the end of life is approaching.* Socrates spoke his final words, according to Plato, when gradual cooling progressed from his feet and legs into the groin (Donaldson, 1980).

Decreased Consciousness

As death draws near, a person's energy is increasingly drained by even the simplest activities of everyday living. Time between naps becomes shorter and shorter. Morning may not bring any sustained periods of wakefulness. Energy to speak is diminished. Most people come to a point of not being able to rise out of bed. Some move slowly into a coma, becoming more and more difficult to arouse.

Normal level of consciousness is determined by a delicate balance of oxygen and carbon dioxide and chemicals interacting with the nervous system. At the end of life, the heart, lung, liver, kidneys, or nervous system often fail to maintain this balance, and the brain is no longer able to maintain alertness. The level of consciousness descends downward either slowly or quickly. First comes sleepiness and indifference, and possible disorientation. As consciousness drops, the person may respond only to shaking or pain and may no longer talk. A comatose person no longer can control any body function. The person may hear you but has no way to make the body respond.

Level of consciousness often varies from hour to hour. Just when we decide that people have become completely unresponsive, they may awaken to smile, squeeze a hand, speak. The dying have some control over the extreme energy it takes to arouse themselves when a situation is compelling. For instance, a 36-year-old woman lay for days in a deep coma with her eyes fixed open and staring. Her eyes needed to be protected with the regular application of artificial tears. On the evening before her death, her close family gathered with the parish priest to celebrate a family mass at her bedside. During the communion, she began to weep and her eyes shed many tears. She died shortly thereafter. Her family never stopped talking to her; they believed she heard them. *Speak to a dying person as if each of your words can be heard.* Choose your words with care.

Disorientation

Dying people gradually lose touch with ordinary reality. They may lose track of time, often living in a past moment. They may mistake the place for a place in the past or for whatever is familiar. Other people may be misidentified, perhaps confused with each other. The person may have conversations with people from the past or hear voices or see a reality not apparent to you or me.

The physiological cause is the same as for reduced level of consciousness, namely the imbalance in blood and chemicals affecting the brain. Many people believe that another underlying cause of disorientation and apparent hallucinations is that the dying are actively making a transition to another reality that will occur after death, that they are reorienting to a new time and place, a separate set of visions. When disorientation is distressing, it is helpful to remind the dying person of what is really going on in the present moment: the time, the place, the loved ones nearby. As attention to the present moment fails, you may have to repeat yourself a great deal. Do not deny the person's visions, but respond honestly by offering your own observations. If disorientation is causing fearfulness or restlessness, it is especially important to maintain a *calm presence* at the bedside, and sedation may be desirable.

Restlessness

It is not unusual for the dying person to begin to toss and turn, to pick at the bedclothes. This may be due to toxic chemicals and inadequate cerebral perfusion and hypoxia. Restlessness may also be due to pain, a full bladder, a full bowel, or drugs causing excitability. Pay attention to verbalized complaints, or to picking and rubbing over one area. Analgesics and/or attention to bowel or bladder may be needed. Evaluate drugs, especially those with anticholinergic or extrapyramidal side effects at high doses.

Protect the person's safety. Arrange the bed so that a distressing fall does not occur. Siderails are conventionally pulled up on a hospital bed; these give some people security though others resent the barrier. It is best to have someone frequently at the bedside to ease fear and continually reorient the patient.

Severe restlessness is exhausting to family and patient; calming medication should be tried. At home, plan ahead by having a small quantity of an injectable sedative, preferably Vistaril or Benadryl, ready in the home cupboard or dresser drawer.

Vital Sign Changes

Temperature, pulse, respiratory rate, and blood pressure are indicators of a person's well-being and dying. In the hospital, these are ritually obtained every 4 hours or more often in a seriously ill person. The predictable pattern in dying is an increased pulse rate that is often rapid and irregular as the failing heart struggles to pump adequate blood to the periphery, breathing changes as already discussed, and there is a dropping blood pressure as less blood moves through the blood vessels. Temperature is often subnormal as metabolism drops, but may be elevated in the presence of an infection or brain tumor. A typical chart might look like Figure 9-1.

Changes in vital signs document the progress of dying. The insertion of a thermometer into the mouth or rectum of the person near death gives us

Time	Temp.	Pulse	Resp.	Blood Pressure
10 P.M.	98° F	104	22	84/40
2 A.M.	97.8	112 irregular	30	64/20
3 A.M.	Not taken	130, irregular; radial weak	26 irregular	52/0 by palpation
3:45 A.M.	Not taken	150, irregular apical	8 with 40 seconds of apnea	Not obtained
3:56 A.M.	Not taken	cannot auscultate or palpate	no breath	

Figure 9-1. Typical chart for a person in the last hours of life.

Table 9-1.   *Signs of Approaching Death: The Last 48 Hours*

- Reduced level of consciousness

- Taking no fluids or only sips

- No urine output, or small amount of very dark urine

- Progressing coldness and purple discoloration in legs and arms

- Laborious breathing; periods of no breath

- Bubbling sounds in throat and chest

---

information to record but actually helps the patient in no way. Changes in vital signs inform us as to how close the end is and thus enable us to make plans, such as calling those who want to be present at the death. For this reason, family members may choose to learn how to feel the pulse, listen to the heartbeat, take a blood pressure, or record temperature. However, they can get the same information from careful observations of the other cardinal signs of the progress of death, as have been discussed. See Table 9-1 for a summary.

Recognizing the Last Days

The nurse familiar with indicators that the final days of life are approaching can be extremely helpful in guiding the plans of patient, family, and professional team. Often a patient has been very ill for a long time but pathology does not predispose to cardiopulmonary failure. The family is urged to plan for "the long haul." Then when signs of cardiopulmonary deterioration appear, it is realistic to begin plans for intensive support in the final days of life.

Case Example: The Beginning of the End

Mrs. Reese was a 74-year-old married woman with metastatic cancer of the bowel that spread to the inguinal nodes, with massive lower-extremity edema refractory to diuretics. She also suffered a growing, fungating, ulcerating lesion over the left iliac crest. Though these conditions had been worsening for months and gradually diminished Mrs. Reese's mobility and normal role performance, the nurse identified no cardiac or pulmonary involvement likely to take her life. Planning involved measures to permit the patient continuing to do "business as usual" and to tape record a life review for her grandchildren.

After several months, the metastatic ulcer began to bleed profusely with each dressing change. Difficulties of ambulation confined Mrs. Reese to living room recliner and commode. She was sleeping more and eating less. At their request, the nurse informed the family of several possible causes of death: hemorrhage, thrombo-embolism, and pneumonia seemed likely. Because of her husband's age and infirmity, the family planned to hospitalize Mrs. Reese when these signs occurred. One evening her breathing became wet and labored, and cyanosis was present in the calves and feet. Since this had been anticipated and plans had already been worked out with the physician and nurse, Mrs. Reese was moved by ambulance to the hospital without flurry or crisis. Palliative measures were initiated on admission to include continuous low flow oxygen, atropine .6 mg every 4 hours, Vistaril 50–100 mg every 4 hours prn, acute restlessness or dyspnea, aspirin suppositories grains 10 every 4 hours prn fever, and unrestricted family visiting. The patient died two days later.

MANAGING DIFFICULT PROBLEMS
AT THE END OF LIFE

In contrast to the last section, which described common landmarks in the final path of life, this section explores problems that are less universal but are frequently confronted in the last days, such as infection, pain, bleeding, and seizures. Uncontrollable pain, bleeding, and seizures at the end of life are greatly feared by patients (Schubert, 1982), and they need reassurance that these events are rare and controllable.

Infection

Dying people are highly susceptible to infection. Almost half of cancer patients die from infection (Inagaki, Rodriguez, & Bodey, 1974). They are immunologically deficient, making them prone to the usual pathogenic organisms in addition to invasion from opportunistic fungi or protozoa. Tumor obstruction and infiltration predispose to infection. As the dying person becomes more weakened and immobilized with associated statis, pneumonia and urinary infections threaten. Microbial invasion is also made more likely with the damage to skin and mucous membranes that comes with surgery, catheterization, venipuncture, and suction.

The development of fever in the last days of life is a challenge to clarify palliative versus aggressive treatment goals. Treatment of an identifiable infection may simply mean an antibiotic course, or it may mean multiple invasive procedures (blood culture, sputum culture, x ray, serologies, spinal fluid culture) when the fever is of unknown origin. Antibiotics chosen for the more resistant infections can be highly toxic. The nurse has a responsibility to help the patient, family, and health care team to clarify goals and consider risks versus benefits. *Patient and family should know the signs of infection and should be actively involved in the decision to treat or just control symptoms.* They may choose to treat the infection if the patient's wish is to keep fighting for life, or if unfinished business remains, such as a family member who has not yet come to say farewell. Often a terminal infection is untreatable, despite the most vigorous investigation and therapy.

The development of an infection may be welcomed by patient-family when the dying has been long and lingering with overwhelming disease present. Palliative goals involve the control of fever and other discomfort from the infectious process. The fever need be treated only if it is causing the person some distress. Cover the person lightly with bedclothes. Two aspirin or acetominophen (Tylenol) are antipyretic; aspirin suppositories may be effective for someone who cannot swallow. Bathe the person with cool water if this brings comfort. Do not use cold water or alcohol baths to lower temperature; they usually cause more discomfort than relief.

Pain

A patient with a history of good pain control will seldom have new trouble with pain in the last few days. Generally, medicine can be given by mouth until the person cannot swallow. Then injections of morphine or methadone or narcotic suppositories can be used (see Chapter 8 for a discussion of switching from oral analgesics). Lamerton's (1979) study of 600 home deaths noted that 40 percent of dying patients with pain will need to have pain controlled by one or more injections before death; the rest never need to switch from oral administration. At home, a small quantity of injectable narcotic should always be ready for the last hours or days of a person who has previously required around-the-clock oral narcotics. Either the family or friends must be trained in injection technique, or a nurse must be easily available. Anticipatory planning avoids the family crisis that occurs when a person stops swallowing at 2 A.M. on Sunday; it is difficult to obtain a written physician prescription at that time, there may be no neighborhood pharmacy that carries injectable narcotic, and there may be no one who is skilled to administer an injection.

As the person slips into a coma, with accompanying "natural anesthesia," it is common to reduce analgesic cautiously. The dose is carefully titrated to nonverbal indicators of pain: moaning, grimacing, tossing and turning, rubbing body parts. Always question dramatic reduction of narcotics in the comatose patient because of the risk of narcotic withdrawal as well as the breakthrough of severe pain.

Bleeding

Loss of blood is sometimes a precipitating factor in death. Coagulopathy is common with impaired synthesis of prothrombin or production of platelets. Blood vessels are weakened by eroding tumor, inflammation and infection, atherosclerosis, surgery, and ulceration. Frequently blood leaks slowly into body tissues or cavities. Weakness and breathlessness are precipitated by the resulting anemia.

Occasionally, a dramatic loss of blood causes death. Martinson (1971) notes, however, that overt hemorrhage has been rare in the experience of home care for the dying child. And the M.D. Anderson Hospital study of cancer deaths showed an only 7 percent incidence of fatal hemorrhage, a low statistic attributed to the prophylactic use of platelet transfusions. (Inagaki,

Rodriguez, & Bodey, 1974) Fatal hemorrhage can cause a cerebrovascular accident, massive hematemesis and melena, hemoptysis, hematuria, vaginal bleeding, blood accumulating in the peritoneum, or blood loss through open wounds or stomas.

In the event of dramatic hemorrhage, death can occur quite peacefully with gradual loss of consciousness. The difficulty comes with trying to maintain a calmness at the bedside when we are all so conditioned to be horrified in the presence of large amounts of blood. The ideal approach to anticipated massive terminal bleeding is to maintain continual vigil at the person's side, and to give sedation to control apprehension and restlessness. Analgesia may be needed if blood is accumulating to cause pressure on pain-sensitive structures. Ice and pressure can be tried over bleeding sites, and topical anticoagulants can be applied to wounds and oral mucosa. Disposable tissues and towels are used to soak up blood and quickly removed before their accumulation causes a distressing appearance. Some hospices quietly bring out red blankets to absorb the blood.

Quietly watching a person bleed to death requires maturity and courage even on the part of the experienced hospice nurse or physician. In situations where bleeding is a predictable cause of death, it is helpful for family to discuss ahead of time how they will approach this. Some will feel most secure with hospitalization if hemorrhage occurs.

Seizures

Convulsions are rare at the end of life, but many people fear their occurrence as a dread "uncontrollable" event. Dexamethasone to reduce intracranial pressure, anticonvulsants, and barbiturates can be used to control seizure activity. When a terminal course has included significant seizure activity, the family is taught to understand what to expect during a seizure. The patient is protected from injury with head turned to drain vomitus and prevent aspiration. As death nears, some patients-families may choose slight seizure activity over heavy sedation (Martinson, 1981).

THE DEATH VIGIL

The Dying Person

As death nears, the dying person withdraws from active involvement in everyday living. Some prefer to continue surrounded by daily life by remaining in the living room, on a sofa, recliner or hospital bed. Most will, however, withdraw into the bedroom and into their own world. The last days of life are not a time to expect much verbalization, even from the fully conscious person. Affairs need to be put in order way before this time.

It is helpful for those who surround the dying person to say whatever has not yet been said to heal old hostilities; openly to express hurt and willingness to forgive. Reminiscing about past experiences together is helpful to both the dying and the survivors. Mourners may choose to share their future plans for living after the death occurs. The dying person should not be expected to express opinions at this time. What is said should not demand a response.

Even in Coma

Hearing is the last sense to be lost. Narcotics do not affect hearing (Halpern, 1982). Those who arrive after the person has lost consciousness should be encouraged to make their peace verbally. Assume that the person is fully present. Intervene when anyone switches to casual speech that considers the person near death as a body only.

The Environment

Much can be done to create a peaceful environment. Unless specifically requested, darkening the room and remaining hushed is not necessary. Instead, that which the person finds beautiful and satisfying can be nearby. One social worker spent her last evening in the living room while wine was being sipped, oil paintings discussed, and Beethoven played on the stereo. In contrast, a 21-year-old druck driver died on his sofa with a marijuana water pipe on the coffee table, the Moody Blues playing on the stereo, his teddy bear propped up across the room, and a half-eaten cheeseburger beside him.

Waiting for Death

As everyone sees clearly that death is very close and that release may be welcomed after the long struggle, the last few days often seem to take forever. Family and other caregivers may begin a tiring vigil at the bedside. The longer the lingering, the greater the strain on everyone.

The timing of death remains a mystery. Often it seems that a person can delay death by continuing active investment in the activities or unfinished tasks of this life. Nevertheless, the end eventually comes. When loved ones have been very involved in the vigil awaiting death, they may become preoccupied with the hope that they can be present *at the moment of death itself*. In reality, it is common for people to die in just the moment when a spouse, child, or friend has left the room. Help families understand this and realize that it is their persistent help and everyday sharing that count, the harvest of a lifetime. They need to realize all that they *did* do with the person.

If the person lingers long, poised between life and death, it is helpful to consider what might be holding the person back. People can put all their will into surviving if unfinished business remains. Try to figure out what needs saying or doing. What friend or family members have not yet said goodbye? Some family members may want to give the person permission to leave them. At one family conference around the bedside of a dying 43-year-old mother, a teenage son spoke: "I want you to know that I've decided to go back to school and get my diploma, just like you want. You can go now, Ma. I don't want you to live like this. I'll be o.k."

Some experienced hospice practitioners have tried visualizing a place of peace and rest for the dying person. The image depends on what has been meaningful in the dying person's life.

Meditation for One Who Is Lingering

Imagine going to a favorite beautiful place: a mountain, a beach, a garden, the woods. You feel totally comfortable and rested in this place. Explore the sounds and sights of the environment. A clear and radiating light surrounds you here and there is total peace.

In his new work, *Letting Go,* Boerstler (1982) describes a dramatic technique called "co-meditation" in which the person near death is assisted to achieve a calm meditative state. The one requirement of the patient is that she or he listen to the guide's voice. Following progressive relaxation instructions (see Chapter 7), the guide begins to breathe with the patient. "Ahhh" is sounded with exhalation, and the patient is invited to join in making this sound if she or he wishes. For rapid or irregular breathing, breaths are counted from 1 to 10 and then repeated. Boerstler claims that co-meditation will rapidly slow respiration and thought to achieve a peaceful state.

The Spiritual Journey

Mystical teachings of the major religions emphasize fostering a special quality of awareness at the time of death. Hindu scripture describes a person's dying thoughts as influencing his or her spiritual journey after death. In great detail, the Buddhist *Tibetan Book of the Dead* instructs the dying person in the recognition and union with the Clear Light. The Eastern tradition requires chants and meditations before, during, and after death to assist the person to avoid the suffering of reincarnation and instead experience union with God.

Medieval Jewish Law required the gathering of ten men (a minnion) to be present to read the Psalms, to pray, to light candles, and to pronounce a blessing and rend their garments at the time of death. For a Jew, "afterlife is said to be a reunion and all of life a preparation for it" (Heschel, 1974, p. 64).

For centuries, the 23rd Psalm has provided comfort at the bedsides of the dying as have the following verses from Isaiah:

Fear not for I have redeemed you; I have called you by name, you are mine. When you pass through the waters I will be with you; and through the rivers, they shall not overwhelm you; when you walk through the fire you shall not be burned; and the flame shall not consume you.—Isaiah 43:1–2

Medieval Christianity stressed conscious decisions at the time of death, with much use of imagery depicting the emissaries of heaven and hell struggling around the deathbed. Family and clergy gathered for final goodbyes, to vigil, and to pray. Theological debate continues to this day as to whether conscious deathbed repentance and conversion or the moral and spiritual choices of a lifetime determine journey of the soul after death. In the twentieth century, the death denial of western society has affected the church powerfully. However, faithful Christians of all creeds continue to find strength and blessing by gathering, praying, and reading scriptures that comfort the dying and surviving:

Let not your hearts be troubled; believe in God, believe also in me. In my Father's house are many rooms; if it were not so, would I have told you that I go to prepare a place for you? And when I go and prepare a place for you, I will come again and will take you to myself, that where I am you may be also.—John 14:1–3

Behold the dwelling of God is with men. He will dwell with them, and they shall be his people, and God himself will be with them; he will wipe away every tear from their eyes, and death shall be no more, neither shall there be mourning, nor crying nor pain any more, for the former things have passed away.—Rev. 2:3–4

Boerstler suggests that his co-meditation technics can be used to achieve spiritual peace, regardless of religious affiliation. Following the meditative state induced by attention to breath, he suggests repetition of a sacred word or verse with each exhalation. The words are chosen for their past or childhood meaningfulness. If the person is Christian, Boerstler (1982) suggests, the Jesus Prayer of the Heart might be chosen: "Lord Jesus Christ, have mercy on me." Jewish patients might use the ancient "Sh'Ma" ("Hear, oh Israel, the Lord our God, the Lord is one.") Buddhists might use "Om Mani Padme Hum." This chanting can be done by the family and played back on a recorder. The comatose and/or sedated patient is believed to be able to hear.

Following is a nondenominational prayer for peaceful death, for reconciliation or union with God, and for healing of sorrow:

Dear Lord, Father, Mother, Saviour, Creator, Spirit, Divine Presence, Light Within (Choose the most fitting based on religious heritage): Bless us all in this time of passing, especially our loved one, _____, who is soon to leave us. Please guide (him/ her) to know your light and truth and come into your full presence. Help us all who are gathered in love and caring to let (him/ her) go. May our grief be healed as we move into a changed life. We thank you for all that is love and life. Amen.

Many people who have no particular religious conviction will find comfort in reminders of the eternal rhythms of all that lives, the endless circles and seasons of birth and death, decay, and sustaining life again from soil and water. Ohiyesa, a Dakota Indian physician, in 1911 described his peoples' celebration of the unity and mystery of life:

In the life of the Indian there was only one inevitable duty...the daily recognition of the Unseen and Eternal. His daily devotions were more necessary to him than daily food. He wakes at daybreak, puts on his moccasins and steps down to the water's edge. Here he throws handfuls of clear, cold water into his face, or plunges in bodily. After the bath, he stands erect before the advancing dawn, facing the sun as it dances upon the horizon, and offers his unspoken orison.... Each soul must meet the morning sun, the new sweet earth and the Great Silence alone."*

Where Will Death Occur

A comfortable, dignified, loving environment can be created in either hospital or home. To stay at home and comfortable, the following elements are essential: family motivation to try, family members' awareness of their own limits, supportive professionals, and availability of a support network from friends and community. It is wise to plan for the long haul, twice as long as anyone thinks the person will live. Exhaustion and emotional tension will be the worst enemies of the caregiver (see Chapter 13 on ways to help family cope and develop a support network). Most people can be kept very comfortable at home. The problem with the job is the hours; one or two family caregivers alone will have trouble maintaining a 7-day around-the-clock work week.

If there is any money saved or other source, now is the time to use that financial reserve to buy private-duty nursing. A night shift is especially helpful to enable family to sleep. A good agency will send only mature skilled people into the home of a dying person. Private-duty care is costly ($300 daily or more for 24-hour, R.N. bedside care in 1982 in Seattle). Many insurance companies cover a portion of the cost of licensed nurses, if the physician orders a skilled level of care that demands procedures like injections, dressings, irrigations, oxygen. Most dying people do not require this technically complex care but do well with good basic bedside care that a mature and compassionate nursing aide can provide. Insurance, however, seldom covers this.

If there are no funds available, help the family to call on "natural helpers" from their community. Teach the family to ask for help and to be selective. Some might choose to eliminate people who talk constantly and those who hope for last-minute religious conversions. Others might welcome such people. Again, sleep is precious. Encourage family members to ask Aunt Emma to sit at the bedside and knit so they can catch a few winks at night. Maybe a concerned neighbor can come in while her children are still in school to permit an afternoon nap. Nurses teach and prepare those who are relieving the family. Specially prepared hospice volunteers are of great help to provide respite.

*From McLuhan, T.C. *Touch the earth.* New York: Promontory, 1971, p. 36. With permission.

If emotional reserve and family–community resources are exhausted, recommend hospitalization for the last few days. Some people will on their own choose hospitalization to conserve everyone's energy and to obtain what they believe will be better care. Help them become aware of the rights and advantages of hospitalization. Family members should be allowed to be present in the hospital at the bedside day and night. Physical symptoms should not be allowed to get out of control. The person has a right to refuse any of the usual hospital routines: temperature taking, forcing of food, insertion of IV's, urging to get up and walk, electronic monitoring, resuscitation. If they do not want life prolonged by dramatic measures, a living will should be signed way before the time of last hospital admission.

Many hospitals are now setting up their own hospice teams to go to the bedsides of persons dying throughout the hospital or in separate hospice units (see Chapter 16). Even without a hospice program, most contemporary hospitals have professionals on staff who serve as advocates for those who seek a peaceful and comfortable death of their own choosing.

For many in our society, the question of death at home or even in the hospital has become a moot point. Lengthy terminal courses and family inability to provide care have necessitated nursing home placement where death is often prolonged over months and years, with gradual loss of selfhood. Family may be faithful visitors, occasionally present, or estranged and conspicuously absent. The challenge of the nursing home nurse is to maintain a personalized approach in the last days of life both in his or her direct attention to the individual and in teaching, supervising, and supporting nonprofessional caregivers to work constructively with their own grief and to slow down to stay at the dying patient's side and care. This requires a lower patient load for staff who have patients very close to death.

Diagnosis of Death

Traditionally, death has been defined by the cessation of breath or heart beat. In the absence of life support technology, the best indicators of imminent death are found by cardiopulmonary assessment. Death can be expected within the hour if the extremities are cold and cyanotic, if the breathing is very irregular with long periods of apnea, if the pulse is very weak or cannot be felt, if the blood pressure is very low or cannot be heard. Some people will gradually deteriorate in all these areas. Others will only have some of the signs before breath stops. Note the time of death immediately. Loss of bowel and bladder control often occurs immediately before death. This may not even be noticed until straightening linens afterward.

Immediately after death, the eyelids may remain slightly open; the jaw will relax and keep the mouth open. It may be easier for loved ones to look upon the person's body if the eyes are gently closed and the head propped up by a towel roll or small pillow so that the mouth closes.

For contemporary professionals, the cessation of cardiac or respiratory function has become an automatic herald to start cardiopulmonary resuscitation. The more technological the environment, the more likely resuscitation attempts will proceed. The easiest solution is to clarify patient–family–medical choices beforehand and to request physician documentation in the patient record. This is more difficult to achieve when there is any question of reversing the patient's condition by aggressive resuscitative care.

If life support technology continues the breath with a respirator and the heart with drugs and pacemaker, death is then legally defined using the following criteria: absence of response to external stimuli; lack of spontaneous muscle movement, including respiration; absence of all reflexes; collapse of arterial blood pressure; flat electrocardiogram and electroencephalogram (Thompson & Cozard, 1981). The decision to remove support technology becomes an agonizing moral and legal question, for that which is begun is not easily undone. Individual personhood is lost in the technological order.

When death occurs at home, with symptoms controlled and families prepared, many will choose not to call for medical or nursing help until after the death has occurred. When symptoms and emotional distress are a problem in the moments preceding death, it is best if the family has a lifeline to a helping professional who can advise them or come over. This is one of the essential services of a hospice program. Without such service or because of stress and a need to feel that everything has been done, some families may respond by calling an ambulance or dialing 911 for emergency help from trained paramedics. Remember that they will try to restore life to the dying unless nurse or family inform them of other wishes.

Immediately Thereafter

Family should do what they feel is comfortable and appropriate at the time of death. Many will want to gather around the bed to pray, meditate, cry, be silent, reminisce. Some will want to leave the bedside to regain their own balance. Many caregivers with long experience of being present at the moment of death tell us that they continue to feel strongly the presence of the person, sometimes outside of the body but still lingering in the room. Since this is felt by people of a variety of faiths and no official faith, there is certainly no harm in assuming that the person might still be present. Final words and goodbyes can be spoken.

Some people will choose to hug, caress, bathe the body, though others will find this fearful and strange. It is a normal way of working through the finality of death and should not be discouraged. The funeral home need not pick up the body right away if there are still family members who have not come or need more time at the bedside to grieve. An electric blanket can be used at home to keep the body from getting cold to the touch. The pressure in a hospital to remove the person's body to the morgue is often great. Family members have a right to the last time together.

A checklist of whom to call right after death should be prepared beforehand. See Figure 9-2 for a sample family plan of action after death has occurred.

The legal ramifications of a home death vary significantly from community to community. In some places, the police must always be notified and the medical examiner must briefly inspect the deceased. Nurses and families in these communities plan ahead with police and medical examiner to eliminate trauma for the family when a death is medically expected. In many places, the police need not be called and the medical examiner need only be notified but need not investigate in the case of anticipated death under physician management. Usually the funeral home will assist in expediting all these procedures. It is vital that the nurse know the law regarding a home death in his or her community and advise families accordingly. A local service-oriented funeral director is an excellent source of information for planning. The family should be encouraged to begin coordinating with the funeral home chosen before death.

Figure 9-2. Sample after-death check list

---

1. Call Uncle Bob and Mrs. Rodriguez (phone numbers).
2. Call the Heaven's Gate Home (phone number) and tell them the time of death. Make arrangements for Joseph's body to be taken away in about an hour.
3. Call Dr. Christianson (phone number).
4. Call Pastor Solace (phone number).
5. When Uncle Bob gets here, let him call everyone else while I go and sit with Joseph one last time.

REFERENCES

Boerstler, R. *Letting go.* Watertown, Mass.: Associates in Thanatology, 1982.

Donaldson, N., & Donaldson, B. *How did they die?* New York: St. Martin's, 1980.

Halpern, L. Dialogue with Hospice of Seattle Team. May 19, 1982.

Heschel, A. Death as homecoming. In J. Riemer (Ed.), *Jewish reflections on death.* New York: Schocken, 1974.

Inagaki, J., Rodriguez, M.D., & Bodey, M.D. Causes of death in cancer patients. *Cancer*, 1974, *33*, 568–573.

Lamerton, R.C. Cancer patients dying at home. *The Practitioner*, 1979, *223*, 813–817.

Martinson, I. Understanding of the process of dying and the death event itself. *Hospice Education Program for Nurses*. Washington, D.C.: U.S. Department of Health and Human Services, 1981.

McLuhan, T.C. *Touch the earth*. New York: Promontory, 1971.

Shubert, V. *Anticipatory guidance for family caregivers to manage the last few days at home*. Workshop presented at the Advanced Symposium on Care of the Terminally Ill, Seattle, February 26, 1982.

Thompson, L.M., & Cozard, W. Is life living? Defining death in a technological age. *Death Education*, 1981, *5*, 205–214.

Zerwekh, J. The Dehydration Question. *Nursing 83*, 1983, *13*, 47–51.

1. T		*6. F*	
2. T		*7. T*	
3. F		*8. T*	
4. F		*9. T*	
5. F		*10. F*	

10

Grief and Bereavement

Answer the following questions True (T) or False (F). Answers appear on the last page of this chapter.

1. *The five stages of grief described by E. Kübler-Ross have been valuable in helping counselors recognize normal patterns of response.*

2. *The best way to handle anger in grieving patients is to point out how their complaining and resentment show a lack of appreciation for all that is being done to help them.*

3. *When a patient truly accepts impending death, a deep depression will be present.*

4. *Reminiscing with a bereaved person stirs up all kinds of good memories that are best forgotten.*

5. *Hospice bereavement programs are by definition available to all close family and friends of the patient for a year or until no longer necessary.*

6. *Bereaved family and loved ones are particularly vulnerable to physical and psychological stress and resulting illness.*

7. *The primary care nurse has the ultimate responsibility for bereavement counseling.*

8. *It is good to use drugs that keep the bereaved from having to deal with the reality of death during the first weeks when the stress is high.*

9. *There is no point at which the bereavement team has the right to decrease the dependency of the bereaved on their support.*

10. *Bereavement counseling can help a person set realistic goals for a reintegration into a fulfilling social life.*

We must set the model that mourning is not an illness, is not a weakness, is not a self-indulgence or a reprehensible bad habit, but rather, mourning is an essential psychological process which must be recognized and facilitated.*

GRIEF IS A NORMAL reaction to the profound feelings that accompany loss. We are all vulnerable to these feelings. Grief reactions vary among people and are not reserved for death alone. People must cope constantly with loss—the loss of home, employment, friends. The feelings of loss that occur with divorce, being passed over for an expected promotion, the departure of a grown son or daughter from home, and retirement, may be devastating.

As health care professionals, we constantly see individuals who, while ill and hospitalized, have lost their sense of home and independence. Life-threatening illness may have brought with it a number of losses, including loss of mobility, of attractiveness, of body parts, of functions, and of sense as well as a host of symbolic losses relating to self-esteem. Each of these losses, depending on individual perceptions and sensitivities, will prompt its own grief response. The patient who is dying, and the family who watches, will have been through many such losses.

There are several kinds of grief. *Preparatory grief* is experienced by the patient who understands she or he is dying. This loss, which is of the whole universe and being as the patient has known it, is the most comprehensive. The person must mourn the loss of everything and everybody, including the loss of a future.

Deep grieving may occur in patients who begin to lose a sense of significance in the family. They may be removed from the family home, institutionalized, and visited irregularly. They and relatives may grieve profoundly at this time. Emotions may scarcely surface when death occurs, for in terms of separation, it has actually already occurred.

The family and loved ones, as they observe the physical decline toward death, will experience *anticipatory grief.* If the patient is in significant pain or

---

*Farmer, Patrick J. Bereavement counseling, *The Journal of Pastoral Counseling, 15,* 32, 1980.

distress, this can be a deeply disturbing period for those who love him or her. If symptoms are well controlled, if spiritual and social anxiety is resolved and communication is kept open, this can be an extremely valuable and healthy period of bereavement. It can allow for the beginning of adjustment to the ultimate separation. Complete family resignation to the separation—for example, when there has been a long period of chronic disability—may be emotionally healthy for them, but cause great pain and loneliness in the patient who senses that she or he has already been forgotten.

Following the death of the patient, a period of *bereavement* follows for those to whom the patient was significant. The person who has died met personal needs that cannot immediately be transferred to other people or activities; as a result the bereaved person may find himself unwilling or unable to acknowledge his loss. Even if the person is willing, the patterns of emotional outreach continue to repeat as if the dead were not really gone. The desire to talk with the person who is no longer there cannot be turned off immediately. Sexual needs do not cease with the death of one's mate. Life goes on, with its emotional needs and established patterns (Jackson, E.N. 1971).

There is also a cessation in the ability to "give to" the deceased, and the bereaved may feel great guilt over failures of the past. Concern can focus for years on slight problems or oversights in the past relationship, and severe arguments or offenses can cause tremendous frustration and guilt.

Therefore it should be evident that the emotional and psychological events of the past are often more important in the grief process than the physical. William Rogers (1963) advises us that "grief is not the result of what happens to the loved one. It is rather the result of what happens to the bereaved. Something of a great importance to the individual, something that is part of his psychic life, has been torn out, leaving a great pain, the emotion which we call grief" (pp. 19–26).

In view of the foregoing, it is not difficult to understand such emotional responses on the part of the bereaved as sorrow, fear, guilt, anger, and loneliness and such somatic symptoms as nausea, disorientation, change in appetite, nervousness, restlessness, and sleeplessness. It is in every sense the whole person who is caught up in the grief, and if we are to counsel wisely we must consider the whole person.

THE PROCESS OF GRIEVING

The German word for mourning, *Trauerarbeit,* translates as "grief work." Grief is a normal working-through process of a loss the individual has experienced. But even though the normal process of grieving may in time be resolved, there are ways in which those who grieve may benefit from the help of specially trained professionals and nonprofessionals. Such people can provide valuable support to the bereaved in dealing with the following four major kinds of changes that often occur in the grieving person:

- Deeply painful sadness
- Loss of interest in everyday living (other than concerns that recall what has been lost)
- Decline in activity, functioning, and social interaction
- Loss of the capacity to love

For some, of course, these grief attitudes are "self-healing" as they are overcome by the reality of a continuing and challenging life with other goals, friends, loves, and aspirations.

The classic study of Erich Lindemann following the tragedy of the Boston Coconut Grove Fire in 1944 brought to the attention of social and medical scientists the characteristics of acute grief. Lindemann (1944) interviewed over one hundred patients and survivors of the fire and outlined an apparent and predictable syndrome with both psychological and somatic symptoms. The nearly consistent reactions Lindemann described included the following:

- Sensations of somatic distress, which included a feeling of tightness in the throat, choking with shortness of breath, need for sighing, an empty feeling in the abdomen, lack of muscular power, and an intense subjective distress described as tension or mental pain
- Intense preoccupation with the image of the deceased
- Strong feelings of guilt
- A loss of warmth toward others, with a tendency to respond with irritability and anger
- Disoriented behavior patterns

The British psychiatrist, Colin Murray Parkes has described a number of psychoemotional phases in grieving. Parkes (1970) states that the first response is often an overall "numbness," followed by a period of holding onto or reuniting with the lost one. He calls this latter phase "yearning" and includes in it "searching" and "protest." Elements of the protest state are often anxiety, fear, restlessness, and an irritability directed toward both oneself and others. Such irritability can result in outbursts, particularly at those who encourage the mourner to accept or forget the loss. The third phase described by Parkes is one of "disorganization," in which the bereaved person may show no interest in the future or even in the activities of daily living. This may last from weeks to months, but typically, according to Parkes, lasts about a year. According to Granger Westberg (1982), the ten phenomena listed in Table 10-1 are likely to appear—not necessarily in the order shown—in normal grief.

Parkes also describes several components of more severe reactions. For example, in what he calls "identification phenomena" the person may adopt

Table 10-1. *Elements of Grief*

- Shock that cushions the blow temporarily
- Emotional release
- Depression, accompanied by strange thoughts and loneliness
- Physical symptomatology
- Panic
- Guilt—both neurotic and justifiable
- Hostile resentment
- Inability to return to normal activities
- A gradual awakening of hope
- An adjustment to reality as a person acceptant of the loss

Source: From Westberg, G. *Good grief.* Rock Island, Ill.: Augustana Press, 1962. With permission.

"traits, mannerisms or symptoms of the lost person, with or without a sense of his presence within the self." Pathological variants of grief also include an excessive, prolonged or distorted period of mourning (Parkes, 1972).

Following the normal reactions to grief, there may be a gradual decline in mourning and a re-entry into the social activities of everyday life. There is a reestablishment of personal contacts, hobbies, and occupations are reestablished and the person becomes willing to look toward growth and a future.

Nurses, counselors, ministers and others who assist the bereaved should be aware of these normal and predictable components of the process. Two widows who, with humor and no illusions, describe their own unpreparedness and the lack of understanding in those around them state, "Most people think you are suffering when you are in shock, and think you are recovering when you are suffering" (Kreis & Pattie, 1969, p. 36).

THE STAGE ANALYSIS OF GRIEF

The varying reactions of patients to the imminence of death have been conceptualized as forming a series of "stages." A great disservice has been done, however, both to the originators of the stage concept and to the patients and families who continue to face death. Too often it has been assumed that the "stages" described are meant to be consistently sequential. Counselors have tried to fit a person into a certain stage rather than listen carefully to the person's needs; such tactics show little understanding of the original intent of the research. The purpose of defining the "stages" was to suggest a pattern through which individuals move back and forth, over varying time spans. Not all people will pass through every stage, and some will respond in previously undefined ways. Once the stage concept is properly understood, however, its use may well enable one to become a better counselor.

In one of the most thorough studies of patient grief, Elizabeth Kübler-Ross (1969) identified a pattern of five stages through which the more than four hundred dying patients she interviewed appeared to pass in coming to terms with their dying: denial, anger, bargaining, depression, and acceptance. These stages, which are discussed in the next five sections, may be seen in families and others who mourn dying patients as well as in patients themselves.

Denial

Denial is the avoidance of the truth of death's probability. Patients may not really process the information given them in the prognosis—they may go on speaking and acting as if they will soon be well. Or the fact of the probability of death may be met with a bold counterattack, such as, "No, it can't be. We'll find another doctor, another hospital." Just as the body goes into physical shock when it is assaulted, the human psyche goes into shock when confronted with the possible loss of self. Patients or loved ones may at first appear dazed and unaware of what is happening; they may feel a kind of numbness. In some cases, when the numbness starts to wear off, denial may actually be therapeutic. It may allow the person to adjust gradually to the news rather than be overwhelmed by it. It can also take the form of an emotional outburst directed at those who would present the true facts or of withdrawal in order to escape confrontation.

Anger

Anger may be the most intensely felt reaction of all. There is recognition of the fact of death and all its resulting losses. Something of great value has been lost, and someone, something must be to blame. Such anger may be discharged at God, the health care providers, family, self, or just the world in general. The rage of "Why me?" is frequently aimed at the closest target—the nurse.

Wound up in this anger there may also be guilt. There is guilt for not having lived fully, now that the end is near. And the loved one who is left behind may feel guilt for still having a life. Or there may be guilt and frustration in not having done all or said all the good that one would have wished. After a person loses someone close, it is quite common to dwell on what "could" or "should" have been said or done.

Sometimes bereaved people feel anger—anger at the dying person for "going off and leaving me"—and then guilt when they recognize the anger for what it is. Anger then may be turned on themselves.

Bargaining

At some point many people will accept the fact of loss but attempt to stall or manipulate the outcome. Bargains will be struck with God or whoever the person feels is in control, to change or at least detain the inevitable. If one bargained-for point seems to have been granted, such as living until a favorite child arrives, another and yet another may be made without end until the person realizes the futility of such "deals."

Depression

Unfortunately, the fact of impending death cannot be ignored forever. Frequently, for the patient, a deteriorating physical state is evidence of the approaching end. This response may become a silent sadness, terribly painful and lonely, and sometimes unrecognized as deep suffering.

For a bereaved loved one, the loss may not become real until the funeral is over, the friends and relatives have left, and she or he is left alone to cope with the empty place the deceased used to fill. In varying degrees there may be unresponsiveness, confusion, tearfulness, loneliness, and lack of concentration or interest. There may be an almost morbid preoccupation with that which is lost. Such a preoccupation can lead, in the extreme, to an actual search for the lost person; in a less dramatic form it may surface as a holding onto an object, such as a picture, an article of clothing, or a toy, to which the person now dead had attached meaning.

Parkes (1970) reports that there may be a significant group of bereaved people who actually "see" or "hear" the person who has died. Almost no one is prepared for such hallucinations—or for that matter, for many of the very strong grief responses one may go through. People's reactions may seem to them out of character, out of control—even marginally insane. It can all be very frightening unless someone is there to counsel the person as to the universality of many of the feelings.

Acceptance

Acceptance is not resignation (which may be part of depression) or "giving up." It is not the admission of defeat. It is instead the ability to overcome the grief, to accept the life that is left, and to reenter the everyday world on the new terms. In the dying patient acceptance may bring a peaceful feeling and the posture of separating himself or herself from all but one of two of the closest persons. Often farewells, either thinly veiled or very direct, are said to others and then those relationships are not maintained.

In the bereaved, attachments are slowly broken, and new investments of self are made in others and in the future. Slowly, for the person left, the guilt in enjoying life without the other subsides. "The old loss is not forgotten, but merely put in a special place which, while allowing it to be remembered, also frees the mourner to go on to new attachments without being pathologically tied to the old (Rando, 1980, p. 141).

REACTIONS TO LOSS AND GRIEF

Physiological Reactions

Illness may occur by chance in a person who has recently lost a very significant person, but very often it can be attributed to the stress of the loss and the grief. Several studies have revealed a high incidence of grief-related illnesses—enough to validate the possibility of the existence of a causal relationship. Lindemann (1944), in a study of 41 colitis patients, discovered that over 80 percent of his subjects had developed this condition shortly after the loss of an emotionally close person. Parkes (1964) focused a great deal of his attention on widows and concluded that bereavement can affect physical health. He found a close association between the anxiety and grief of a major loss and complaints of "somatic anxiety symptoms, headaches, digestive upsets, and rheumatism," particularly in widows and widowers in middle age. Even certain life-threatening diseases, such as coronary thrombosis and hematological cancers, were suspected of being aggravated by major losses. It is becoming generally accepted that extreme stress puts demands on the body's defenses and immunities to the extent that predispositions to disease may be able to challenge a person's system. Certainly strong grief provides a radical increase in the level of stress due to social, physical, and emotional changes. In a study by Parkes (1972), 4486 widowers had a death rate 40 percent over the expected rate for married men of the same age. According to Parkes, a major portion of this increase was due to heart diseases, specifically coronary thrombosis and arteriosclerotic heart disease. A study by Rees reported significantly higher mortality in a group of people who suffered the loss of a very close person than in other groups. And in fact, the closer the relationship, the higher the rate of mortality. (Rees, W.D. & Lutkins, S.G., 1967.)

According to Rando (1980), a mourner may exhibit any one or a combination of the numerous physiological reactions listed in Table 10-2. An illustrative case, cited by John J. Schwab, describes a 38-hear-old businessman who had been hospitalized for attacks of chest pain that simulated

Table 10-2. *Psychophysiological Reactions to Loss*

Anorexia
Gastrointestinal disturbances
Loss of weight
Inability to sleep
Crying
Tendency to sigh
Lack of strength
Physical exhaustion
Feeling of emptiness and heaviness
Feelings of "something stuck in throat"
Heart palpitations and other indications of anxiety
Nervousness and tension; inability to sit still
Loss of sexual desire
Psychomotor retardation
Decreased sensory acuity
Shortness of breath

Source: From Rando, T.A., 1980. Concepts of Death, Dying, Grief and Loss. *Hospice Education Program for Nurses.* DHHS-HRA81–27. D.C.: Department of Health and Human Services, 1981.

myocardial infarction seven or eight times within the year after his father's fatal heart attack.

Case Example: Heart Attack As Sign of Grief

The patient's chest pains, we ascertained, were a patterned response to making decisions about the business. His father had started the business many years earlier, and the patient had been a junior partner for about fifteen years. The father was a domineering, self-made man who kept the son in a very inferior position and did not allow him to participate in decision making. The son had chafed about this restrictiveness and had often had fantasies about what he would do with the business after his father died. In the year before the father's death their relationship had deteriorated and the son had begun to express his overt hostility. After he was able to talk about his hostile feelings toward his father and his sense of relief rather than grief at the father's death, his fears about a heart attack subsided. He expressed ambivalent feelings of guilt, hostility, affection, and sorrow. After he was able to grieve his "heart attacks" did not recur.*

Emotional and Psychological Reactions

A number of psychological manifestations of grief occur. Parkes reports that memories "of the deceased were characteristically clear visualizations of

---

*From Schwab, J.J. *Grief: Therapeutic interventions.* Paper presented at Kent School of Social Work Conference on Death and Grief, Louisville, Kentucky, April 1, 1976.

the dead person as he was when alive. Usually he would be in his accustomed place in the room and the memory would be so intense as almost to amount to a perception. A similar clarity was often present in memories of his voice or touch, 'I can almost feel his skin or touch his hands.'"†

Hallucinations and illusions of the dead have long occupied a place in myth and folklore. Robert Burton, who quotes from many classical sources in *The Anatomy of Melancholy* (1621), described the sense of the presence of the dead person. Widows in Parkes' studies frequently thought they heard or saw their husbands at some time during the first month. While many widows report sensing the "nearness" of the husband, a few actually experienced transient hallucinations. According to Parkes, "One widow repeatedly 'saw' her husband coming home through the door in the fence; another was upset by a hallucination of her husband sitting on a chair on Christmas day" (Parkes, 1970, p. 453). Both widows did recognize the experience as a hallucination. Parkes (1970) concludes that—in whatever form or degree—sensing a presence may "reflect the urge to look for and, in some sense, to find the lost person" (p. 453).

Unresolved grief reactions are often seen by psychiatric consultants who work with extreme behavioral changes such as serious alcoholism, hasty marriages and divorces, semi-stuporous depressive states, and conversion reactions in which the individual develops symptoms resembling those of the deceased (Schwab, 1976).

There is also often a preoccupation with objects and places associated with the deceased. Treasured possessions may be gazed at constantly and evoke great sadness. After a time there is a tendency to avoid looking at such closely associated items as clothing or photographs. Over a longer period of time—a year perhaps—the grief these items evoke gradually subsides.

Social Reactions

The social reactions to grief appear most often as a loss of normal patterns of conduct and changes in individual social habits (Lindemann, 1944). A general restlessness may drive the mourner to a constant flurry of activity in order to keep from ever having time alone, or time to think. Although many activities are excellent outlets for physical and emotional stress and provide good exercise, misdirected and frenzied activity is a way of running away from dealing with painful thoughts and emotions.

For very young adults, *delinquency* can be a substitute grief reaction. In a review of fourteen cases by the California Juvenile Probation Department where the onset of delinquent behavior was extreme, sudden, and unprecedented, a death in the family had occurred in each case. In no case had severe antisocial behavior occurred before the death. When the youths were

---

† From Parkes, C.M. The first year of bereavement. *Psychiatry,* 1970, *33,* 444–467.

counseled through a normal bereavement process, most of the behavior problems disappeared (Shoor & Speed, 1972).

Marital problems may occur between husbands and wives who are grieving differently and do not understand how their partners "could possibly act that way." A stoic may not understand tears; a silent mourner, a desire to talk about the loss. Behaviors such as drinking too much, staying up all night, or taking long drives alone may isolate one's mate. If a son or daughter has died, husband and wife may blame each other—or themselves—for the circumstances of the death. They may say, "If (she or he) had just locked the cabinet, checked the crib, found a doctor earlier." If left undiscussed, such resentments and recriminations can erode the strongest of marriages. If an illness has been prolonged, psychic and physical fatigue may already have decreased patterns of affection and sex or leisure time. There may also be severe financial problems. The longer these feelings smoulder unexpressed, the greater the potential for divorce.

FACTORS THAT AFFECT GRIEF REACTIONS

Many factors influence an individual's response to the death of someone. To achieve a better understanding of the kinds of reactions we have been discussing, let us look at some physical, psychological, emotional, social, and religious influences on personal grief.

Physical Factors

One of the most common modern influences on the grief response is the drug. Many medical professionals are quick to prescribe drugs to quiet and minimize the anxiety of loss and grief. Mild sedation can certainly be used to advantage for example, to prevent over-exhaustion or long-term insomnia. But drugs that sedate the mourner to the point where she or he is unable to experience the loss may be very harmful. If the bereaved are heavily drugged throughout the initial period of normal mourning, the funeral, or the visitations by relatives, they may miss the opportunity to vent and share their pain at precisely the time they can receive support and help. They are then left to confront their pain, alone and even in socially misunderstood ways.

The bereaved may experience other physiological changes that ultimately affect the grief response, such as altered taste, gastrointestinal upsets and physical exhaustion from restlessness and inability to sleep. Since a great deal of energy is needed to work through grief, such physical weaknesses may decrease the person's ability to cope. Even the most well-adjusted person may find an "impossible" personal problem easier to face after a good night's sleep or a relaxing dinner.

Psychological Factors

Psychological influences are complex and extensive. A person's coping style is fairly consistent, however, as Rando points out.

In most cases, the coping behaviors that one utilizes throughout life in other stressful situations do tend to form and will generally be those she or he selects to cope with the crisis of loss. "Similar to the dying patient, the individual will grieve (and the dying patient will tend to die) in the same manner in which the rest of life has been conducted."*

If the bereaved has always been a person who used support resources openly and has worked through other crises by facing them, she or he will probably follow the same pattern even with a more severe problem. The best guide then to prepare for a person's reactions to an anticipated bereavement is to gather information about how she or he has reacted to a loss in the past.

Coping skills are also affected by an individual's general level of maturity, intelligence, and learned strategies from dealing with other loss. Past experiences with similar losses do not necessarily decrease the pain but they do provide knowledge about what is happening now, how one may feel next, and what resources may help. Past experience also offers some assurance that pain does, in time, subside.

Emotional Factors

Perhaps the most profound influence on the way a person responds to a loss is the depth of the emotional tie between that person and the person who has died. The extent and intensity of the human bond between people defies definition, no matter how we may try—by role, relationship, duration, or any other way—to value such a relationship. For example, friends may be far closer than sisters or brothers; a brother may be more strongly bonded to a sister than to his own wife. Such relationships vary over the years, shift, and are replaced. There are many very important youthful relationships that diminish over the years until the loss is scarcely perceived. In other cases the news of an old friend's death can be felt deeply if that friend once provided great affection. It is sometimes surprising to people just how much emotion is still there for someone they have not seen in years. And the emotion may be confounded with a bittersweet memory of another era—one perhaps now lost for the bereaved as well.

---

*From Rando, T.A. Concepts of death, dying, grief, and loss. In *Hospice Education Program for Nurses.* Proj. Director, Henry, H.O. DHHS-HRA81–27. Washington, D.C.: Department of Health and Human Services, 1981, p. 145.

Parents are emotionally bound to their children in different ways also. It is not uncommon for one child to be far closer to the mother, another perhaps to the father. Spouses may, or may not, really love one another deeply and emotionally. There may be a very significant loved one outside of the marriage. If we pre-judge the depth of emotion by labeling relationships— "wife," "son," "friend," "girlfriend"—we will fail to appreciate many persons' grief.

Social Factors

The ways in which one person is socially dependent on another will affect the grief experience. Each of us relates to others in both a personal and a social context. Therefore, we may, on the social level, be someone's nurse but on the personal level, his or her friend. A woman may be to her mate, on the social level, a wife and on the personal level, a lover. There are relationships that exist primarily on only one of these levels. A valued employee may relate to many only through his or her role in society as an employee; a friendship may be basically personal.

It is difficult to lose a relationship that fills either a personal or a social role. But when the person has filled both, it can be devastating. For example, a mother of three children may lose each personal relationship when the first and second child move away from home. When the third and last child moves away, the mother may feel she is losing her societal role as a mother, and her nurturent and protective role. It is not, to paraphrase Shakespeare, that she loved the first children less, but that she loved motherhood more.

The loss of a mate is, for similar reasons, also tragic and difficult. The surviving mate loses his or her role and function as social partner, protector, provider, and at the same time the object of his or her deepest love and affection.

A number of other social factors influence grief. These include the bereaved's religious and cultural background. The expression of bereavement is to some extent a set of learned behaviors and is guided by tradition, the memory of the mourner of other family members and the rituals of one's culture and religion. The belief system held by the bereaved concerning the meaning and purpose of death affects the comfort with which she or he accepts that outcome in self or someone significant.

Another variable in accepting the social sense of any death is timeliness and circumstance. The death of one's child (regardless of the child's age) often provokes a more intense grief response than, for example, the death of a parent or of an elderly spouse. It does not make sense that a young person— someone who is your child—should die before you (Rando, 1980).

Several factors that may help the mourner to make sense of a death involve social circumstances:

- The location was good; the person died where she or he wanted to.
- The bereaved was able to participate and/or be of help.
- The deceased had a fulfilled life.
- Personal and business tasks were completed.
- The deceased showed an inner contentment and acceptance—she or he was ready to die.
- All that could be done medically and spiritually was done.

It is in these very important aspects of the death environment that the hospice program is so invaluable. The experiences which become the last weeks or months of the patient's life can often be guided to a positive and rewarding conclusion.

Religious Factors

People are not usually very far away from questions of faith, religion, or the meaning of life. The hospice interdisciplinary team should make every effort to keep the dialogue between patients and their minister, priest, or rabbi open and productive. Individual team members should not be afraid, however, to consider spiritual questions with patients and their families. It may be very helpful for the nurse, for example, to listen carefully to his or her patient's religious questions, doubts, fears, and beliefs. Such listening may in fact be the most helpful part of spiritual counseling. A woman was once asked what she would like most from the hospice team members. Her response was, "someone who looks like they are trying to understand what I believe" (anonymous, 1979). It is important to note that she did not ask that someone have all the necessary expertise to answer all the questions she had, or even arrive at an understanding of her beliefs. She really just wanted someone who would *try*.

AREAS OF RELIGIOUS CONCERN

It is helpful, when one is asked to share in a discussion of spiritual issues, to have some understanding of the issues with which people may be dealing. Clergy are quite familiar with the concerns about which, almost universally, people want to speak. The patient and family may have the greatest confidence in their pastor, priest, or rabbi because of his or her education and statement of faith and the position she or he represents in relation to what that person considers holy. This may be true even if such a relationship has existed at no other time between the individual and the clergy.

Paul Puyser (1976) has outlined areas of belief about which both dying patients and bereaved families might question hospice team members. These areas include the person's view of (1) what is sacred; (2) providence, or divine will; (3) faith; (4) grace, or forgiveness; (5) repentance; (6) communion, or sharing; and (7) the purpose of life.

What is Sacred

A person may hold certain things sacred, or holy. Whatever it is that the person regards as sacred should be accepted and openly discussed. The degree to which people are in touch with what is held sacred will often determine their anxiety about it. If that which is revered is loved and loves or is approachable in return, people will often find joy in the belief. It may for example be helpful to share with them your attempt to understand their version of what is sacred. If that which is sacred is feared, denied, or has proven itself unworthy of respect, people may seriously doubt everything. This may well occur when a life is being "taken away." They may turn to others for reassurance, in doubt or disillusionment. They may be searching for options in which to believe (Puyser, 1976).

Providence, or Divine Will

Those who are experiencing tragedy or loss often wonder about the intention of the divine being toward them (Puyser, 1976). They want to discuss how others regard the will of their God. They question whether that will is one of benevolence and love or vindictiveness and anger. Whether or not this will is trusted or accepted will determine to what extent the person trusts and accepts what is happening in his or her life (Baker, 1975). Whatever people believe about a divine purpose either within themselves or through a divine being, the trust and security they feel in the hospice team members can greatly increase their ability to retain hope in a life or death with meaning.

Faith

The way people understand and relate to that which they consider holy is often expressed as faith (Puyser, 1976). If faith is strong, the person may derive from it a sense of hope and comfort. If the person has not experienced faith, there may or may not be an anxiety over that which never was. Perhaps the greatest discomfort is caused in those who once had faith and have lost it or who feel somehow that they should have more faith than they do. They may feel guilty, betrayed, or both. Still others who have always expressed, and still express, a deep faith may be shaken or angry if that faith provides less comfort than they think it should. Allowing people to explore past feelings and events that have affected their faith and to openly discuss faith may (1) reinforce and comfort those of strong faith, (2) decrease anxiety in those who are searching and uncomfortable, and (3) remind some that faith has continued through other bad times (Saunders, 1981).

Grace, or Forgiveness

People who believe in a divine being or purpose may have beliefs about their need to be forgiven for not having always followed that purpose. The way they respond to such perceived guilt is based to some extent on the degree to which they believe in grace, or forgiveness (Puyser, 1976).

What the individual who seeks forgiveness may wish for is a blessing from someone of the clergy. It is seldom possible for a layperson to reassure another of the presence of grace and the gift of their God's forgiveness. This blessing may require also the taking of sacraments. Real peace of mind will come through the priest, minister, or rabbi who brings these sacraments and confirms the mercy and acceptance of the person's repentance.

The hospice team member who is asked by a dying person to hear his or her sins can contribute, however, to the person's peace of mind by being kind, patient, and nonjudgmental. The team member who does not convey a sense of shock or condemnation will have a positive effect on that person's self-image and his or her courage to live or die in peace.

Repentance

People who are suffering from a loss frequently feel the need to repent. They may be sorry for what they have done in the past and simply want to live differently in the future, or they may want to work out some form of restitution for wrongs committed. Telling about or admitting the source of perceived wrongdoing may be enough (Puyser, 1976). Or people may want to do things that the team member can help them complete. This may mean speaking to or writing to someone, in a patient's behalf, or paying back a debt. Helping set realistic goals for reconciliation or repayment and then fulfilling them can be very important in restoring satisfying relationships with friends, family, and the religious community or being in which they believe.

Communion, or Sharing

The sense of communion many people long for has a great deal to do with being cared for and being a part of all humankind and a caring universe. The positive side of this is seen in the person who draws strength from this kinship; the negative may be seen in those who feel alienated or isolated by their grief (Puyser, 1976). Some people may feel singled out for trouble, and the experience needs to be worked through with someone who can, by listening, reaffirm a person's belief that she or he is not on the outside of everything. It is extraordinary how effective the whole hospice community is at fulfilling the role of the caring society and restoring faith in humanity through its simple concern with each individual's needs.

The Purpose of Life

Those who are very ill and their families may find it almost impossible to find any purpose in life. Whether they believe that such purpose comes from an ordered universe or a divine being or is within each person's striving to do each given task as well as she or he can, there is little visible evidence that life is worthwhile when grief is deep. The team member can be very helpful in restoring the person's confidence in old purposes and encouraging the development of new ones when the grief is again manageable.

Meeting patients on their spiritual ground takes courage. Patients often feel that no one will face directly and nonjudgmentally the questions they want, but fear, to ask. Often the person who succeeds in being of real help is the one who comes to this meeting openly, without set patterns of religious response. Such people's compassionate attempt to share feelings and struggle with difficult concepts may be most valued because they are just being themselves.

THE CHILD AND BEREAVEMENT

When someone close to the family dies, parents commonly are uncertain of the role that children should play in the period of bereavement and particularly in any cultural or religious services. It is important that a child of any age receive the supportive, empathic concern necessary to including him or her in the event. The questions asked should be honestly answered. Attention to the needs of the child should be regular and consistent (Barnes, M.J., 1978).

It is important to understand what children, considering their degree of maturity and past experience, do understand. Stories, music, art, and games can all be used to help reveal the range of knowledge and emotions held by the child. Suspicion, guilt, fears for their own death, and a host of other unanswered and incomprehensible questions may surface, if they exist, so that they can be worked through. Almost without exception, children should not be "sent to a distant relative" or shuffled off to their own rooms each time the topic of either impending death or recent death is to be discussed. To whatever extent children are included in the family structure and sharing, they will be comforted and more secure. If there is no such family security, the counselor should attempt to construct an outlet for questions and a support system of concern.

Lies should not be told. To say "She has gone far away" or "he is lost to us" or "She is asleep" can eventually create fantasies and misconceptions far more painful. One hears pitiful little stories; for example, a young boy fought desperately to stay awake each night as a reaction to being told that a little cousin had "gone to sleep forever." One father tells of his daughter, Stacy, coming home and joyfully announcing after her first day in kindergarten that she had *"found* Betsy"—the first child whose death the parents had always explained by saying "we lost Betsy when she was only a few days old."

Children are sometimes kept away from religious and cultural services. While any child's reluctance to participate should be honored, even young children should have an explanation of the purpose and meaning of any service, and should know that they will be included if it is their wish. Irene Moriarty explains the possible need for a child to be involved in family traditions in the following way.

She concludes that the children in the family each had a relationship with the deceased and will feel the loss and separation. These feelings of loss and separation will be reinforced if children are excluded from sharing this significant family experience. Attending the service dispels some of the mystery and superstition with which children surround death. If excluded children may allow their vivid imaginations to create troublesome pictures of what has happened. By attending the services, the children gain the support of the extended family and friends. Older children may want to invite their own friends and school mates to create their own support system at the services.*

While such services, rituals, and family traditions may be painful confrontations with the reality of death, it is in that confrontation that their healing power lies. Children should not be excluded, even if they are limited in understanding, from this potentially honest and supportive experience.

RECOGNIZING ABNORMAL GRIEF REACTIONS

Grief can be abnormal, either by the absence of any overt mourning or by the distortion or exaggerated intensity of mourning. It is important to note that there is a tremendous range in individual reactions. An evaluation of a person's reaction must always take into account the person's personality and past behavior. One man's "alarming disappearance" may be another man's "fishing trip" each time the pressure is great and he wants time alone to think.

---

*Moriarty, I. Sudden death: Pastoral presence with the bereaved. *Journal of Pastoral Counseling,* 1980, *18,* 45.

A *wide* departure, however, from what is both individually representative and generally acknowledged as common response is reason to request immediate specialized counseling support.

Lindemann (1944) classified "abnormal" grief as either (1) a delay or absence of normal grief reactions or (2) distorted grief reactions. In the latter category Lindemann included a number of behaviors that, when carried to an extreme, are abnormal. If some of these seem familiar it is because they are distorted versions of those less intense and normal grief reactions listed in the preceding section. Individuals may be involved in constant activity without recognition of the loss they have experienced. They may mimic symptoms seen in the final period of the deceased's illness, or develop a psychosomatic illness. There may be social isolation lasting for several years. Others may become hostile toward anyone connected with the care of the dying person by laying blame or finding unreasoning fault. Some maintain stoic or controlled formality overlying a hostility that occasionally surfaces. Particularly disturbing are those who begin patterns of irresponsible and self-destructive actions, such as giving away one's home and personal effects, spending savings, or taking on a destructive relationship. Finally there may be insomnia, anorexia, or a depression marked with despair, feelings of worthlessness and selfchastisement. Lindemann emphasizes that if a suicide threat is stated, it should be taken seriously.

In his study of unresolved grief, A. Lazare (1979) outlines many social and psychological reasons why people fail to grieve at the time of death. For example, the death may have occurred through drugs, suicide, or recklessness and be hidden from the public. Or occasionally it is not known for sure that a person is dead and so the grief remains unresolved. Such grief remains buried for months or years, and then sometimes appears later in a distorted form. Let us look at some of the reasons that are applicable to the situation of the person with terminal illness.

Reaction to Loss Removed in Time or Space

As our society travels more, and as families and friends live at greater distances from one another, people are more often removed from the actual time and place of death. Thus there are fewer actual support systems for an individual who sustains a loss. Word of a death comes by wire—by a phone call—sometimes even through an incidental story. Often it is only after the death has occurred that someone learns that there was ever a life-threatening situation. The distance and expense may be too great for everyone to gather for a service or final memorial.

In the short story, "The Agreement" (see Appendix 10-1), a young teenager writes of such displacement and of the disjointedness of the modern family's time of grief.

Reaction Conditioned By Need to "Stay Strong"

At the time of a death, many responsibilities are imposed on a family. Most immediately there are calls to inform others, medical releases, funeral arrangements. Later there may be a will, a house to close, possessions to be sold. There is often one person who is implicitly or explicitly regarded as "the strong one" who makes most of the decisions and who cannot "fall apart." This person may be denied the opportunity to grieve because of the role she or he must play in helping everyone else.

Reaction Conditioned By Individual Psychological Factors

People have a multitude of mindsets, predispositions, and psychological problems that either delay or distort grief. Even though such factors may cause almost impossible problems for the person, they are uniquely human and not too difficult to empathize with. For example, the bereaved may have regarded the lost person as a part of themselves. Admitting the death would be losing a part of oneself. Or, the bereaved may have strong negative feelings that they are afraid to confront in the way grieving would demand. Sometimes people fear that admitting grief would bring back another earlier loss that is unresolved.

THE HOSPICE BEREAVEMENT PROGRAM

One of the finest aspects of total hospice care is the bereavement service provided to the family and/or those who have been responsible for care after the death of the patient (this service, when explained to the patient, can also bring him or her a great deal of peace of mind). The Standards of Care advise that this service should be available to the bereaved for a period of one year after the patient's death or until it is evident that such help is no longer needed or wanted. The hospice bereavement program is unique in that it reaches out to the family unit after all the medical teams, visitors, relatives, and others have withdrawn.

Working with the bereaved is a challenging, sometimes frustrating, yet often rewarding task. Table 10-3 lists some characteristics needed by the person who takes the responsibility of helping someone through the grief process. Figure 10-1 offers a very valuable set of do's and don'ts, entitled "A Decalogue for the Concerned Caregiver."

Some bereavement services can be carried out through a regularly scheduled meeting for those close to the deceased. Such support groups can provide an opportunity for peer group association, for listening, and for sharing memories, experiences during the illness, and many other normal

Figure 10-1. A decalogue for the concerned caregiver.*

DO NOT

1. Avoid the subject of personal death in your discussions. The mental health of us all is not the denial of tragedy but the frank acknowledgment of painful separation.

2. Wait for the occurrence of death by not preparing for that inevitable moment in life. Encourage others to plan for the necessary details of funeral director, cemetary, wills, insurance, organ transplantation. And formulate your own plans as well.

3. Discourage the emotions of grief. Anger, tears, guilt, despair, and protest are natural reactions to family disorganization. Never be so cold to human feelings that you do not accept the emotional reactions of those who hurt.

4. Close the door to doubt, questioning, and differences of opinion. Respect the other's unique personality for in the long run it is he or she who must discern the meanings to the questions of life and death.

5. Tell a person (especially a child) what he or she will later need to unlearn. Avoid fairy tales, half-truths, and circumlocutions. Honesty is the only policy. The word "truth" in Judaism is *Emet.* containing the first, middle, and last letters of the alphabet.

DO

6. Share (but not legislate) your religious convictions as to *faith, God, immortality, prayer, life,* and *death.* But have more concern for the welfare of the bereaved than for the "protection" of religious institutions.

7. Spend time with responsive listening to the needs of the mourners. The dedicated caregiver is a perceptive listener to the spoken word and an astute discoverer of the nonverbal communication.

8. Make referrals to other supportive people. There are times when even the best-informed and well-intentioned are simply inadequate. Seeking further help from a therapist is not an admission of weakness but a demonstration of strength and love.

9. Remember that the process of adjustment to death is longer than the funeral. The height of depression is six months after death! Make frequent visitations and encourage when possible widow-to-widower programs.

10. Be human. It is not wrong to express your own emotions of grief...to shed a tear...to physically and spiritually touch a person in pain. Regardless of theology employed, emotional tones are transmitted. Just remember the words of Thornton Wilder: "There is a land of the living and of the dead and the bridge is *love*—the only survival, the only meaning."

*From Grollman, Rabbi E.A., *A Practical Guide for the Living:* Boston, Beacon Press, 1974.

Table 10-3. *Skills of the Bereavement Counselor*

Listening conscientiously

Accepting the discomfort of the person in pain

Tolerating both progress and regression in the bereaved

Accepting nonjudgmentally the perceptions and beliefs of the bereaved
Staying in the situation constructively and maintaining interest even when the process
is slow

feelings which are held in common. Such a regular assemblage also provides a
forum for the expression of appreciation to the hospice program at a time
when it can be most important to those who feel they have been on the
receiving end for months.

One bereavement counselor also points out the need for socializing
within these or special-event groups. Those bereaved who have, in addition to
the personal loss, also lost a social partner may have almost no (acceptable to
them) social life left. The parties, picnics, or holiday celebrations can be
genuinely fun and thus provide affirmation that it is okay to laugh again.
Hopefully the hospice social gathering will become a stepping stone back into
an individual social life.

There may also be a need to provide help to the bereaved about legal and
financial matters. When the deceased has been the one who generally
managed such matters, the new responsibility can be devastating. Details of
Medicare, inheritance taxes, property transfers and sales, wills, lock boxes
and Social Security are a few of the problems of survivorship that without
advice can be confusing—particularly coming on the eve of such sadness (see
Chapter 11).

Determining the Needs of the Bereaved

Bereavement support should be, without qualification, available to all
hospice families. It is a mistake to assume that persons who have carried
through nobly in patient care will do the same now for themselves. And some
families may not verbalize a need for comfort because they feel "the hospice
has already helped so much." An initial assessment can be made by the nurse,
counselor, chaplain, or trained volunteer who has been particularly close to
the bereaved. A report or form can be filled out confidentially by this
professional as a means of screening for potential problems and alerting the
hospice to a person's needs. Most hospices prefer not to submit the family to
questioning regarding their feelings at this point.

The following groups of people were found by a study at St. Christopher's (Parkes, 1978) to be at special risk during bereavement:

Table 10-4. *Areas of Inquiry in Assessing Need for Bereavement Counseling*

- Key person or persons to receive bereavement support—their relationship to patient
- Desire of bereaved for support and/or counseling
- Help that is already available
- Description of the family unit; is it supportive?
- Financial condition
- Activities and employment
- Health status
- Level of grief, anger, guilt; significant reactions
- Social outlets
- A subjective evaluation of how the bereaved will cope

- People of low socioeconomic status
- Housewives or those without employment outside the home
- Those with young children at home (who may themselves be at risk)
- Those without a supportive family or with a family who actively discourage the expression of grief
- Those who showed a strong tendency to cling to the patient before his or her death and/or to pine intensely for the patient afterwards
- Those who express strong feelings of anger or bitterness before or after the patient's death
- Those who express strong feelings of self-reproach

Families with a history of psychiatric illness or suicidal tendencies should also be carefully followed. Assessment forms are available from many community hospice programs or can be developed to fit local needs and resources. Many of the forms include the areas of information about the bereaved listed in Table 10-4.

Bereavement Visits

First visits to the bereaved should be unpressured and reassuring. They should not convey the attitude of a research project on grief, or the implication that the bereaved is expected to behave in a certain way. If the counselor is part of a bereavement team and not known to the family, time for the family to develop trust should be allowed. Even though a new relationship must be developed when the bereavement team–specialist is used, there are certain advantages: (1) the patient–family load does not fall on the care team; (2) a bereavement counselor may have special skills, understanding, and experience to guide him or her; (3) a person designated to provide bereavement support can more consistently view this as a primary responsibility; (4) some families have difficulty "letting down" in front of the care professionals and volunteers who were so dedicated and competent.

It is important for the bereaved to understand that time alone will not heal grief. They have to deal with it, to work it through. The health care professional can encourage the mourner to accept help during this time by emphasizing the normalcy of using a person trained and experienced in grief and bereavement. The bereaved may need to hear that it is a sound and healthy decision, not a psychotic one, to use a trained counselor to help resolve the anger, guilt, or despair that often accompanies a deep loss.

Also, the consoler and counselor can recommend reading resources. Many people find relief in the recognition that their feelings are shared by many who mourn. There are many excellent books but some of the most useful are listed in the reference list at the end of the chapter. In addition, many people find helpful the handout, reproduced in Figure 10-2, that the Royal Victorial Hospital Palliative Care Unit routinely gives to close family members or friends after the death of a patient.

At some point, perhaps after six or nine months, the intensity of grief may diminish. It becomes important for the counselor to help the bereaved formulate new goals and establish a fulfilling social life. The person may actually need permission to stop grieving. Traditional rituals and memorials at the one-year anniversary also serve the function of calling an acceptable closure to bereavement.

Occasionally people will use their loss as a way of withdrawing permanently from life. This is particularly likely in those who have always lacked confidence and have never had a circle of friends or fulfilling work. They may have been in the mainstream of life only as a partner to the deceased. With that incentive gone, there is nothing to encourage them. The counselor, cold as it may seem, will need to make continuing support conditional upon the person moving toward the accomplishment of realistic and mutually developed goals.

Getting Back Into Life

People may say they are "fine" before they have actually resolved their grief. After a certain amount of time they may feel that they ought to shape up, or they may want to please others who are concerned. A number of factors can be used to measure the extent to which an individual is resuming patterns of everyday life. It is important to consider the person's past patterns in comparisons of his or her present behavior.

In addition to hospice staff there are organizations associated with churches, community centers, hospitals and other caring agencies that provide continuing group support for the bereaved. A local listing of such groups should be provided to each family-mourner. An initial contact might also be made, if the bereaved wishes it to be done.

Figure 10-2. Dealing with grief*

This checklist highlights a few important matters to consider during bereavement. Each person is different, so beware of readymade solutions. The following are suggestions to consider—they may or may not fit your situation.

These suggestions may be considered under the headings: Psychological, Physical, Social, Economic, and Spiritual.

Psychological

Everyone needs some help—don't be afraid to accept it.

Although you may feel pressured to put on a brave front, it is important to make your needs known by expressing your feelings to those you trust.

Often numbness sees us through the first few days or weeks. Don't be too surprised if a letdown comes later.

Many people are more emotionally upset during bereavement than at any other time in their lives and are frightened by this. Be aware that severe upset is not unusual and if you are alarmed, seek a professional opinion.

Whether you feel you need to be alone or accompanied—make it known. Needing company is common and does *not* mean you will *always* be dependent on it.

There is no set time limit for grieving. It varies from person to person, depending on individual circumstances.

Physical

It is easy to neglect yourself because you don't much care at a time of grief.

You are under great stress and may be more susceptible to disease.

It is especially important not to neglect your health.

Try to eat reasonably even if there is no enjoyment in it.

Although sleep may be disturbed, try to get adequate rest.

If you have symptoms, get a doctor to check them out.

If people urge you to see your doctor, do so even if it doesn't make sense to you at the time.

Social

Friends and family are often most available early in bereavement and less so later. It is important to be able to reach out to them when you need them. Don't wait for them to guess your needs. They will often guess incorrectly and too late.

During a period of grief it can be difficult to judge new relationships. Don't be afraid of them, yet it is usually wise not to rush into them.

Someone who is not too close to you but who is willing to listen may be particularly helpful.

No one will substitute for your loss. Try to enjoy people as they are. Do not avoid social contacts because of the imperfections in those you meet.

Figure 10-2 (continued)

Sometimes, in an effort to stop the pain of grief, people turn toward replacing the lost person (e.g., adoption of a child, remarriage) too soon. It is hard, though to see new relationships objectively if you are still actively grieving, and this kind of solution may only lead to other problems.

Try to make clear to children that sadness is perfectly normal and that neither theirs nor yours need be hidden. It is important that periods of happiness be enjoyed and not cause guilty feelings.

Economic

Avoid hasty decisions. Try not to make major life decisions within the first year unless absolutely necessary.

In general, most people find it best to remain settled in familiar surroundings until they can consider their future calmly.

Don't be afraid to seek good advice. Usually it is wise to get more than one opinion before making decisions.

Don't make any major financial decisions without talking them over with experts.

Having a job or doing voluntary work in the community can be helpful when you are ready but it is important not to overextend yourself.

A job will not fulfill all your needs and you should not turn to excessive involvement in work. Relationships with family and friends should not be sacrificed in an effort to keep busy.

Spiritual

Personal faith is frequently a major source of comfort during bereavement.

For some, however, maintaining faith may be difficult during this period of loss.

Either reaction may occur, and both are consistent with later spiritual growth.

*Adapted from Mount, B. and Ajemian, I. *The Royal Victoria Palliative Care Unit Manual*. New York: Arno Press, 1980. With permission.

In conclusion, bereavement counselors must be aware that not all of those they set out to help will work through their bereavement normally. Some will do quite well with little help. A few will flatly refuse the support. Others will turn to a friend outside the hospice team or cling dependently to the primary care nurse or physician.

Yet no family should be left unapproached, and a continuing offer of support should be kept easily accessible to families for a year. The scenario can change: a last child moves away, a job is lost, an illness occurs. Suddenly the formerly well-coping bereaved may be overcome again by accumulating losses. Some checking back periodically should be conscientiously done even with families no longer in an active support stage.

REFERENCES

Baker, J.A. *Why should this happen to me?* Address given at St. Christopher's Hospice, London, England, 1975.

Barnes, M.J. The reactions of children and adolescents to the death of a parent or sibling in Sahler, O.J.Z. (Ed.), *The Child and Death,* St. Louis: C.V. Mosby, 1978, pp. 185–201.

Burton, R. in Parkes, C.M. The first year of bereavement. *Psychiatry,* Washington, D.C., *334,* 1970, 444–467.

Farmer, P.J. Bereavement Counseling. *The Journal of Pastoral Counseling,* 1980, *15,* 32.

Grollman, E. A dialogue for the concerned caregiver, in Concerning Death: A Practical Guide for the Living, Boston, Beacon Press, 1974.

Jackson, E.N. *When Someone Dies,* Philadelphia: Fortress Press, 1971, p. 12.

Kreis, B., & Pattie, A. *Up from grief.* New York: Seabury Press, 1969.

Kübler-Ross, E. *On death and dying.* New York: The Macmillan Co., 1969.

Lazare, A. Unresolved grief in Lazare, A. (Ed.), *Outpatient Psychiatry: Diagnosis and Treatment.* Baltimore: Williams and Wilkins, 1979, 498–512.

Lindemann, E. Symptomatology and management of acute grief. *The American Journal of Psychiatry,* 1944, *101,* pp. 141–148.

Moriarty, I. Sudden death: Pastoral presence with the bereaved. *Journal of Pastoral Counseling,* 1980, *18,* pp. 41–49.

Mount, B., & Ajemian, I. *The Royal Victoria Hospital Manual on Palliative Hospice Care.* New York: Arno Press, 1980.

Parkes, C. Effects of bereavement on physical and mental health—A study of the medical records of widows. *British Medical Journal,* 1964, *11,* 275–79.

Parkes, C. The first year of bereavement. *Psychiatry,* 1970, *33,* 444–467.

Parkes, C.M. *Bereavement studies of grief in adult life.* New York: International Universities Press, Inc., 1972.

Parkes, C.M. Psychological aspects. In C.M. Saunders (Ed.), *The management of terminal disease,* London: E. Arnold, 1978.

Pruyser, P. *The personal problems in pastoral perspective: The minister as diagnostician.* Philadelphia: Westminster Press, 1976.

Rando, T.A. Concepts of death, dying, grief and loss. Project Dir. Henry, M.D. In *Hospice Education Program for Nurses.* DHHS-HRA81-27. Washington, D.C.: Department of Health and Human Services, 1981.

Rees, W.D. and Lutkins, S.G., Mortality of Bereavement. *British Medical Journal,* 1967, *4,* 13–16.

Rogers, W. The pastor's work with grief. *Pastoral Psychology,* 1963, *14,* 16–26.

Saunders, C.M. The moment of truth: Care of the dying patient. In *Hospice Education Program for Nurses.* Project Director Henry, M.D. DHHS-HRA81-27. Washington, D.C.: Department of Health and Human Services, 1981.

Schwab, J.J. *Grief: Therapeutic interventions.* Paper presented at Kent School of Social Work Conference on Death and Grief, Louisville, Kentucky, April 1, 1976.

Shoor, M., & Speed, M.H. Death, delinquency and the mourning process. In R. Fulton (Ed.), *Death and identity,* 1972.

Westberg, G. *Good grief.* Rock Island, Ill.: Augustana Press, 1962.

1. *T*	6. *T*
2. *F*	7. *F*
3. *F*	8. *F*
4. *F*	9. *F*
5. *T*	10. *T*

Appendix 10-1   The Agreement

"Hello, Michael?"

"Dad, is that you?" Michael picked up the phone and carried it into the living room. Smiling, he continued, "Hi Dad! I'm glad you called; it's been a long time. How is everything?"

"Mike, I'm afraid I have some bad news."

"Grandpa—" Michael broke off suddenly, realizing what had happened.

"The funeral will be in a few days. I'll call you once it's over. Would you like me to put your name on the flowers with mine?"

The thousand miles between them was greater now than ever. It seemed to Michael that he might as well be listening to a story about different people in another time. This should upset me, he thought to himself repeatedly, but the whole situation seemed too distant to deal with.

"Michael?" His father began the conversation. "Hey, Mike are you okay?"

"Uh, yeah, I'm fine. Listen, anything you want to do with the flowers and stuff is fine with me. Call and tell me how everything went, okay?"

"Mike, I know how rough this must be for you, I realize that you and Grandpa were really close, and I'm awfully sorry you can't be here."

"Yeah, I'm sorry too, Dad. Is Grandma okay? Tell her I'm sorry and I still really love her."

"Alright. Are you sure you'll be okay?"

"Yeah. I'm fine. I'm really sorry. "Bye, Dad."

Michael put down the receiver slowly and sat on the couch, looking at his reflection in the coffee table top. He sighed deeply and put his head in his hands, but no tears came to his eyes. There were more than a thousand miles between him and his grandparents. He couldn't even begin to understand what had happened. Because he had never had an older brother, and his father had always been on business trips, Michael's grandfather was the one to take him fishing, camping, and all the other activities fathers have an unspoken responsibility to do. His grandpa was always the first one to notice if something was bothering him. And, like a brother, the first one to tease him, about a girl or anything else Michael happened to be making a fuss over at the time. When Michael was to move from his home in Boston to a new one in Los Angeles when his parents were divorced, he had felt sorrow at leaving his friends and father, but not so much as he had at leaving Grandpa. Now Grandpa was gone forever, and all Michael could feel was a kind of guilt for not being there.

Outside the rain had stopped and the sun was drying the sidewalk. Michael could hear several of his friends shouting for him to join them in a pick-up game of baseball at the schoolyard. Taking a deep breath, he stood up and leaned out the window. He called out to them, "I'll be there in a minute—after I get my stuff. Meet me there." He turned to reach for his equipment as his mother called down the stairs to him.

"Michael, who was that on the phone?"

"Uh, that was Dad. Grandpa didn't pull through the operation. He's dead. Is it okay if I go play ball up at school? I'll be home by six for dinner."

"Michael—" his mother came running down the stairs.

He turned away not wanting to face her and pretend to be upset. More than anything, Michael just wanted to get out of the house and into the sun. There was nothing here, a thousand miles from home.

"Michael, Honey, I'm really sorry. I know you and Grandpa were very close."

He touched his mother's shoulder in a comforting way, as though she had suffered the loss. "It's okay, Dad and I talked for awhile, and I feel better now."

"Are you sure? Is there anything I can do?"

"I'm sure. Where's my bat?"

"Your bat? You don't have a baseball bat here."

"Sure I do. Grandpa and I play all the time. What do you think I hit the stupid ball with, my hand?" he snapped impatiently.

"Michael, that was Grandpa's bat. Don't you remember the agreement? He bought it on the condition that you'd play with him once in a while. You two used to play three or four times a week. He was the one primarily responsible for making you the best shortstop in the league, you know."

"What do you mean it's not my bat? That's a stupid agreement." Michael's controlled attitude had turned to rage as quickly as the news of his grandpa's death had come.

"Michael, you left it purposely, promising you'd always be back to play with him."

With increased anger Michael shouted, "Why didn't you remind me to bring it? You knew I'd find a place to play with it out here. Now it's all the way across the country, just sitting there. Why did you let him keep it? How am I supposed to play? I might as well just forget it! It's too late now anyway!"

"Michael, someone else will have a bat," she offered.

Now almost in tears, Michael had completely lost control of himself. "No! I want that one. Nothing else will work, and I can't exactly go back and get it, can I!"

Michael stood trembling, tears streaming down his face. He let his glove fall to the ground as he leaned against the wall, slowly sliding down and sinking his head into his hands. He looked up and said with genuine understanding, "I can't go back and get it from him, can I?" Silently, his mother knelt down and held him gently as if in protection from the reality that had wrapped itself about the boy and was draining him of spirit.

by Lynnell Major

11

Social Decisions and Social Support

Answer the following questions True (T) or False (F). Answers appear on the last page of this chapter.

1. *Hospice patients do not want to be bothered with financial matters.*

2. *There is plenty of time after the death to think about funeral preparations.*

3. *An executor has the power to distribute an individual's estate if there is no will.*

4. *Funeral services function in many valuable support ways.*

5. *Life insurance benefits are available to a surviving spouse only if the policy premium is paid in full.*

6. *The hospice staff and volunteers can best function to provide social support to a family when other friends and relatives do not retain much responsibility.*

7. *Informal social support can come from a variety of areas, including neighborhood, workplace, and church or synagogue.*

8. *One way to support those who need to build their self-esteem is to ask their opinion and then listen carefully to their ideas.*

9. *Very practical tangible help like food or transportation cannot be as supportive as counseling or personal help.*

10. *The hospice staff should include informal support-group persons among those to whom they give positive feedback about roles and responsibilities.*

Tranquil talk was better than any medicine; Gradually the feelings came back to my numbed heart.*

T HE DYING patient tends to make fewer and fewer social decisions. There are reasons for this. The patient may feel the weakness and passivity created by disease, drugs, or emotional pressures. She or he may be physically isolated by confinement to bed, chair, or dwelling. Informational isolation may come from a desire on the part of caregivers, family, or friends not "to bother" or not to include the person in "trivial" matters when she or he is under other more obvious pressures of illness or pain. Or it may be that social decisions and planning that imply a future without the dying person are simply too hard, too painful to bring up.

A great deal can be done to minimize the anxiety aroused by the confusing legal and financial matters that often must be dealt with after a loved one's death. It is particularly important that mates, business partners, or others who share financial holdings or legal contracts discuss, while both are in reasonably good health, the actions that must be taken on such matters at the death of one (or both), person(s). Such pre-death arrangements reassure the survivors that the wishes of the deceased were at least heard and understood. The survivor understands what the deceased had planned, is educated as to the nature of resources and/or liabilities, and thus has to make fewer unexpected or uninformed decisions.

KEY SOCIAL DECISIONS

In the midst of the emotional pain and fatigue of caring for a loved one who is dying, the family must deal with a number of practical matters. Some measure of relief from the personal pain, however, for both the patient and the

---

*Po Chu-I. *Ninth Century Chinese Poems.* London: George Allen and Unwin, 1946.

caregivers, may derive from "setting things in order." A dying person often feels relief in knowing that his or her legal, social, and financial concerns are being resolved.

Any number of people can help in this area including social workers, accountants, or family financial or legal counsel. The nurse should be supportive in coordinating these services so that the patient and family can conveniently arrange such affairs as the will and estate, funeral arrangements and burial plans, and survivors' financial resources.

Will, Executor, and Estate

Unless there are special extenuating circumstances, everyone should have a will. When people die without a will (referred to as dying *intestate*), their property is distributed according to the laws of the state in which they have resided. Such laws, which tend to divide property among close heirs and by a set formula, are often entirely inappropriate and not at all what the deceased would have prearranged.

Thus a will, prepared when a person is capable of making such choices, is the best way to assure that property will be distributed as she or he wishes, with few exceptions. (Some states limit gifts to charities and have varying rights for the benefit of a surviving spouse.)

At the time the will is written, an *executor* is named as the person who will administer the estate. The executor is often a person held in high regard by the decedent whose duties include collecting the decedent's assets, paying expenses and debts, settling estate taxes, and generally assuring that the estate is distributed according to the terms of the will. If no such person has been named by the deceased, an administrator is designated by the court. The authorities of such an administrator are fixed by statute (Ross, 1974).

Distribution of the estate may be directed through a will in a variety of ways. Unless an estate consists only of very limited and simple resources, the will should be prepared by someone—an attorney or financial advisor, for example—with proper training and experience. With proper counsel, it is possible to minimize the hazards of improper or untimely distribution and decrease federal estate taxes and the inheritance tax applicable in most states. Trusts, joint holdings, gifts, and marital deductions can sometimes be used to lower the tax burden (Ross, 1974).

Funeral and Burial Arrangements

Funerals can accomplish some healthy and positive results:

- Survivors are enabled to reflect on the good and meaningfulness of a person's life.

- Caring people can draw together as a resource and strength for one another in time of grief.
- Organized purposeful activity can be a tribute or memorial.
- In a setting that encourages full attention to mourning but reaches a conclusion survivors can give expression to their grief and then begin to move on to a time of healing.

The benefits of funerals have been recognized throughout history. There is evidence that the Neanderthal, over 60,000 years ago, buried their tribal members with flowers. Over the centuries, the Chinese have left small colored prayer papers on the marked graves, and the Indians cremate the dead in ceremonies of honor. Early Hebrew religions and ethical concepts have become the basis of much Western burial practice (Raether, 1974).

Too often funerals are arranged within hours of death. In such instances the sound advice of good friends, reputable funeral directors, or consultants is most necessary. With guidance and encouragement from a hospice team member, however, some, if not all, of the funeral and burial plans can be assumed by the family itself. The wishes of the dying person can then be known—not just inferred from past remarks.

A family, acting with the best intentions, once buried its grandfather in full military uniform, under a marker outlining his World War I service record. They did this based on someone's memory of his remark about the dignity of the televised funeral of a head-of-state. A great deal of regret and anguish resulted some months later when family members uncovered a diary kept by the old man in which he recounted his grief and guilt over having participated in a war and his desire never to be remembered for that part of his life.

In many situations hospice teams have supported families in their planning of the way the patient is to be honored and remembered, to the great satisfaction of all involved. In some cases, a patient has written a special message of thanks to be read or a song to be played or has selected personally significant readings and music. Far more often than when the dying person is not involved, a service so planned is a true celebration of the person's life (Raether, 1974).

Whether the patient wishes to be involved in the planning or not, arrangements considered in advance of the death are often more moderate in cost. There is less chance that families will buy more expensive caskets and services than they can actually afford or make choices with which they are later dissatisfied. the temptation to make purchases emotionally, out of a desire to do "the best" or to make up for unspoken apologies or love, can be more productively channeled into other expressions of concern.

The stable family supported by a hospice team member who is knowledgeable in funeral planning can work with a funeral director and/or the family spiritual advisor to make necessary arrangements (see Table 11-1).

Table 11-1. *Some Necessary Funeral and Burial Arrangements*

- Removal of the body to the funeral home
- Filing of death certificate and burial permit
- Selection and purchase of burial site and casket or urn, or donation of body to science
- Selection of place, time, and format of service
- Details such as flowers, transportation, music, guest book, notes of appreciation
- Filing of claims for Social Security, Veterans or Union benefits and insurance
- Direction in selecting a memorial marker

Families are permitted certain choices that they do not always know about. It is *not* required by law in all states that a body be embalmed, buried in a vault a well as a casket, and placed in a designated cemetery.* The choices of whether to view the body and of the number of days that may elapse before burial are also to be made by each family. The important issues are whether the service suits the financial, cultural, ethnic, and spiritual preferences of the family.

Thoughtful counsel may also forestall choices that may later be regretted. For example, what at the moment suits the financial, cultural, ethnic, and spiritual preferences of the family may seem to be a warm or whimsical tribute or memorial inscription may prove over time to be less than tasteful (Winters, 1975).

Survivors' Life Responsibilities and Income

Advice should be obtained regarding the dying person's business affairs. If the person has been employed, it is important to find out if she or he is entitled to a pension or life insurance benefits that can now be directed to the beneficiary. Someone needs to talk to the employer for an explanation of company policy.

A dying person who has owned his or her own business should be included in the consideration of what is to be done with the business after death. If there has been a partner in the business, the dying partner may have a contractual arrangement with him or her that needs to be discussed or, as pointed out earlier, together they may need to outline an arrangement. Considerations may include the survivors' right to purchase the deceased partner's interest, the rights of the surviving spouse, or the need for liquidation (Ross, 1974).

---

*Specific state regulations should be checked.

If at all possible, it is wise for the dying person and survivors to select an advisor who is mutually trusted and respected. Decisions about sales, leases, or rentals should be formulated slowly and responsibly rather than out of the fear the survivor sometimes feels in those first months alone. The truth of the old adage, "Act in haste, repent at leisure," is too often confirmed. A careful assessment of what assets and income the survivor can reasonably expect will also reduce such fears.

Several forms of income need to be assessed: social security benefits, civil service benefits, veteran's and/or serviceperson's benefits, stocks and investments, financial accounts, and insurance policies. There will be forms to be filled out, claims to be submitted, and policies to be interpreted. An informed advisor who can help realistically evaluate the financial and legal situation is invaluable in minimizing delays, mistakes, and losses.

Providing Direction

Having legal and/or financial expertise does not necessarily make one a good advisor. There are four main areas in which the nurse, social worker, or other health care professional may be able to help the patient and family to interact effectively with their legal and financial advisor.

Establishing relationships and roles of persons involved.   In general, the legal and financial advisor will be known well to the patient-family. It bears repeating that in many cases the advisor will function quite adequately without a hospice team member's help. If this is not the situation, however, and if the family asks that a team member help out, it is best to be present at a meeting of all parties as an observer, at least at the outset. Occasionally the team member may act as a facilitator, but only in very extreme circumstances will she or he take an advisory or advocate position. The hospice team member can be very helpful in seeing that the patient's and family's concerns are addressed. She or he can help them prepare information and questions in advance of the group meeting, assistance that is both cost- and time-effective.

Identifying and clarifying central concerns.   The patient-family may be confused and disorganized. It is often unclear what the priorities are when one is under emotional strain or lost in details. The team member can help the patient-family focus on the most important issues, clarify problems, and list alternatives that the advisor can then address. The team member can offer realistic evaluation of options provided by circumstances. For example, an advisor may advocate selling a home or business that the team member recognizes as the survivor's greatest source of purpose and fulfillment. It should be remembered that much of this information is confidential. Patients and families have a right to expect that all financial and business conversations and records will be treated as confidential. It is distressing that professionals often seem to regard information outside their discipline as less confidential than their own. An attorney who would never discuss details of a client's financial status will volunteer at great lengths a description of his or her failing health; a nurse, who has never discussed a patient's reactions to physical pain may describe to a friend the pain brought about by financial anxieties.

Assessment of patient–family's strengths and resources.   Positive features of family unity, skills, talents, and desires may be integral to determining the course of the survivors' abilities to cope with their changing life style. What may seem to be an appropriate financial decision, for example, establishing a trust for a widow so she will not have to "concern herself" with financial matters, may actually be very limiting to a person who might later need to liquidate certain assets to begin her own business. It may be necessary to explain to those determining the financial future of the survivor that immediate symptoms produced by present grief—such as anxiety, guilt, poor impulse control, inability to plan and manage rationally, and withdrawal—should pass with time. Options for future control and growth should be left open.

Ongoing support and mobilization.   After the patient-family have made some decisions about the legal and financial future of the survivors with their advisor, the team member can support and help fulfill those choices. If she or he has been included in the planning stages, it is relatively easy to understand incoming information, clarify paper work, and keep anxiety levels at a minimum.

In the event that a real financial crisis is judged to be developing, the hospice team may be able to provide comfort and counseling and, perhaps, generate community support. Informal groups of friends, neighbors, and office mates as well as formal agencies and churches can be mobilized to provide both short-term and long-term assistance. The social worker on the team can be invaluable in developing such linkages for service and support.

SUSTAINING AND DEVELOPING SOCIAL RESOURCES FOR A FAMILY

Hospice teams need to remember that the support network for a patient and his or her family is larger than their team. It ordinarily will involve a variety of friends, business associates, relatives, and casual acquaintances. Most will provide positive input, but some may be quite negative. No matter what their input, however, these people may be perceived by the patient to be important.

Too often a treatment team focuses its energies on doing things for the patient and family. It may be more important to develop a support system that helps the patient and family do things for themselves. One spouse related the following story of what he called "the terminal team."

That hospice group was always right there when we needed them. They didn't bug us, but neither the nurse nor the counselor ever left us alone to deal with frightening things. And the volunteers—we had help with shopping and taking M____ to scouts. They were fantastic. Maybe they were too good. Don't get me wrong; I'm extremely grateful, but after B____ died, even though the counseling (a bereavement program) continued, it was kind of like losing a second family—a second bereavement. No one had ever been good to us like those hospice folks. Then they were gone too.

Without criticizing what was obviously a close and caring situation from which this family benefited, it might be wise to consider this man's remarks.

It really is not possible, even with good bereavement services, to continue after the death the close attention and affection a team may provide a family while someone is dying. It is usually not even necessary. Many families have an established social network capable of sustaining them except under extreme conditions like a period of terminal illness. These networks continue to function in whatever ways they can throughout the illness and team intervention period, and they quickly snap back in place when the team withdraws.

Some families, however, have small or less well-defined support groups that are unsure of how and when they should help. As they see the hospice team, including volunteers, helping, providing, advising, they withdraw even further. They do not ever become involved at a level that gives them any real understanding of the family's needs. When the period of crisis and bereavement follow-up has passed, there is no legacy of sharing or understanding in this support group for permanent help.

The supportive services of the hospice team are not being criticized here. Nor is the fact that the primary concern of the care team and bereavement program is the dying patient and his or her family. In fact, some friendships between hospice families and staff remain for life. However, the majority do not. Therefore it is essential that within the social context, hospice team members see one of their chief goals as developing and sustaining the natural social support systems of families.

TYPES OF SUPPORT SYSTEMS

Caplan (1974) describes three types of support systems that can become mutual-help groups. Hospice teams need to help families develop whichever of the following resources may be available.

1. Neighborhood-based, informal arrangements for the delivery of helping services
2. Primary-group networks composed of kith, blood, and pseudo-family ties
3. Community gatekeepers such as physicians, counselors, and members of the clergy

Caplan also urges professionals to help create support groups and mutual aid groups that will continue to be available to survivors for as long as they need them (Caplan, 1974).

The phrase *natural support system,* used by professionals to designate these supportive groups, has numerous definitions and connotations. It can stand for any variety of individuals and organizations in, for example, the workplace, neighborhood, marketplace, family, and church or synagogue. One does not need to be an expert in social systems to recognize that some family and/or friends do not merit the designation "natural support system." They may function only under the strong influence and encouragement of others or perhaps never under any circumstances (Gottlieb, 1982).

SOCIAL ANALYSIS OF THE SUPPORT SYSTEM

Support should be measured by quality, not quantity. An analysis of an individual's amount of social interaction—for example, number of persons visited, church contacts, visits received, family interactions, telephone calls—may be far less important for the dying patient than the quality of those interactions. Again, it is a very individual matter, but the dying person may derive great satisfaction from the quiet presence of one or two of the closest and dearest people.

A family, however, has some very specific social needs that are present throughout the periods of illness and death but also carry into the bereavement stage. It sometimes is very difficult for the hospice support person (e.g., social worker or bereavement coordinator) working with the family to determine how much people around the family are really helping them. Questions can be asked in order to determine the extent of support an individual is receiving (see Table 11-2).

THE COMPONENTS OF SOCIAL SUPPORT

No definition of social support is universally accepted (Carveth & Gottlieb, 1979). Cobb (1976), however, has delineated three areas of support for an individual's interpersonal life:

Table 11-2. *Assessing the Extent of Support Being Received by a Survivor-Family*

The hospice team member could ask the family member how many times in the past four weeks someone has provided the following types of support:

Personal feelings

Listened to you speak about your
  feelings
Tried to cheer you up
Told you about his or her feelings
Shared a secret confidence
Other:

Material or physical support

Loaned you more than $25
Gave you money
Gave you an object (valued at $10 or
  more) that you needed
Provided you with a place to stay
Provided you with transportation
Helped you get something done
Other:

Advice:

Told you what she or he did or might
  do in a situation
Provided information you needed to
  make a choice
Helped you set a goal or sort our
  priorities
Other:

Self-esteem feedback that builds

Agreed that what you want to do, say,
  or choose is right
Told you that you are competent,
  successful, or just "doing well"
Asked your opinion
Told you that she or he likes you just
  the way you are
Other:

Social participation

Accepted your invitaon to do something
  or go somewhere
Invited you to do something or go
  somewhere
Included you in an ongoing group or
  organization
Other

Negative feedback

Made you angry
Criticized you or your actions
Created a situation that made life more
  difficult
Other:

Source: Based in part on Barrera, M. Inventory of Socially Supportive Behaviors (ISSB) Arizona Social Support Interview Schedule (ASSIS). In B.H. Gottlieb (Ed.), *Social networks and social support,* Los Angeles: Sage Publications, 1981.

1. Emotional support: information that one is cared for
2. Esteem support; information that one is valued
3. Network support: information that one "belongs" to a community of mutual concern and responsibility

A stable social support system can provide the personal community necessary for tangible support, recognition of valued identities, problem solving and adaptive behavior under stress. The personal friends and relatives of a family, members of a hospice team, and members of other hospice families in a support group setting can all fill these roles.

Tangible Support

Although there are several ways people can be of help to families, the usefulness of tangible social support in times of illness or crisis is immediately apparent. Support with the activities of daily life, such as running errands, child care, meal preparation, and transportation, is highly valued when one is involved in a serious problem. In fact, all the emotional support in the world ("caring and sharing") may not be as helpful on one specific afternoon as picking up the children in a family and taking them out for pizza. Such an outing may provide husband and wife with a moment of privacy and the children with a needed afternoon of laughter and release. Both sides will be relieved of the guilt of enjoyment at this serious time of crisis. Volunteers particularly may fill a most important role by providing ongoing, practical, tangible respite and by keeping the household functioning in as nearly a normal way as possible. Social activities designed to relieve boredom can also serve as distractions from pain. Such activities can not only provide the diversion necessary to distract the patient from his or her pain but can help to reestablish to some degree the former quality of the patient's life (McCaffery, 1979).

Recognition of Valued Identities

The need to care for a dying person often casts people in new and unfamiliar roles, such as nurse, counselor, financial manager, or housekeeper. Caregivers may be very insecure about how successful they are in performing these new tasks. Support individuals can verbally acknowledge or reinforce these new identities by socially commenting to the person that she or he is "a terrific nurse," "a very efficient bookkeeper," or "an excellent source of support for the patient." Less explicit forms of support may involve interactions such as asking the person's opinion or accepting his or her ideas about the new role. Such behaviors imply to the caregiver that she or he is doing things well.

Hospice team members can also influence the degree to which friends and relatives remain helpful and active through similar positive feedback. They should be encouraged to participate in helpful ways; information can be shared with them and validation offered of the roles they play. The attentions of real friends can sometimes reduce the isolation that accompanies the feeling the family may have of being the only ones ever to have had to carry such a heavy burden (Levy, 1976).

Problem Solving

A person's social support system can also help in problem solving. Friends and helpers can listen to ideas, thus serving as a sounding board that may help a person put his or her ideas in order. Articulation of a dilemma and its possible solutions frequently helps a person to do the following:

- Recognize what she or he does not clearly understand (If it cannot be stated, it may not be understood).
- Spot areas of illogic or lack of rationality (Having to present an idea objectively so that someone else can support it is difficult if it is based on emotion, not on fact).
- Clarify the idea in relation to past stated values or philosophies (The idea, once stated, may not "sound like the person" to someone who knows him or her well; inconsistencies can then be recognized).

If the listener is responsive and shares ideas she or he may offer the following:

- Additional facts or observations (sometimes these may be erroneous or based on misconceptions).
- New perspectives on or priorities for the basic choices or issues
- Different goals or tactics of problem solving
- Reinforcement; for example confirming that there is or is not a problem, or that the course being followed is correct or should be changed.

It should be noted also that simply confiding in someone or sharing problems is a socially satisfying activity.

Stress Reduction

Serious physical illness and the prospect of death represent serious threats to any relationship. Close members in the relationship may experience physical illness or symptoms, frustration, and interpersonal conflict (Klein, Dean, & Bogdonoff, 1967).

The extent to which family members are stressed may also correlate with the degree of support they receive from both the patient and others around them in their support system. It is very helpful if the patient can be counseled, despite the drains of the illness, to provide some emotional return to those supporting him or her if only through gratitude or encouragement to those involved in the individual's social orbit (Goldenberg & Goldenberg, 1980). Some patients may exhibit social detachment and may not provide such feedback. Or a patient may believe that the cost and effort of self-disclosure to his or her social group may be greater than the benefits. She or he may be correct, but more usually the social detachment may have the effect of alienating the person from his or her social support, straining interactions or eroding trust (Harker, 1972).

Stress also is related to the emotional status of those in one's social support network. Therefore, social support in the form of calmness, caring, and reassurance may reduce anxiety and decrease debilitating emotion or stress. It follows also that a negative social support system can be detrimental to the ability of a patient and family to cope with a life-threatening illness (Garrity, 1973; Hyman, 1971). Families and patients definitely assess the threatening quality of a situation based on the emotional states of individuals around them (Schachter, 1959).

THE IMPORTANCE OF THE VOLUNTEER

Patients, even though they are dying, may continue to need social relationships whether with a professional caregiver, a relative, a lay volunteer or a neighbor who can provide them with the opportunity to share reactions and meaningful affection. According to Klagsbrun (1971), "The kind of meaningful contact a patient requires at this time must come from a warm sensitive person who offers the patient a sense of security he longs for. This can only come from a person who is strong and secure" (p. 944).

The most valuable volunteers are those who spend time with the patient and family, offering nonjudgmental emotional support and all varieties of practical help with daily living. Volunteers who become the greatest resource to a family and who themselves are most fulfilled are often motivated by a desire to serve, to share, and to learn. They are emotionally mature and warm and listen to patients' views with respect. They are dependable team members

Table 11-3. *Components of a Training Program for Volunteers*

- Exploration of trainees' thoughts and feelings about dying, death, and grief
- History and philosophy of the hospice movement
- The family as the unit of care
- Concepts of terminal illness, cancer, aging
- Pain: spiritual, psychological, emotional, social, physical
- Role and function of an interdisciplinary team member
- Creative strategies for helping patients and families; the role of the volunteer
- Listening skills
- Patient perspectives on grief and dying
- Community resources
- Recognizing and coping with one's own stress
- Criteria for volunteers who work with the hospice program that are specific to the particular program, agency, or affiliate

who are willing to use their talents and skills in flexible and creative ways. Finally, they can find humor and value in self and circumstance (Markey, 1980).

The education program to prepare volunteers for the experiences they will face must be comprehensive, thorough, and sensitive. The purposes of the education, to prepare volunteers to work within the hospice team and to support the family structure require an extensive content. A survey of the volunteer training programs of well established hospice programs reveals that they share many of the components listed in Table 11-3. In addition, most programs recognize the need for on-going continuing educational programs, volunteer support activities, and volunteer participation in team meetings.

REFERENCES

Barrera, M. in Gottlieb, B.H. (ed.). Social networks and social support. Los Angeles, Calif. Sage Publications, Inc., 1982.

Caplan, G. Support systems. In G. Caplan (Ed.). *Support systems and community mental health.* New York: Basic Books, 1974.

Carveth, W.B., & Gottlieb, B.H. The measurement of social support and its relation to stress. *Canadian Journal of Behavioral Science,* 1979, *11,* 179–188.

Cobb, S. Social support as a moderator of life stress. *Psychosomatic Medicine,* 1976, *38,* 300–304.

Garrity, T.F. Vocational adjustment after first myocardial infarction. *Social Science and Medicine* 1973, *7,* 705–717.

Goldenburg, I., & Goldenburg, H. *Family therapy: An overview.* Monterey, Calif.: Brooks Cole, 1980.

Gottlieb, B.H. (Ed.). *Social networks and social support.* Los Angeles, Calif.: Sage Publications, Inc., 1982.

Grollman, E.A. (Ed.). *Concerning death: A practical guide for the living.* Boston: Beacon Press, 1974.

Harker, B.L. Cancer and communication problems: A personal experience. *Psychiatry in Medicine* 1972, *3,* 163–171.

Hyman, M.D. Disability and patient's perceptions of preferential treatment. *Journal of Chronic Diseases,* 1971, *24,* 329–342.

Klagsbrun, S.C. Communications in the treatment of cancer. *American Journal of Nursing,* 1971, *71,* 944–948.

Klein, R.F., Dean, A., & Bogdonoff, M.D. The impact of illness upon the spouse. *Journal of Chronic Diseases* 1967, *20,* 241–248.

Levy, L.H. Self-help groups: Types and psychological processes. *Journal of Applied Behavioral Science,* 1976, *12,* 310–322.

Markey, K. Volunteers in palliative care. In B. Mount & I. Ajemian (Eds.). *The Royal Victoria Hospital manual on palliative/hospice care.* New York: Arno Press, 1980.

McCaffery, M. *Nursing management of the patient with pain.* Philadelphia: J.B. Lippincott, 1979.

Raether, H.C., Slater, R.C. The funeral and the funeral director. In E.A. Grollman (Ed.). *Concerning death: A practical guide for the living.* Boston: Beacon Press, 1974.

Ross, M.H. The Law and Death. In E.A. Grollman (Ed.). *Concerning death: A practical guide for the living.* Boston: Beacon Press, 1974.

Schachter, S. *The psychology of affiliation.* Stanford, Calif.: Stanford University Press, 1959.

Winters, I.R. Choosing a memorial. In E.A. Grollman (Ed.). *Concerning death: A practical guide for the living.* Boston: Beacon Press, 1975.

1. F	6. F
2. F	7. T
3. F	8. T
4. T	9. F
5. F	10. T

12

The Family as the Unit of Care

1. *The impact of a terminal illness falls primarily on the patient.*

2. *The mark of a healthy family response to a dying member is the ability to set other matters aside and focus on the patient's needs until his or her death.*

3. *A crisis intervention model is appropriate with families dealing with a terminally ill loved one.*

4. *Children need simple information about an illness and death based on an understanding of their developmental stage.*

5. *After a death, if the members of the family continue performing in the same roles they had before the death, the family system will remain in balance.*

6. *A family who cares for a dying loved one at home, talk openly, and express their emotions freely can deal with all their grief before the death.*

7. *A change in one family member affects each other person and the family system as a whole.*

8. *A small family who have a realistic perception of the crisis of a terminal illness and adequate coping skills but lack sufficient situational support will have difficulty dealing with the care needed.*

9. *Family members whose relationships are enmeshed will have difficulty accepting help from community resources to supplement their care of the patient.*

10. *The hospice visiting nurse should not frighten the family by outlining possible symptom progression as the patient gets closer to death.*

It's hard enough to know I'll have to leave my family soon, without losing them before I die. They haven't deserted me, even though I've been this sick. Their love for me, and the time they spend with me every day makes me realize how precious they are. Relationships can't be measured in length of time together, but in a look or a touch that takes only an instant and lasts for an eternity. We're all frightened and sad and angry, but being together and loving brings us joy and happiness and peace too. Thank God for them.

—Anonymous

IN MANY illnesses, we as health care providers tend to think of the illness as primarily affecting the ill person, and we look to family and friends mainly as a support system for that person. But when an illness affects a person's ability to function in his or her normal roles for any length of time, or when profound changes threaten even the continued existence of the person, the integrity of family and friends as persons may be threatened too. The unit of care for a dying person must include both that person and his or her family.

Facing the loss of one's life raises many questions and issues that intimately affect the people one loves and depends on. Unfinished business in relationships must be dealt with or ignored; the impact of the inevitable role changes must be faced; the question of how the loved ones will exist after the death arises; and the need for help and support from others must be accepted or denied. Family members are involved in each of these areas and must face the loss of an important part of their lives at the same time they are caring for or supporting the ill person and maintaining their own lives.

Family-centered care has many important advantages. It increases the psychosocial support available to the person who is dying. It encourages more open statements available to the person who is dying. It encourages more open statements of the emotional agendas each family member has which, when unstated, can lead to confusion and problems. It decreases the psychological and physical "casualty rate" of the family and helps avoid family disorganization and fragmentation during and after the illness and death (White, 1981).

As our culture holds less tightly to strictly defined family units, *family* has come to mean those persons the dying person identifies as important to him or her. This may include or exclude blood relatives, partners, friends, co-workers, and even pets. Health care professionals may not deal directly with each family member, but they must not forget that each is an inextricable element in the dying experience. When blood relatives are excluded by the patient, they may need extra support and information from the caregiving team. We need to explain to the patient that because the family is the unit of care, we will support each family member at the same time that we accept the patient's right to relate or not relate to people according to his or her wishes. Often as death grows nearer a reconciliation is desired or accepted by both parties.

As a consequence of changing family patterns in our culture, we are now dealing with many single-parent families, with remarriages that blend two family units and give children four parents, and a multitude of other life-styles including childless couples, group living that comprises all levels of intimacy-noninvolvement, unmarried couples, or homosexual partners. Conflicts can arise when the family units caring for the dying person include a traditional nuclear family and a more newly chosen, nontraditional "family." These groupings may have different values and different beliefs about who should have more decision-making power. These problems can arise also between a patient's grown children and his or her "new" wife or husband.

When threatened with the loss of a loved person, the family must deal with many newly imposed challenges, as well as with their normal (and normally sufficient) responsibilities and interests. The dying experience is almost always a new one, even for family members who have experienced other deaths. The newness may comprise a different relationship or role, a different environment (mother died in the hospital; my husband is staying at home), or a different level of involvement (my sister was primary caregiver or supporter for mother; I am the primary person for my husband). So the family member has many roles: learner in a new and potentially frightening situation; continuer of ongoing life and responsibilities; caregiver and/or supporter; griever for an unwanted impending loss; decision-maker–crisis intervener with the patient; and anticipator of a vastly changed life after the death.

The family is a system comprised of individuals, with both individual and group needs when one member faces death. The caregiving role of the family is important, whether the patient is at home or in an institution. Special issues arise when the family includes children, and these are explored in the final section of this chapter.

THE FAMILY AS INDIVIDUALS AND SYSTEM

Like any system, a family is greater than the sum of its parts, and that is what makes family-centered care so exciting and at times harrowing! Individual needs cannot be isolated from relationship needs within the family.

The relationships between wife and husband, parent and child, sibling and siblings, all interact. Families create a balance for individual and relational needs; anything affecting the balance of the system affects each individual. Any change in one individual affects every other person and the system as a whole, forcing the others to change also (White, 1981). And what could have more of an impact than a terminal illness? This places unasked-for, acute demands on the family in terms of caring for the ill person or arranging for and coordinating care, rearranging priorities in personal lives, dealing with multiple emotions raised by the illness and expected death, and being involved in difficult decisions. Each member must also come to terms in his or her own way with the meaning of the illness and death, and the new beginning necessitated by the loss of the loved one.

When assessing a family system, one must look at the identity, responses, and needs of each member and of the family as a whole. The nurse can be helpful to the family if she or he understands the family's *characteristics and identity*—how they communicate, how they relate to each other and to the rest of the world, and what their beliefs and values are. Against this background the responses and needs of the family can be understood and positive coping styles can be encouraged. Needs of the family system when dealing with a life-threatening illness include the need to know *who will be involved* and how; the need to *continue each member's own life* and that of the family at the same time they care for the dying person; the need to *maintain balance in the family system;* and the need to come to terms with the *meaning of the illness, death, and subsequent family reorganization.* We will be exploring each of these areas in the next several sections.

Intervention centers around the concept of enabling the patient and family to do what they want to do to meet their goals. This involves information-giving, teaching, joint goal setting and problem solving, advocacy, and adequate support to the system. In home care, this demands 24-hour-daily access to a nurse (shared among a team to avoid nursing burnout). In addition to counseling and spiritual support, volunteers are most important, as we noted in the last chapter, in helping family members with tasks they cannot complete or staying with the patient while the family shops, visits friends, or rests. Family goals and directions are honored; the care team starts with them where they are, and helps them get to where they want to be. Persons or families "in denial" are there for a good reason. It is advisable not to confront but to establish a reliable and trusting relationship where the family feels safe; then one can invite them to explore other elements in their thoughts and feelings. Some families will not talk directly about "depressing" or "negative" things, but will communicate on other levels; one must learn to hear these two. For example, a man may express great anger toward the medical system instead of revealing rage at his illness and dependence. Or a woman may be completing her will at the same time she talks about being well in a few weeks. Another person may be more than usually touched by a visit from a relative who lives far away. The nurse can speak with persons about both sides they are expressing.

Basic assumptions about intervention with families with a dying loved one include simple but powerful elements. The *relationship* between the patient-family and a nurse is effective in giving, for example, an initial measure of pain relief secondary to anxiety reduction, if the patient believes the nurse is *capable* and will hold herself or himself *accountable* for symptom relief. These things need to be directly stated to patient and family, and then demonstrated to be true. Assuring the patient and family that the whole *family* is the unit of care serves to relieve each of them of concerns that the family will overdo and become exhausted and unable to cope. Keeping the understanding that the patient-family have control and that *self-determination* will be respected by the nurse is important.

Recognizing when to refer families to counselors on the health care team or to long-term therapists can be a challenge. Be clear as to your goals; are they to support the family through the crisis of a dying member? If so, refer families with longstanding or multiple serious problems who need help to restructure relationships. If a family does not accept a referral, be clear about your own limits in the helping relationship.

When dealing on a personal level with family members about their feelings, beliefs, and contributions, *accept* each person where she or he is. *Affirm* family members' feelings, and accept their different coping styles. Assume that at all times each person is *doing the best* she or he can. Know that *no one can take away a person's painful feelings;* the only way out of felt pain is to go through it. We can be *witnesses* and walk beside people, but we cannot lift the load from them. Focus on *enabling* the family to learn, cope, and help each other. Help the family with *joint goal setting,* assisting them to share their feelings and desires, then negotiating shared goals.

Family Characteristics and Identity

In assessing the family system, the nurse must try to understand each individual's feelings and reactions and the roles she or he performs; then the nurse can begin to see how these all blend and interact. Suppose, for example, that a wife and mother of three is dying. The daughter may feel loving, or guilty, and may want to give her mother personal care; the husband may be immobilized by this impending loss and sit holding his wife's hand; one son may be an organizer and doer, taking care of financial matters and coordinating the helpers; another son may flee. In a family such as this, each member has different coping styles and meets different needs, and they may not understand or accept each others' responses or appreciate their varied contributions. In addition, the roles each person has traditionally performed affect the way each is treated by the family. If the father has always been active and in charge, the children may push him to fulfill the decision-making role when he feels unable to do this. If the women have always been the caregivers, the whole of the care may be left to the daughter, leading to her exhaustion and resentment. The fleeing son may fill a most important family role, that of scapegoat. In situations involving the painful loss of a loved one, anger at the "irresponsible" behavior of one person can distract the rest of the family from the pain of the loss and the need for reorganization of the family (White, 1981).

To further complicate the picture we have painted, the roles the mother has always played are now either diminished or lost, and the family must adapt to the loss and reintegrate those roles into the smaller family. Keeping the patient as actively involved in the family as possible helps both her and the family in the gradual transition. Although the focus in this chapter will tend to be on the other members of the family, the patient will be assumed to be included in statements about "the family."

Before looking at the family as a system, let us consider briefly the commonalities in individual responses when a loved one has a life-threatening illness. In fact, family members' responses are similar to the patient's: How will this affect my life? It's been forced on me. Why me? Why now? And, I must deal with this and then start over. Related feelings include disbelief, anger, resentment, depression, love, tenderness, acceptance, or anxiety and insecurity about the impact on roles, self-image, and identity.

Cultural differences are clearly vital in understanding the family. Often the family is the best resource for learning how cultural identity affects the response to a terminal illness and death. One needs to ask questions about the areas where assumptions are often made according to one's own background (See Chapter 4).

A brief look at some family system theory will assist in organizing one's thoughts about the assessment of the family. Virginia Satir's (1972) and Salvador Minuchin's (1974) descriptions of family relationship styles can be very helpful in assessment and intervention. Consider Table 12-1, which summarizes the major characteristics of each of these family therapists' family types and their possible responses to a dying loved one. A patient in a family that represents Satir's *closed* family system for example, which involved protective communication styles, might say, "I don't want to tell the family I'm dying—or angry—it will just upset them." Each family has rules that govern how the family should act, what they can feel, what can be expressed or not expressed, and what kinds of relationships are acceptable with those outside the family. In closed family systems these rules are unclear and not stated, but they are rigid and discussion about them is prohibited.

Somewhat differently, Minuchin's *enmeshed* relationships characterize families where boundaries between members are weak and unclear. In an extreme case, for instance, a daughter might say, "Mother is the only one who understands me. I don't want to live if she dies." *Disengaged* family relationships, on the other hand, involve great distance: "Our family never did much together anyway; I can't take the time to take care of every little need of Dad now."

Minuchin's *normal* family or Satir's *open* family system characterize families with direct and clear communication and rules; separate individual identities, with neither isolation nor excessive dependence between members; a flexibility allowing for change in the system and in family roles; and supportive relationships both within and outside the family. These families can accept help from persons and agencies outside the family and can move toward adapting to new roles and meeting all members' needs in the face of changes demanded by life-threatening illnesses.

Case Example: A Mixed Family System

A couple in their eighties had been married and had had a very close relationship for 30 years. This was a second marriage for each, and now the wife was dying of lung cancer. The husband's investment in life—his active involvement in his business and his interest in family and friends—was founded on his wife's enthusiasm. He felt she was his meaning in life, and he did not know what he would do without her. As his wife became sicker and less responsive, though he did not want her to suffer he resented her increased sleeping, wanting her awake and talking. He avoided conversations about her wishes with respect to arrangements after her death and spoke to her of daily life. Until his wife needed heavy care he took excellent care of her, and he declined any assistance from counselors, chaplain, or volunteers. When a nurse did begin regular visits, he would wait until she completed her transactions with his wife and then would talk with the nurse about the beautiful antiques in the home.

In contrast to the husband, the woman's daughter sought out conversation with her about her desires for the time before and after her death, and they spoke openly about many areas. The daughter had to balance her own time between her mother and her own growing family. She wavered often but did manage to set limits on the time she spent in each home. The daughter accepted help from nurses and volunteers, exploring her feelings as well as the care needs.

The husband had an enmeshed relationship with his wife, and had a closed communication style, at least while the nurse was present. The daughter–mother relationship was more open, neither enmeshed nor isolated. Both of these family members were able to offer great support, comfort, and care to the patient, but in very different manners. The daughter organized and took care of business; the husband loved and nurtured.

The nurse's role was different with the husband and the daughter, according to their needs. More direct conversations were held with the daughter concerning her feelings about the loss of her mother, the difficulties in juggling the needs of two families, and plans for terminal care and for the funeral. The nurse respected the husband's desire to limit direct communication and numbers of outside helpers and enjoyed discussions of antiques with him, forming a trusting relationship around this

Table 12-1. *Theories of Family Systems*

Theory	Relations among Family Members	Relations with Outside World	Possible Responses to Terminal Illness
Minuchin			
Enmeshed	High dependency High involvement, belonging Emotional symbiosis Diffuse boundaries between family members Low autonomy	Strong boundaries between family and outsiders	Difficulty accepting outside help Intense response to one member's stress Difficulty separating from dying person Becoming overloaded and unable to adapt to stress
Disengaged	Weak bonds Absence of structure Low dependency, belonging Rigid boundaries between family members Autonomous	May be strong boundaries	Difficulty accepting outside help Difficulty requesting help Difficulty organizing and caring for ill members (Only high stress situations activate family support)

Normal	Strong, individual identities Reliance on each other Flexibility; ability to adjust roles	Flexible boundaries; relating to others and accepting help is acceptable	Ability to adjust roles to meet new needs Ability to accept outside help Ability to share feelings, support
Satir			
Closed	Resistance to change Indirect communication Unspoken, unclear family rules	Restricted	Difficulty changing roles and rules as needs and abilities change Difficulty accepting outside help Difficulty expressing feelings
Open	Change accepted as normal Direct, clear communication Flexible rules to meet changing needs Communication about family rules High self-worth	Direct access to supportive relationships outside family	Ability to accept help from outside Ability to adjust roles and rules to meet new needs Ability to share feelings, support

Source: Minuchin (1974); Satir (1972).

area. She applauded his excellent care for his wife, and when the care became too heavy for him, assisted in hiring a private duty nurse. When death was near, the husband was willing to talk about the loss, but again indirectly, mostly sharing about the death of his first wife. He was able to find comfort from the fact that he survived that loss; he would also survive this one.

Who Will Be Involved

Given the multiple and varied definitions of membership in families, the "who" question can be either quite clear or confusing. People vital to the care and comfort of the patient and in need of support and teaching will be found among the nuclear family, extended family, and in the social network. Added to this are the health care providers. Once the significant actors are identified, the desired and actual role of each must be clarified.

For example, a difficult situation was created when the parents of a dying young man arrived from across the country, expecting to be central in care and in making decisions with or for him. The young man had close friends who knew him well and who were the ones he preferred to have care for him and whom he trusted to honor his preferences. In these circumstances it was vital that the patient's preferences and choices be identified and written down or communicated to all active participants before he was too weak to lead in decision making. This young man's parents stayed in his hospital room most of each day after he was unable to communicate, instructing the nursing staff to restrict other visitors. But those restricted visitors were the close friends he loved and wanted beside him, feeling closer to them than to his parents. Tact and support were needed in dealing with both the parents and friends, helping them to work together on the same team, not as competitors. Fortunately, in this situation, a nurse who had known the patient over several admissions was able to help the family to a graceful compromise, so that their son's wish to spend time with his friends could be fulfilled. They realized that a final gift to their son was to "share him" with his friends.

Even when dealing with a family where the actors are clearly defined, as in a closely-knit nuclear family, one must take nothing for granted. Assumptions that apparently uninvolved family members are unaffected by the illness are obviously false in theory, but it is easy to lose track of this fact in practice. I recently worked with a family in which the father had a degenerative neurological disease and needed total care. The wife and daughter gave all the care and described the son as unavailable, uninvolved, and unreliable. Both children were grown and lived near the parents. The son did not come to any family conferences held and did seem to be out of the picture. Then one day I received a call from him asking for a visit when he entered the hospital for surgery the next week. The purpose of the visit was to get information about his father's illness and prognosis, to begin expressing his pain about this, and to look for support. Apparently the son had been the "identified patient" of the family, the one who always was the sick one, and he was unable to ask for help until he was in the sick role himself. I learned in that visit how involved he was with the family; he called his father daily, his mother twice a day, and visited every other day!

Demographic data, such as age, sex, religion, occupation, ethnic origin, and education level, are important to the extent that the data provide insight into people. Such information can help guide us in the search for individual and family personality, values, beliefs, and capabilities.

Family identity and ability to respond to a terminal illness can be explored by learning how the family has dealt with crises in the past. Were the past crises similar to the current life-threatening illness? In what ways? What roles did each person play? Who made the decisions, and how? What resources were the family able to accept and use? One value of living through tragedies is the learning that can come from the process. Ask the family what they learned and compliment them on surviving, assuring them they can survive and grow from the current experience too. If the roles they each played in the previous crises were effective and met the family's needs, they can adapt those roles to the present situation. Or the nurse can help the family identify new roles and behaviors that will be helpful in meeting the specific needs of the current situation, and the members can share the tasks. For example, one person could coordinate schedules for visiting nurses and friends who visit the home or bring dinner or sit with the patient while the family goes out; another might spend special time with young children in the family; a third might be in charge of financial and insurance planning; and a fourth could make sure the family sits down together and shares information, feelings, and support.

It is important to help the family make use of the assistance offered by friends and available from community resources. In terminal illness, with its multiple effects on each person in the family, resources become vitally important. Each person will need emotional support, plus help perhaps in daily tasks such as child care, while the parent is visiting or caring for the patient, or homemaker services. Help may be needed to evaluate financial resources, including income, insurance, and eligibility for additional assistance. Remember that families who have never used outside resources *may* be unable to use them now, and may decline efforts at networking.

Families need to know just who from the health care team will be there for them and exactly what each will offer. At home: who will teach them the care they will be giving? Who will help with difficult decisions? Who will be there at three in the morning if they have a crisis? Who can be with the patient while they do the shopping? In the hospital: Who will be constant for the patient and family? Who will answer questions about changes? Who will really include the family in giving comfort-oriented care? Who, among all the changing faces, will really know the patient and be there for the family?

Caring for a Loved One and Continuing One's Own Life

The illness and dying of an important loved one is such an extraordinary process that families often focus all their resources on giving care and support to that person; they may put themselves on "automatic" for continuing their regular day-to-day activities. This will work for a short time, but longer periods demand that individual and family needs be met. This is one reason for increased strain on the family system in long-lasting terminal illnesses. Children must still be raised with love and attention; work goes on; daily successes and failures must be acknowledged; food and clothing must be obtained. The nurse's role is crucial in legitimatizing the family's need to focus on other needs besides the patient's and to identify realistic limits they must place on how much they can do. They often feel quite guilty if they don't spend every waking minute for the patient. Alternatively, they might spend excessive time and energy for the patient, neglecting other family needs, and then wonder why the family is falling apart, or why they feel resentful. Each person must determine how much focus to give to each area. If the need to be with the patient necessitates some neglect of other family members' needs, such as children, the nurse can help the family plan for others in the family or for friends or agencies to help meet those needs.

When friends are caring for a dying person, limit-setting can be difficult as friends weigh their love for the patient against the level of commitment they feel willing and able to make. If they are uncertain about the latter, the added element of wondering whether "I want to continue doing all this for my friend" complicates the picture when the going gets rough. These friends need an objective listener and supportive ear, as well as encouragement to share with the patient.

The family often neglect simple maintenance needs such as shopping, eating, recreation, adequate rest, or worship in the name of caring for the patient. Friends or volunteers can help with some; for the rest the family must come to terms with the fact that even though one person is dying the rest of the family must continue living. If the ill person is part of a sexual partnership, the illness will certainly have an impact on this area. The loss of an active sexual relationship may add stress particularly to the well partner. It also can evolve into a new tenderness and deep relating through more gently holding and stroking the loved person. Often for the patient sexual relationship needs go through a transition, with more emphasis on the need for love, closeness, and holding. If the couple can talk openly about their needs and feelings, they can work out ways of meeting their needs that are acceptable to both. Remember that sexuality involves more than sex. Appearance and grooming, as well as maintaining life roles compliment the need for physical contact in one's sexual self concept (Taylor, 1983).

Other family life changes can compete with the life-threatening illness. Consider the normal life changes the family is experiencing during the time of the terminal illness; is there a new marriage or birth, retirement, or children leaving the home? If so, this will intensify the adaptational needs of the whole family. The family whose mother was hospitalized for an expected terminal stay the same day her daughter was admitted to the same hospital to deliver her first baby had much to deal with. The mother improved enough to go home, the daughter and her new family moved in with her to care for her until she died and dealt with the beginning and end of the life cycle under the same roof. Two other deaths had come to this family within the last year, making it even more difficult to combine the joy and challenges of a new baby with the difficult care and pain of loss of the mother. Fortunately, the communication patterns in this family were open and supportive, and they could be clear about each person's needs. They were also able to accept needed help into the home.

The family juggles yet another set of sometimes conflicting roles. They are care providers and/or coordinators for the patient (see the next section), and they are also the recipients of care in their role as part of the family, the unit of care. In open or normal families, people can both give and receive. In enmeshed, closed, or disengaged families, especially those with strong boundaries between themselves and outsiders, family members may not do well with one or the other of these roles. Caring for or sitting with a dying person is a very intimate experience; if it is not in the family's history to do this, it will be difficult. It is also an experience involving feelings of helplessness, difficult for most people. It is true that the family cannot save the person from dying, but the nurse can help them identify things they *can* do that help with the person's comfort, and can repeat often what a good job they are doing. In the hospital, such caregiving can include turning every two hours, frequent mouth care, massages, reading aloud, sitting quietly, holding hands, talking, bringing favorite treats. At home the family still have feelings of helplessness, often centered around the issue of food ("I can't get her to eat!"), but there's always much they do that can be pointed out to them as vitally important.

Maintaining Balance in the Family System

In every family there is a certain balance, or normal way of operating, and a particular set of roles are distributed among all the family members. If something disturbs this balance, such as the addition or loss of a member, there is a strong internal pressure toward finding a way to reestablish the original roles and balance. The alternative to this is to change the system identity and give up or change some of the traditional functions of the family members. The choice is difficult.

The need to make these adaptations comes at one of the most difficult of all times, when the family faces a painful loss and has the additional burden of caring for a patient at home or making many trips to the hospital to support him or her. The family must absorb or lose the roles of the person who dies. If the mother was wife, lover, friend, breadwinner, supportive confidant, primary housecleaner, and disciplinarian of the children, the family has many roles to absorb. The patient will still be able to fulfill some important roles, even though in a less energetic manner: a confidant can still listen, a lover can still hold hands, a disciplinarian can advise. The family can make a gradual transition together. Most healthy families start this work before the death, having the flexibility to trade roles when appropriate. More troubled families must contend with a more rigid approach to roles; the inability to reassign roles makes it difficult to meet individuals' needs, and risk of current and future problems is high.

Case Example: When a Mother Dies

Let us compare two families with young and teenage children; in both cases, the mother is dying of long-term cancer. The first mother planned the transition of the major parenting role to her husband, who had taken an early retirement so he could be home with her and the three boys. The patient taught her husband to cook the meals the children were used to, referred them to their father for permission to go out with friends (a role she had always played), stayed in bed until they'd left for school so they would get used to leaving the house with only one parent to kiss, and told the children that they would be fine with their father. She spent time with each of them at other times in the day, times of warmth and intimacy, but she also encouraged time spent with extended family.

The second mother did not trust her husband's judgment with the children and never relinquished her role as disciplinarian. She had her mother do the cooking. This patient never talked with her children about her dying or reassured them that they would be all right with their father. In this family the son was ill often, the daughter worked around the house constantly, and the father was overwhelmed and depressed.

The first family grieved and went on with their newly adapted lives; the second family grieved and searched painfully for ways to meet their individual and joint needs. The first family adjusted to role changes needed; the second had to begin learning new roles during the initial painful bereavement period.

Nursing intervention for the first family centered mainly on supporting the dying mother in the loss she felt, assuring her of the wisdom of her chosen course, and encouraging her to stay actively involved with her family in other ways. The rest of the family did not feel the need to explore things in depth with the nurse or a counselor, focusing their support needs within themselves and the extended family, thus building the changing relationship they would need later. The second family also declined social work involvement. The nurse attempted to help the mother and her family adapt to new roles and encouraged the patient figuratively to hand her husband the reins by reassuring the children that they would be fine with their father after she died. This mother chose not to do these things, as was her right. Instead, in response to the family's request for help with this, the nurse kept the children informed of their mother's status and talked with the husband and children about how things would be after their mother died.

If a nuclear family has difficulty replacing some of the roles of the dying person within its own system, someone from the extended family or social network can sometimes help fill such roles (if the nuclear family does not shut itself off). The nurse can help the family to sort this out and can relieve the family's sense of guilt if they are unable to meet all needs from within their family. Friends and neighbors can be excellent confidants, chums, problem-solvers, and, at time, cooks and housecleaners. This of course necessitates a redefinition of the family grouping temporarily, and a commitment on the part of friend or neighbor. Extended family members can often give more intensive short-term help, and may be able to make long-term commitments if they live nearby.

Finding Meaning in Illness, Death, and Transition

Coming to terms with the meaning of the illness and loss of a loved one is a long-term and often elusive task. This is an individual need for the patient and each family member; it is also a need of the family as a system. It is a continuing process, beginning when the life-threatening illness is discovered and perhaps never completely finished, though a resolution or direction is usually worked out by the end of the first year after death occurs. Anticipatory grief (see Chapter 10) is part of this process, as is finishing unfinished business with the dying person, planning for oneself and the family after the death, and the working-through of grief during the bereavement period. The happenings, process, and resolution of the illness and loss will come up in memory at pertinent times in the family's life, as reminders of the loved one, the loss, and as a grounding for further growth. Families can retain a real sense of receiving a legacy of love and of learning from the person who died.

The search for meaning in the experience often leads people to reexamine their beliefs, their sense of self, and their roles. It involves people's feelings and ways of coping.

Family belief systems that affect the way the system deals with a dying member include religion or spirituality, beliefs about themselves and the world, and beliefs about death. Clearly, the family's religious or spiritual beliefs and community can offer great support and meaning through a difficult time as well as in good times. Learn about the type, depth, and level of support each member experiences from such beliefs; Stoll (1979) offers a helpful guide to spiritual assessment. Assist the family to gather their friends for needed help. People not identified with an organized religion may have deep spiritual beliefs and practices that they do not readily discuss. Those with no identified spiritual belief system may nevertheless have convictions in the same area that they may call "philosophical" or "just a common sense" wrapping up of things. This spiritual/philosophical resolution is often expressed in people's individualized ways of finding meaning in their experiences. "This has brought us closer together," or "I've learned to live one day at a time and really can see the trees and appreciate my friends." It can also take place in the process of a life-review.

Beliefs about self and the world form basic approaches to new situations and often predict whether those approaches will be successful: "Am I capable; can I learn new skills during a stressful time?" "Mother was hospitalized after Uncle Jake died; can our family survive another crisis?" "Will the medical system lie to us again like they did with Uncle Jake?" "We've always been self-sufficient; is it a failure if we let strangers help us?" Depending on how these questions are answered and on the family's response to the challenges inherent in coping with a terminal illness, the members and the system can learn and grow immensely. If the nurse and other members of the team can offer a supportive, consistent, and capable environment, it will help enable the family to increase their coping skills. This view of the care team as *enablers* is a most vital one in assisting the family to grow.

Values and beliefs about death often are the subject of unspoken family rules, and the nursing intervention often consists of helping the family identify what those beliefs are. Once exposed to the light of day, myths about death may explode; for example, "It's a punishment," or "It's because I was promiscuous in my twenties." When painful myths are released, the comfort of personal or spiritual beliefs may be realized. The more open the family can be with each other and with the care team the more reinforcement there is for the positive effects of their beliefs.

Approaches

The interventions we have been exploring are based in large part, on a crisis intervention model. The request for help from the family is not for counseling for long-term behavioral change but for support and assistance in dealing with a relatively short-term crisis situation. A life-threatening illness certainly fulfills the criteria of a crisis, for both the ill person and for the family. It is a threatening situation that is not readily solved by the family's customary problem-solving or decision-making methods and that this leads to disequilibrium, anxiety, tension, and difficulty in thinking. Successful dealing with the crisis can lead to psychological growth and increased competence, whereas the sense of being unsuccessful can result in anxiety and feeling threatened and ineffectual (Wilson & Kneisl, 1979). Crisis intervention is focused on immediate problems. It is developed with the patient and family, being consistent with their life-style, their values, and their current level of thinking, behaving, and feeling. And it is time-limited and realistic. Crisis intervention respects persons as able to grow and to control their own lives (Wilson & Kneisl, 1979).

Situations of terminal illnesses that last longer than a few weeks do not fall within the definition of "crisis," as crises are time-limited. In such long-term situations, increased demands and stress become the status quo. Intervention is aimed toward similar goals as in a crisis situation, focusing on the current situation, planning changes, and utilization of resources that will relieve the sense of being over one's head. The nurse needs to acknowledge to the family the challenges and difficulties of the extended time involved and to convey the hospice team's appreciation of all the family is contributing in the long-term care of their loved one.

In assessing family coping abilities in the stressful situation of a terminal illness it is useful to evaluate the presence of "balancing factors" (Aguilera & Messick, 1978). The first such factors is a *realistic perception of the event:* does the family see clearly the implications of the illness and prognosis and of their decisions regarding home care versus hospital care or "no life-saving measures"? The second factor is *adequate situational support:* Does the family have enough time, knowledge, and energy to fulfill their decision to take care of the patient at home, or can adequate additional support be generated and accepted from friends and helping agencies? The third factor is that of *adequate coping mechanisms:* Can the family deal with the physical care and the emotional impact of the illness and impending death? Identification of a lack in one of these three areas guides the intervention.

Figure 12-1. Questions for those who help*

1. Should I take this terminal diagnosis seriously or disregard it and try to go about business as usual?
2. Am I willing to discuss the diagnosis and the decisions it compels with the person I care about?
3. What are my current responsibilities?
4. What are my current needs and capabilities to help? What could I do best? What are my limitations?
5. What could I realistically offer the dying person over time?
6. What are my own sources of strength and support? How can they be enriched?
7. Am I willing to actively listen to the dying person and assist with his or her choices, even though they may be different from my own?
8. Am I willing to share my needs and feelings with the family and both give and receive support?
9. Am I willing to learn the skills needed to provide physical care for this person? What are my physical limitations?
10. What are my true motives for helping this person?
11. How much can we as a family do, what are the priorities, and are we wiling to accept help from outside?
12. Who among friends, family, and community connections can we find to share the responsibility and the opportunity to help?

*Developed by Joyce Zerwekh, 1982.

Table 12-2 *Framework for Assessment and Intervention for Family with Terminally Ill Member*

Patient–Family Need	Nursing Assessment	Nursing Interventions
To know who will be involved	Identify available resources within family, social system, community resources	Resource identification Problem solving
	Identify strengths, weaknesses, and availability of family (including past crises and family's coping mechanisms)	Advocacy Networking Information giving
	Identify level of need for resources from both within and outside family, and ascertain ability of family to accept help	Coordination of health care team Assisting family to coordinate helpers Family conferencing
To care for the loved one and continue family members' lives	Determine how realistic family's perception is of illness, prognosis, and care needed	Active listening Problem solving
	Identify family's joint capabilities, fears, and limitations in respect to caregiving	Information giving, teaching, caregiving measures Negotiation Affirmation
	Identify individual and family needs affected by caring for patient and family's ability to adjust roles or recruit help to meet those needs	Teaching about needs and balances Values clarification Family conferencing Assisting with realistic goal setting

Goal	Assessment	Intervention
To maintain balance in the family system	Identify historical roles of patient and family members Assess openness, role flexibility, dependency-isolation, level of communication and methods of coping in family Assess patient's ability to relinquish roles and others' ability to absorb them Assess communication and decisionmaking patterns	Active listening Problem solving Assisting exploration of roles and desired readjustments Values clarification Family conferencing Conflict resolution Possible referral to counselor
To find meaning in the illness, death, and transition.	Assess family's and individual's beliefs in the areas of spirituality, self, and the world (including strengths and weaknesses) Identify patient "legacy" available to family Identify role or life changes necessitated by illness and death of loved one as well as goals	Active listening Values clarification Teaching normal grief Possible referral to counselor, spiritual advisor Bereavement support Assisting evaluation of desired—necessary changes Identification of support system Assisting exploration of new learning and strengths and of patient's "legacy"

261

A useful guide for family members in assessing their own abilities and realistic involvement in the care of a terminally ill loved one is offered in Figure 12-1. Table 12-2 presents guidelines for the use of a nurse in working with a family in which one member has a life-threatening illness. It contains a summary of assessment and interventions for each of the four family needs identified in this section: the need to know who will be involved, to care for the loved one and continue their own lives, to maintain balance in the family system, and to find meaning in the illness, death, and transition.

THE FAMILY AS CAREGIVERS

In the hospital or nursing home we invite the family to become part of the interdisciplinary care team. At home, the family invites us to join their caregiving team, and decides how active a role we will have. These two basic facts explain much of the difference between the varying caregiving roles the family assumes in each setting.

Family Role in the Institutional Setting

In an institution the family needs to be invited in specific ways to become involved in the comfort and care measures given to the patient. The goal is to help the family to feel involved both with the care and with the team, without becoming overburdened or feeling that family members are left holding the bag. This involvement diminishes their sense of helplessly sitting by and watching and thus may prevent them from withdrawing from the patient. We have all seen the family who sits always at the foot of the bed, talking with visitors and nurses about the patient almost as if she or he were not there. It is an art to include the family in the hospital care team, and it is beautiful to see when it works. The family stays involved, perhaps bathing or massaging the patient, if that is meaningful, bringing favorite foods, giving mouth care or skin care, keeping track of time for position changes or for symptom-management medications, and discussing changes and decisions with the patient, physicians, and nurses. This sense of inclusion is most helpful in allowing the family to talk openly among themselves about the illness, impending death, and future plans, and to accept support from friends and staff. In addition to decreasing the family's sense of helplessness, this arrangement enables them to feel useful, and they are aware of the gift of caring and comfort they give their loved one. Many hospitals arrange an extra cot or empty bed in the room so family can stay the night; particularly touching is the husband or wife who slips into bed with the patient to hold the person while she or he falls asleep.

Coordinating versus Doing

When a family is deciding whether they can care for their loved one at home and agonizing over the decision because the care is beyond their capabilities or schedules, the nurse can assure them that it is not always necessary to *do* everything themselves, but that they can *coordinate* the care and *assure* that it is done. The same assurance can be given family members whose other responsibilities keep them from doing as much as they would like. Guilt raises its powerful head in these situations, and people lose their objectivity. Assurance from a nurse "who knows" helps them accept that they are doing all they can and that coordination of friends, family, hired caregivers, or hospitalization is a reasonable and wholly acceptable alternative to doing it all themselves. Families near exhaustion can identify with the admonition that if they work to the point of exhaustion or illness they will leave the patient high and dry.

The location of the patient can be a hot issue when patient desires and family capabilities clash. If the patient wants to be at home but the family is exhausted and feeling stretched beyond their limits, the nurse can talk with the patient about a gift of respite to the family while she or he goes into the hospital for a few days (or whatever the need is). The family can then discuss whether they just need a rest or whether they cannot resume the home care again, and they can negotiate and plan together. If the patient is in the hospital wanting to go home and the family fears they won't be able to handle it even though they'd like to, the nurse can discuss the benefits of a trial period. Even if things do not work out, the family will have given a gift to the patient of some more time at home. This idea seems to avoid the succeed/fail trap for the family.

The Family at Home

At home, the family is responsible for the care of a person, the nature of whose disease—including its progression—often is not known to them. Moreover, they rarely already possess the caregiving skills they will be using. In addition, many families assume that good care is vigorous and *cure*-oriented and that therefore better care is available in the hospital than at home. They need educating as to the nature, symptoms, and predicted progression of the disease, along with learning the skills necessary for *comfort*-oriented care. Discussing the "natural" and expected progression of the disease toward death often reassures the family and prevents them from developing frightening images of the illness raging out of control and producing alarming and unmanageable symptoms. The capable nurse who assures the family that we "together can anticipate and manage the symptoms that arise" helps create a relaxed and competent family team (see also Chapter 7).

Fears about caring for a loved one at home affect family members' ability to function well, and these fears guide the nurse in interventions. Schubert (1982) studied areas of family fears and identified such fears as giving inadequate care, making a mistake (e.g., undermedicating or overdosing, or hurting the patient when moving him or her), not knowing what to do in emergencies and at death, and worries about other family members.

Here again, the goal is to *enable* the family to do the things they would like to do for the patient. The nurse can teach caregiving skills as well as assessment skills that facilitate simple decisions regarding medication administration and knowing when to call the nurse or physician. Families need simple, specific information given in a reassuring manner about anticipated symptoms, the probable manner of death, and their role in each of these areas. Suppose for example, that a patient with lung cancer is hypoxic, dyspneic on any exertion, and intermittently confused and that he is expected to die within a week. The style of explanation the nurse uses will depend on her judgment of the family's capacity to understand the strictly medical aspects of her explanation and of their emotional capacity to deal with the information she provides. One approach might begin as follows:

Joe's lung cancer seems to be moving on, and his lungs just aren't working efficiently anymore. He has to work harder to get the oxygen he needs, so he gets exhausted and short of breath lots more quickly than before, even when he talks. He gets confused sometimes because not enough oxygen is getting to his brain; that causes confusion. It will only happen some of the time, so when he's confused you can acknowledge it, and you can agree that you'll let him know if you don't understand something.

When Joe's lungs aren't working well, his heart also is working harder and is less efficient. As a result, less oxygen and nutrients reach all of his organs, and everything tends to slow down together. He'll tend to sleep more and want to do less, and he'll continue to be more short of breath when he does things. Usually what we see is that people sleep more and sometimes go into a coma (when they're not responding to us, but probably can hear us) for a few hours or a day or two, and then (while sleeping or in a coma) just slip off, and have a quiet and comfortable death. It's very helpful if you can be with him and talk to him, and reassure him if he gets anxious (getting less than a normal amount of oxygen can cause anxiety, among other things) and give him [a particular medication] for acute shortness of breath.... Here's how you tell when you should give it.... You can tell us anytime if you have questions or if something is happening and you don't know if you should worry or not.

There are many variations on this theme, but the reassurance that we expect a peaceful death and that the patient is progressing in the normal fashion toward that end is greatly relieving to the family.

Assessment and Intervention with Families

Assess the caregiving capabilities and the availability and willingness of the individuals in the family system. Are they physically able to give the care needed, and mentally able to assess changes in the patient and to know when to call for help? How can each person's personality and strengths contribute to the caregiving needs? Is one a doer, another a coordinator, another a person who can sit with the patient and talk or listen to music, or hold hands? Can each family member share all these things with the patient? It is often helpful to divide the tasks and to write down a schedule, so everyone knows who is doing what, and when. Some specifics that affect a family's ability to give physical care include their ability to tolerate the sights, smells, or acts involved (e.g., one person may be able to give injections but not to change the dressings on a purulent wound), and the ability of the family member and patient to handle the intimacy involved (e.g., a son bathing his mother). Often, instructions as to the simplest and most efficient ways of helping with basic care needs enable the family to give more comfortable care while reducing their fatigue. For example, bathing a person on a standard double bed can be exhausting! Teaching good body mechanics and transfer techniques relieve caregivers who have hefted patients out of bed for a month and have tried not to complain about their aching backs.

Some families can take care of basic personal care (bathing, toileting, feeding, mouthcare, transfers, skin care, etc.) but lack the confidence or skills to perform more technical tasks such as injections, dressing changes, or decubitus care. Some families give excellent care up to the point of a feared symptom such as acute dyspnea, then lose confidence that they can handle things, and desire hospitalization. This can often be avoided if the nurse anticipates problems and includes the family in plans to alleviate potentially difficult symptoms. When presented in a matter of fact manner, many technical procedures and potentially frightening symptoms can be handled very well by the family—witness the many patients living at home with a Hickman catheter, which must be irrigated, and requiring regular injections of medications.

The family needs to know what the anticipated symptom (as part of the natural progression of the illness) will be like, and *what they can do about* it. For example, the nurse can teach the family about moist-sounding breathing, or "death rattle" (see Chapter 9) and can instruct them in the use of Atropine. Then if necessary, they can inject Atropine to dry the secretions and calm the noisy respirations. Twenty-four hour on-call nursing is essential in this situation for consultation or emergency visit. When families know a nurse is *available 24 hours* a day by telephone or visit, they are able to cope with many things that would otherwise overwhelm them. The nurse should tell the family when to call (when they have questions about physical changes, when anything frightens them, or when they do not know whether a problem is trivial or important) and should explain who will answer their calls (a nurse who has been updated about the patient's physical problems and medications). Emergency availability does *not* replace comprehensive planning, affirmation, and support. Counselors, chaplain, home health aide, and volunteers should be used to help maintain a stable, functioning family unit. Also adding to the family's ability to deal with sometimes difficult care is the knowledge that it will not go on forever. People often need to hear the estimated, ballpark figure for how long the patient will live ("I can do this for two months, but not for a year!").

Learning the signs and symptoms of approaching death (see Chapter 9) helps the family keep perspective and stay calm toward the end. As our hospice home care team has steadily improved in preparing families for what to expect and what to do, we have received increasingly fewer calls requesting the presence of a nurse at the time of death. The calls we do receive are from families in which death occurs within a couple of days after we meet them or from those with especially difficult symptom management problems.

WHEN THE FAMILY INCLUDES CHILDREN

When a family includes children special needs and considerations must be taken into account. The experience of the dying child has been described briefly in Chapter 7. Now let us look at the child in the family, whatever role she or he plays. Again, in assessing children, one must look at them individually at first and then as part of a family system. Then appropriate interventions can be planned.

Basic Needs of the Child as an Individual

Children living through the illness and death of a family member are much like any other children, involved in their developmental stages and tasks, and fulfilling their roles in the family. The nurse should learn the age of each child, the child's past experiences with death, and the degree to which the parents are open, inclusive, and supportive of the child with respect to the death.

According to Adams & Moynihan (1982), five basic needs are common for children of any age (or for any adult, for that matter). First, *children must be given age-appropriate information about the illness and death.* The need is explored in the sections that follow.

Second, *children need reassurance that life and the family will go on,* and they need to know how it will be the same or different. For example, a father might say, "Mommy will be gone, but I'll get you ready for school in the morning, and Aunt Ruth will be here when you get home from school." It's most helpful if the dying parent can tell the children who will take over his or her roles; it helps the children to accept the change. Many children also need to know who will care for them if their other parent should die too (a common fear).

Third, *children must have the opportunity to express their own thoughts and feelings.* The hospice team members should give the children a chance to talk, to do what they want to do; going for ice cream, playing games, drawing pictures can build trust. Questions can start a conversation: "How is your Mom.... What do you think will happen?" Answer their questions, and try to learn how they interpret the things they've been told. Expressing their feelings is most important in working through the experience of the illness and loss of the loved one. Almost any feeling is acceptable and normal. For example, a child may feel guilty because he wishes Daddy were dying instead of Mommy. Reassure him that this just shows how much he loves Mommy and how much he wishes she weren't dying. Feelings that are buried now can resurface later again and again in the person's life, perhaps never understood as the source of the resultant depression or anxiety or inability to form lasting intimate relationships.

Fourth, *children need to be children.* They need to know that the parental role of guidance, love, and discipline will be maintained. Children, especially adolescents, can be greatly helpful in caring for a patient—housekeeping, running errands, and looking after smaller children. People may come to rely on this help, forgetting to give children equal time and encouragement to be children—to play with friends, to test limits, to be unable sometimes to deal with added responsibilities, to giggle in the corner and to have fun too.

Fifth, *children need to feel involved.* Age-related tasks can be found for any child to help the sick person. In one family I worked with the 15-year-old daughter cared for her father after school until her mother arrived home from work, up to and including giving pain shots. The 10-year old daughter did not give shots but massaged her father's hands and feet and helped him wash his hands and face. A younger child could draw a picture, or sit with Dad while they watched TV, or tell him about the day at school, or bring a washcloth, and so on. The knowledge that "I have an important role" in caring for Dad is very helpful to a child. You can ask children what they could do to make Dad more comfortable; their answers will be personal, family-specific gifts. But try to keep them from promising the impossible.

When children are excluded from what's happening with the dying person they often misinterpret events, and their fantasies are usually worse than the reality. "Mommy is spending more time with Johnny and hardly any with me; she must be mad at me." or "They won't talk about what's happening to Daddy and they don't spend much time with me; maybe he and Mommy don't like me anymore and they're going to leave me." They also will tend to act out more. They may regress to an earlier developmental stage (e.g., sucking their thumbs, wanting a bottle, wetting the bed). They may develop a school phobia or become a behavior problem at school or home. Or they may develop headaches, manifest physical symptoms similar to the patient's, become depressed, or have severe separation anxieties. These problems can be minimized if the family share both information and caregiving with the child.

Developmental Stages in Dealing with Death

Developmental stages affect the child and family who are experiencing the dying of a family member in two ways. First, the need to move on in one's development does not stop just because someone is dying; as already pointed out, the child must have the opportunity for experiences and activities that are part of his or her growing. Second, the stage influences the type of information and support the child needs. According to MacElveen-Hoehn (1981) four developmental stages outline the evolution of the child's understanding of death and dying.

0–3 years. Children as young as three can grasp the idea of death (Bluebond-Langner, 1978). The most important issue for this age group, however, is *separation* and *abandonment.* In this stage, children are focused on their own needs and need to know someone will be there to take care of them. Babies as young as six months have been seen to exhibit grief-like behaviors such as withdrawing, eating less, smiling and laughing less, or screaming and yelling.

3–5 years. Children in this period see death as *reversible.* Moreover, they do not think everyone dies, and they certainly do not think they themselves can die. Again, separation is a big issue, and children need to hear that other family members love them and won't abandon them no matter what.

In both of the youngest age groups, it is important to maintain routines and familiar people and events, both before and after the death. This is not the time to send the children away from home. They will do better being with the people who will be with them after the death.

6–10 years. This age group begins to get the idea that death is *final.* The general *concept* of death is understood; they see that lots of things live and then die, or that old people die more often than young. Beliefs about what happens after death depend on the family's beliefs. These beliefs can be helpful in conversation with children as they begin to fear death and to see it could happen to their parents. Magical thinking is very powerful at this age, and children often feel guilty because they believe that in some way they have caused the illness or death. They need reassurance from parents and others that they could neither cause nor prevent the death. Angry feelings cannot kill, anymore than loving feelings can prevent death (Suarez, 1980). Children in this age group have questions about their concepts: Will this happen to me? To you? What happens after death?

Adolescence.   Adolescents know death is *irreversible* and that everyone dies. Being in a state of disequilibrium, moving from child to adult and from dependence to independence, the teenager tends to have a foot in each camp, alternating between the two states. Many adolescents deny or repress their anxiety about death, trying to be grown up. They can discuss specifics and concepts, and often display great wisdom, spiced with swings to "childish" acting out.

When talking with children about an illness and death, the parents or nurse need to be simple and honest. Children can be very literal, and explanations can lead to unexpected reactions (MacElveen-Hoehn, 1981). For example, "Daddy went to heaven because God needed him" can lead to anger at God for taking Daddy when the *child* needed him. "Grandmother went to sleep and didn't wake up" can lead to fear of going to sleep. "He's gone away" can engender a variety of responses; thinking that the deceased will return, or anger that the person chose to go away, or fear that others won't return from a trip.

Helpful information is factual and simple (MacElveen-Hoehn, 1981). For example, if an old person dies, tell the young child, "Grandma's body grew old and her heart just wore out and can't be fixed." If the person died in the hospital, reassure the child: "Most of the time doctors can help people get better, but sometimes they can't fix what's wrong no matter how hard they try." This helps relieve fears that if the child needs hospitalization he or she will also die. If a death is accidental, discuss the need for judgment and for taking care of ourselves to avoid accidents. When death is caused by an illness the child can be told that the person had a disease and because the person's body could not work normally enough, she or he died. Because children may worry about how Mommy will breathe or eat in the coffin, it is important to explain that a dead body feels nothing and no longer needs anything like air or food.

Children should not be overloaded with too many details. Planning for the time of death, however, can help children. One can describe what the person will look like; one can plan whether the children will go into the room and what the family will do. The family can tell the children what to expect at the funeral: where they will sit, and with whom, and whether they can leave. And it is important to explain that some people will cry because they will be missing the person.

Difficult Feelings

Some common fears of children involve the magical thinking or preschool years. Children fear that they are the *cause* of the illness: "If I hadn't gotten mad at Mommy and wished she'd go away, maybe she wouldn't have gotten sick," or "God is punishing me for the bad things I've done." The fear that "it'll happen to me too" ranges from fear that "I'll catch the same disease" to "If God wanted Daddy and took him to heaven, what's to keep Him from taking me too"—or taking Mommy.

Moldow and Martinson (1979) identify problem feelings as negative feelings toward parents for not sharing information, sadness at the loss, anger at parents for giving the children less attention, and *guilt*. Guilt comes in many packages: there is guilt over anger toward the dying person; guilt over the child's inability to take care of the dying loved one; guilt over the child's inability to take care of the dying loved one; guilt over not having been quiet enough, or not doing enough (Suarez, 1980). Suppose, for example, that an adolescent who was angry that her father wasn't available for her when she needed him cannot let this go so that she can be with her father now that he needs her. You might negotiate, by asking what is the minimum the daughter can give her father that's genuine and will not lead to resentment; for example, this might be one hour's time a day or every other day. Then you could ask the father for the ideal and minimum time he wants with his daughter. Their answers might be surprisingly close (Suarez, 1980).

Children who may be expected to have a particularly difficult time with the bereavement include the oldest in the family, because they may be pushed into adult roles earlier. Previous experiences with separation and loss may help or hinder in the child's adjustment, depending on the level of trauma versus the growth in understanding of death and in one's own strengths. The number and kinds of changes they experience after the death, such as moves, changes in routines, or the addition to the family of a new member who takes over a lost parent's role can make the adjustment more difficult.

The Family System

Assess the family as discussed in the section on "The Family as Individual and System." What are the roles of the children, and what roles will be lost when the patient dies? Is the family open and inclusive of the children in the process of the illness? Is the parent able to give enough time, guidance, information, and support to the children? If not, as is often the case, help the family identify a person or persons among family or friends who can commit time to be with each of the children and supply some of their needs. Reassure the children that this attention is meant to supplement the parent's, not replace it.

When it is a child who is dying, a marital relationship may be greatly strained by the need to deal with the other children as well as to care for the dying one. The patient may take all the energy the parents have, and their support and nurturing for the other children and for each other can go by the wayside. In families where this problem appears to be intensifying, a referral for long-term counseling is valuable. A counseling referral is also important for families who are not communicating, although such people are very likely to refuse counseling. Where families are not discussing matters openly, acknowledge to the children that this makes things difficult for them and affirm that they are strong and can surive and learn from the situation (MacElveen-Hoehn, 1981).

REFERENCES

Adams, M., & Moynihan, R. *Issues of children with seriously ill and dying parents.* Paper presented at American Cancer Society Workshop, Portland, Oregon, July 1982.

Aguilera, D.C., & Messick, J.M. *Crisis intervention: Theory and methodology.* St. Louis: The C.V. Mosby Co., 1978.

Bluebond-Langner, M. *The private worlds of dying children.* Princeton, N.J.: Princeton University Press, 1978.

Burton, L. Tolerating the intolerable—The problems facing parents and children following diagnosis. In L. Burton (Ed.). *Care of the child facing death.* London: Routledge and Kegan Paul, 1974.

Cohen, P., Dizenhus, I.M., & Winget, C. Family adaptation to terminal illness and death of a parent. *Social Casework,* 1977, *58,* 223–228.

Hollingsworth, C. Role adjustments in families after death. *World Journal of Psychosynthesis,* 1978, *10,* 13–16.

Kalish, R.A. The effects of death upon the family. In L. Pearson (Ed.). *Death and dying.* Cleveland: Press of Case Western Reserve University, 1969.

MacElveen-Hoehn, P. Children's loss of a parent. Hospice of Snohomish County lecture in Everett, Washington, February 1981.

Marks, M.J. Dealing with death: The grieving patient and family. *American Journal of Nursing,* 1976, *76,* 1488–91.

Minuchin, S. *Families and family therapy.* New York: Basic Books, 1974.

Moldow, D.G. & Martinson, I.M. *Home care for dying children: A manual for parents.* Minneapolis: University of Minnesota, 1979.

Reilly, D.M. Death propensity, dying and bereavement: A family systems perspective. *Family Therapy,* 1978, *5,* 35–55.

Satir, V. *Peoplemaking.* Palo Alto: Science and Behavior Books, 1972.

Schubert, V. Anticipatory guidance for family caregivers to manage the last few days at home. Paper presented at Hospice of Seattle Advanced Symposium on Care of the Terminally Ill, Seattle, February 26, 1982.

Slivkin, S.E. Death and living: A family therapy approach. *American Journal of Psychoanalysis,* 1977, *37,* 317–23.

Stoll, R.I. Guidelines for spiritual assessment. *American Journal of Nursing,* 1979, *79,* 1574–1577.

Stubblefield, K.S. A preventive program for bereaved families. *Social Work Health Care,* 1977, *2,* 379–389.

Suarez, M. Children and Death. Hospice of Seattle lecture in Seattle, Washington, July 1980.

Taylor, P.B. Understanding Sexuality in the Dying Patient. *Nursing 83,* 1983, *13,* 54–55.

White, W.L. Family dynamics and family counseling. In *Hospice Education Program for Nurses.* Publication No. HRA 81-27. Washington, D.C.: U.S. Department of Health and Human Services, 1981.

Wilson, H.S., & Kneisl, C.R. Life turning points. In *Psychiatric nursing.* Menlo Park: Addison-Wesley Publishing Company, 1979.

1. F	*6. F*
2. F	*7. T*
3. T	*8. T*
4. T	*9. T*
5. F	*10. F*

13

Establishing a Community Hospice

Answer the following questions True (T) or False (F). Answers appear on the last page of this chapter.

1. *A hospice program has the greatest chance of succeeding if it is established by physicians.*

2. *If a hospice program is not formed and accepting patients within six months it has little chance to succeed.*

3. *It should be clearly stated from the first planning meeting that a community hospice program must generate all of its own services in order to be consistent with high standards of care.*

4. *Many community hospices have formed planning committees before they had adequate funding to begin patient care.*

5. *One criterion for all members of a hospice Board of Directors is experience in direct patient care.*

6. *Writing a clear goal statement can unite the board in purpose and provide an excellent public education document.*

7. *Agencies and institutions in a community should be willing to provide services to the hospice program without compensation.*

8. *A sound public education program in the community will broaden the program's base of support.*

9. *In order to receive donations an organization must have an IRS tax-exempt number.*

10. *By-laws should be straightforward and general. Specific rules should be addressed in a policy manual.*

One strong characteristic of hospice programs which prosper is a constant concern, above all personal and institutional ambitions for the quality of care provided to patients and their families. *

A NURSE, a minister, a physician—it is not particularly important *who* first perceives the need for a community hospice program. But the manner in which that program is established and the steps that are taken, or ignored, are crucial. The first months in the growth of the community hospice are the most essential for establishing lines of communication, fostering community support, educating professionals in an accurate concept of hospice care, and generally establishing the kind of climate among area policymakers that will enhance the development of the program.

THE CHALLENGE OF BEGINNING

Many people who begin community hospices want to know precisely how long the steps should take, from the first committee to first patient. It is impossible to predict the course of development, but generally experience has shown that a program that utilizes existing professional resources and has sound financial support, such as a hospital or nursing home with personnel and dollars already committed, will develop in about a year. A program beginning in an unaffiliated professional and lay committee that has to generate these services through affiliation, fund-raising, and professional education may need up to three years. Note also that there is a direct relationship between the rate of development and clarity and consensus on program goals and priorities.

---

*Blues, A. Characteristics of a successful hospice program. In Ajemian, I., Mount B. (ed.). *Royal Victoria Hospital Manual of Palliative/Hospice Care.* New York: Arno Press, 1980, p. 60.

The problem of fitting hospice into the bureaucratic maze of American health care without changing its purpose and nature is perhaps the most significant challenge of the hospice movement.

A basic tenet of the community hospice program is the utilization of existing local resources. It is counterproductive to duplicate already existing local agencies and services. It can save time, money, and energy to foster a cooperative rather than a competitive spirit among the groups able to offer excellent care.

Forming a hospice program within a community by interfacing with existing provider agencies and professionals has been likened by one local director to attempting to assemble a plane while it is in flight. Hospice must have a unique involvement in the community because of its very special service. In addition, hospice organizers' management styles and goals must reflect the special needs of their own community. It cannot be repeated too frequently that hospice should not be established in order to threaten the roles of excellent hospitals, nursing homes, or home health agencies. Koff (1980) states that hospices should "develop relationships with these health agencies in order to interpret the unique service of hospice" (p. 137).

Depending on the financial resources of the group, it may be helpful to employ a part-time staff person to coordinate the activities of the planning group. A less expensive alternative would be to appoint a chairperson who does not have other pressing professional or personal commitments.

An initial task of the planning committee should be self-education. They should become well versed in the hospice literature and the experience of other functioning hospice groups. Site visits to near-by operational programs that exemplify a variety of models and settings will be useful. The committee should be in touch with the city, state, or regional hospice association and the National Hospice Organization.

Assessment of Needs

Next, or perhaps to some extent concurrent with self-education, should be the completion of a thorough assessment of needs in the community for care of the terminally ill. It is wise to estimate the following for the community population.

- overall incidence of death
- incidence of death from cancer
- numbers of terminal patients cared for by local nursing homes, hospitals
- numbers of patients traveling to large urban medical centers for on-going care
- occupancy census of local hospitals, nursing homes, home health agencies

The complete needs assessment is also an assessment of the resources already available to meet these needs. Among those categories of agencies and professionals whose input should be tallied against community need for services to the terminally ill and their families are (1) health care provider institutions, agencies, and groups; (2) service agencies; and (3) professional–academic organizations and institutions.

In fact, some or all of the people and institutions listed in Table 13-1 will probably be present and willing to interface (Weigart, 1981). It is possible, however, that these institutions and organizations are already providing service to the limits of their budget and that any additional demand on their services would also have to be supported in some way by funds, volunteers, or materials by the hospice program.

It is also valuable to develop a resource list of available volunteers. For example, does the community include the people listed in Table 13-2? Can their help be enlisted?

The Hospice Concept in the U.S., writes Janet Lunceford, is still struggling for widespread acceptance into our health care system. A myriad of legal and financial problems are yet to be resolved before hospice can be truly

Table 13-1.   *Does Your Community Have These Programs?*

American Cancer Society	Community Senior Citizen Services
American Red Cross	Homemaker Services, profit and
Area Agency on Aging	nonprofit
Tumor Registry	Drug stores:
Vocational Rehabilitation	with delivery services
Visiting Nurse Association	with low-cost pricing policies e.g.,
Department of Public Health Nursing	American Association of Retired
Agencies providing child care	Persons
Church groups	with policy of offering generic drugs
Women's groups	(discount drug service)
Service clubs	Candlelighters
Fraternal organizations	Make Today Count
Loaves and Fishes Site food program	Compassionate Friends
Adult day-care centers	Acute care hospitals
Meals on Wheels food delivery	Out-patient departments
Hot lunch centers	Nursing homes
Various "take-out" food services,	Skilled care facilities
especially with home delivery	Extended care facilities
Grocery stores that permit home	Social Security Administration office
delivery	Community transportation services
Drop-in centers	University extension services, especially
Boy Scouts	handicapped homemaker services
Girl Scouts	

Table 13-2. *Volunteer Resource List*

Clergyperson	Occupational therapist
Child care worker	Pharmacist (with a clinical specialty)
Dance (movement) therapist	Physician
Dentist	Physiotherapist
Family counselor	Play therapist
Gerontologist	Poetry therapist
Lawyer	Psychiatrist, psychiatric nurse,
Music therapist	or psychiatric social worker
Nurse	Psychologist
Nutritionist	Social worker with a medical orientation.

integrated (1980). In spite of the obvious benefits of hospice care to families, patients and health care professionals, it does not fit well into any of the models now identified by licensing and reimbursement plans.*

The Steps

There is, in spite of the complexity of the task, an orderly sequence of steps that should be taken by the developers to assure the on-going existence of the program. This text will define three basic stages: formation, early development, and stability. Formation includes (1) forming a planning committee; (2) assessing needs and resources; and (3) developing goals, writing by-laws, incorporating, and establishing tax-exempt status. Careful attention to all these matters is essential, for a poorly constructed program will continue to plague the project and its implementors. The second stage, of early development, includes the designation of (1) committees, (2) staff, and (3) affiliations. The third stage, stability, encompasses (1) implementation and (2) funding.

FORMATION

Establishment of a Planning Committee

At the outset there should be a planning committee or a task force of interested persons. This group, which may begin as a committee or another agency such as a church, hospital, university, or home health agency, should

---

Lunceford, J.L. Hospice in America. Paper Presented International Conference on Hospice. London, 1980.

make every effort to enlist immediately the advice and help of a multi-disciplinary cross-section of community professionals and lay people. This group should include key individuals from those health care organizations and agencies that will ultimately be involved in providing patient care or staff development.

After this first period of self-education and a beginning needs–resources assessment, it is crucial that the hospice planning committee take time to define its interest and expectations for the hospice program. The answers to questions like these asked early in the planning process are extremely valuable.

- Why do you want to establish a hospice program?
- Where will you get the funding?
- How much time do members of the planning committee really have?
- What services could the hospice provide that are not already adequately provided?

Statement of Purpose

Programs are being started and will more than likely disappear within 18 months because they really never develop a clear statement of purpose. Others have poor reasons to start up such as a desire to compete with another, recently founded institution, to fill vacant hospital or nursing home beds, or to challenge poor care in institutions or shake up perceived medical community indifference. Occasionally it also happens that a single individual wants a hospice in the community and is even willing to fund it in spite of an obvious indication of lack of professional support or need. The time must be right for those who have essential skills to contribute, and the enthusiasm and commitment must be there on a wide basis.

Groups have found that the task of writing a statement of purpose is well worth the effort. It allows people to consider their own feelings about death, their profession, and their expectations for the program—one that helps individuals become aware of their philosophies. A well formed statement of purpose or philosophy will help to keep the group unified in its mission and prevent confusion in its decision making. Such a statement is also an excellent handout for educating the public and the media about what your group intends. People are far more supportive of something if they understand it.

From the statement of purpose should evolve well-articulated long-term goals and specific short-term goals. The literature contains guidelines for the writing of clear, evaluable goals, but we may note that the content of those goals should cover the following areas:

- Admissions criteria
- Services
- Population served
- Size-scope of program
- Fiscal security and reimbursement issues
- Education
- Research and evaluation
- Staff support
- Administrative growth
- Certification and licensing

Along with the goals should be an estimate of the time and resources necessary to accomplish them and responsibility should be assigned for implementation and accountability. The principles outlined in the NHO Standards document should be carefully studied. Without such principles, goals may be vague and the ability to define hospice care elusive. All programs need not be alike, nor like an existing model. But all hospices should demonstrate conformity to the basic hospice philosophy outlined in Chapter 6, "Principles & Standards of Hospice Care."

Formation of a Board of Directors

Once the planning committee has determined a genuine local need for hospice services and has written its goals for the scope of those services, a board of directors can be formed. A board usually comprises a group of 9–12 people selected for purposes of setting policy and devising the means to carry out the objectives of the group as a whole. Officers are elected, such as president, vice-president, secretary, treasurer, and an executive committee may be formed to carry out policy on a daily basis. In a for-profit corporation these board members may actually do the work of the organization and be paid for it. In a nonprofit corporation they must get *no* monetary return on their investment.

Incorporation

Anyone may involve himself or herself in hospice activities, either as an individual or in coordination with others, without actually incorporating. Some definite advantages to incorporation as a nonprofit organization, however, are as follows:

- Eligibility for tax-exempt status
- Security in corporate responsibility for the actions of those in the agency
- Accountability for services and resources within an organizational framework

The laws governing incorporation and tax-exempt status are somewhat complex. Thus it is strongly recommended that a qualified attorney and/or accountant assist the group throughout the process of incorporation.

The nonprofit corporation is an entity created and recognized by the law. The original governmental thinking behind the nonprofit organization was that if an organization were formed with the purpose of providing a service that is good for society, the government could let the organization collect the funds directly from the individual taxpayer. In addition, the government could allow the taxpayer to determine *where* this money went and to receive credit against the taxes she or he would otherwise pay to help the government run the same service.

The basic document to be filed with the state office responsible for the certification, e.g., the office of or Secretary of State, the Corporate Commissioner is an Articles of Incorporation. Most articles or certificate of incorporation require you to set forth the following information:

- Name of corporation
- Period of duration, which may be perpetual
- Purposes for which corporation is organized and membership classes, if any
- Provisions for regulation of internal affairs, including provision for distribution of assets on dissolution or final liquidation
- Address of office and name of registered agent
- Number, names, and addresses of initial members of board of directors
- Names and addresses of all incorporators, those persons forming the original organization. There are variations among the states, so it is best to check specific requirements before writing the document.

The necessary forms and a modest filing fee must then be filed at the state office. When, after several weeks, a copy (marked "filed") is returned to the registered agent, who is the person who is designated for receiving official communications, the corporation exists legally!

After the corporate by-laws are written, an official organizational meeting of the group of incorporators must be held, at which the first official board of directors is elected and the by-laws are adopted. Some groups spend several meetings writing the by-laws before the board is elected.

By-Laws

The purpose of nonprofit corporation by-laws is to provide the basic rules for the internal organization and management of the corporation according to its stated purpose or mission. The by-laws should cover, among other topics, the corporation's fiscal year; the number, place, and dates on which meetings of the board are to be held; voting procedures and quorum;

election duties, and procedures for removal of directors and officers; committees; membership and dues, if any; and arrangements for the keeping of books and other records.

Any provision that is consistent with the articles of incorporation may be written into the by-laws. However, once the by-laws are adopted by a board of directors, the power to alter, amend, or repeal the by-laws or to adopt new by-laws will be restricted to the board unless otherwise provided in the articles of incorporation or by-laws themselves. Such changes can be costly, time-consuming, and cumbersome, so the best by-laws are simple, direct, and general. Also to prevent loss of time and disappointment, check the chosen name for the hospice corporation through the state office to make sure no other organization exists with the same or similar name. Specific rules and procedures that may be subject to change over time should be written as "policy," in a separate policy manual that may not require full board action for alteration. A copy of model by-laws, as proposed in the Model Non-Profit Corporation Act, is available from the American Bar Association or from a state bar association.

Tax Exempt Status of Nonprofit Corporations

Most community nonprofit corporations providing hospice services will want to seek exemption as charitable organizations as described under the Internal Revenue Code—see I.R.C. Section 501(c)(3)—as amended by the Tax Reform Act of 1976, Section 1313(a).

Tax-exempt status exempts the nonprofit corporation from paying income tax on its income. In addition, persons or organizations who make donations to the corporation may deduct those donations when filing tax returns.

Seeking tax-exempt status is best done with the advice of an accountant and/or an attorney. An application must be filed with the District Director of the Internal Revenue Service for the district in which the organization's principal office is located. Several documents will need to be submitted, including a description of the organization's activities, its membership, its organizational chart, and copies of the articles of incorporation and the by-laws. A completed form SS-4 will also be required in order to receive an Employer Identification Number. It is necessary to have this number, which is used for witholding employee taxes, before anyone can be employed by the corporation.

If all is well documented, within several months the IRS will issue a ruling or determination letter. This letter may be issued before an organization has begun providing patient services, if the corporation's purposes are clearly defined. If the hospice is denied an exemption, the decision can and should be contested through the Regional Director of Appeals and within 30 days from

Table 13-3.

- When writing by-laws make them clear and broad, so that small operational changes do not require full board action.

- Write specific organizational, fiscal, personnel, office, and committee procedures in a policy manual. Make sure each employee and board committee member has a copy.

- Check the name chosen for the organization with the state office prior to filing for incorporation, in order to avoid delay. (The name must not be the same as or highly similar to the name of any other organization incorporated in that state.)

- File as quickly as possible for corporate standing and tax-exempt status. It is far easier to receive a positive determination before the organization has a complex history of meetings and activities that may be difficult for the IRS to interpret.

- Do not overlook continued filing with the IRS of correct tax information for the nonprofit tax-exempt organization.

the date of the determination letter. In the appeal, try to determine the basis for the denial and to redefine these areas in your description of proposed services.

At the time of this writing one interesting fact for hospices that have access to some immediate funding is that if the application for exempt status is filed within 15 months from the end of the month in which the hospices were organized, the exemption, if granted, will be retroactive to the date of organization, rather than the date the application was received. In other words, money donated prior to the granting tax exempt status will be tax deductible if the hospice is ultimately awarded tax-exempt status.

Lastly, the hospice board should be aware that even though the organization has obtained its tax-exempt status, it is not relieved of its obligation to file certain reporting forms with the Internal Revenue Service. Table 13-3 provides a helpful checklist of steps in the formation of a hospice program, including such filing of information into the IRS.

EARLY DEVELOPMENT: COMMITTEE ORGANIZATION AND FUNCTION

Even as the board of directors is awaiting a decision on the status of the organization as a nonprofit, tax-exempt corporation, the work of hospice can begin. This may best be accomplished by forming committees for specific purposes. The membership of each committee should include one representative from the board. Committees that hospice groups have found valuable are generally organized by task rather than by profession. Although some hospices still have nurses' committees, social work committees, medical committees and the like, such an arrangement does not support the multidisciplinary communication so essential to hospice care. Some useful committees that can be organized as needed are outlined in this section (in no particular order of importance). Each committee as formed should articulate its specific purposes and responsibilities.

Patient Care Committee

This multidisciplinary committee actively interprets the hospice's standards of care. The committee will be responsible for the range, appropriateness, and manner in which care is provided, records are kept, and care teams are coordinated. The committee should develop a system of team meetings and communication. The board may also assign to this committee the development of a plan for meeting licensure criteria and the establishment of billing services. In the latter function, the committee should of course work with an accountant and with the finance committee.

Intake–Admissions Committee

This multidisciplinary committee may establish criteria for admission, develop and review admission forms, and consult with referring physicians as to appropriate referrals. Admission criteria should consider patient–family needs and the hospice ability to meet those needs.

Finance–Development Committee

This committee is responsible for developing a sound and permanent financial base for the hospice. The committee should stimulate grants, donations, memorials, and community support. It can also handle issues of reimbursement such as requirements through Blue Cross/Blue Shield, Medicare and others. It is wise to have persons with accounting, fund raising, grant writing and financial experience on this committee.

The finance committee, along with the administrator-chairperson, should immediately begin to develop an outline of reasonable and necessary costs associated with the hospice organization even if patients are not paying for services. These should include direct care costs, administrative and overhead expenses and program expenses. When determined necessary for the patient, the hospice should provide, and assign a charge which would be billed if reimbursement were available for the following:

- Home care services, including skilled nursing, home health aid-homemaker, therapy (physical, speech, occupational, nutrition)
- Prescriptions
- Hospital care
- Physician home and office visits

- Durable medical equipment: beds, wheelchairs, orthopedics
- Patient travel from home and institution
- Bereavement counseling
- Patient psychological and social counseling

Realistic fees can be arrived at when the past history of costs is analyzed and a realistic estimate is averaged.

Friends of Hospice Committee

This committee comprises a group of volunteers other than those who will do direct patient care. It is responsible for such necessary activities as fund-raising events, media contacts, good-will benefits, the newsletter and general office management. It is an excellent way for people who may be in an active bereavement stage or who do not want direct patient involvement to participate in the program.

Bereavement Committee

This committee has a special interest in a coordinated program of bereavement and the use of a bereavement counseling team. It is responsible for the evaluation of bereavement care, development of a bereavement training component of the education program, and on-going training for those doing bereavement work.

Counseling–Spiritual Concerns Committee

The function of this committee is to coordinate with the patient care committee the components of counseling and/or spiritual concerns. These concerns are sometimes handled by two separate committees or by a subdivision of the patient care committee. This group will, for example, determine procedures of dealing with patient needs and family conflicts, religious counseling, interface with and education of local religious leaders, and observing and reporting patient/family concerns.

Legislative Committee

This committee will not be the focus of activity in the early establishment of hospice services, but it can have a tremendous impact on the long-range future of the program. It is this committee that will undertake the education of policymakers in the areas of regulation, licensure, reimbursement, and laws regarding provision of services. Be sure to note some restrictions regarding lobbying exist for non-profit corporations and should be checked.

Education and Training Committee

The education and training committee is responsible for the development and implementation of on-going education programs for professionals, lay volunteers, and public. The committee also considers options to develop seminars, workshops, resource materials, library and media presentations, and a speaker's bureau. A special, well-informed subcommittee may be organized to conduct public presentations. The committee should also develop a support program to address staff stress (see also Chapter 17).

Lay Volunteer Committee

This committee is responsible for the development and coordination of a lay volunteer program within the interdisciplinary framework, including the screening and assignment of volunteers. This committee can assume full or partial responsibility for lay volunteer training or share this with the education and training committee.

Research and Evaluation Committee

This committee is sometimes combined with education and training. It is responsible for needs and resource assessment, program self-evaluation, and research into improved therapies. The committee's effort should also be directed at establishing a basic data set for funding requests to support the viability of the hospice. Helpful in gaining support are the following data:

- Projected caseload and costs
- Costs for similar care in other-than-hospice settings
- Patient origin studies
- Use of services
- Patient–family evaluation of services
- Affiliation with, use, and endorsement of existing community services

Other Committees

Other committees that serve a useful purpose in hospice include the following:

- An employee council which is composed of all levels of hospice staff and meets monthly to review personnel practices, policy changes, and problems. This council should make recommendations to the hospice administrator.
- A committee on confidentiality may meet as necessary to review team management of records and to consider requests for research, special trainees, or student involvement.
- Special sub-committees or study groups for *inpatient safety, infection control, pain management,* or *staff stress* may be formed as the need arises.

Quite obviously, all of the committees described in this section are not necessary in the early stages of development, and even after community needs are expressed, for example, some may be combined with others—bereavement with counseling, admissions with patient care, research with education.

Careful attention should be paid to the selection of the chairpersons of all committees. These persons should be willing to devote both time and effort to the organization of their assignments. It is nice if they have professional stature; it is much more important that they have real capability and the desire to work.

As committees begin to develop policy and promote programs, a number of events should occur. Volunteers will be selected and trained, articles and public relation speeches will inform the consumer, professional contacts will be developed, fund-raising will proceed, and affiliations and working relationships will be defined.

HOSPICE STAFF

Nursing and Medical Directors

Great care should be taken in the selection of nursing and medical directors. Frequently the patient care committee chairperson is the nursing director. It is also an advantage, when possible, that the director of nursing be a paid staff member.

The nursing director will perhaps coordinate a nursing staff of registered nurses, licensed practical nurses, and nursing assistants. In some programs the entire care team is coordinated by the nursing director. She or he is responsible for coordination of inpatient and home care including assessment and diagnosis, definition of problems and tasks, and results of the care team. Because it is frequently the nursing staff who is most readily available to the patient, it is this staff who will most often provide information, explanations, and instructions to the patient.

There is tremendous variation in the way medical directors are selected and utilized in the program. Some programs are basically organized and directed by a physician or group of physicians who do all the patient medical care. In other programs, the medical director is both available to care for admitted hospice patients and to work with the patients' own doctor. In yet other hospices, the medical director may be a medical educator and a spokesperson for the group, offering advice and assistance in areas pertaining to therapies, medication, or diagnoses and the like. Each program, legally, should have a medical director who is a currently licensed physician who understands the principles and practices of palliative care. She or he must relate effectively to the patient-family, to their attending physicians, and to the professional community. Reimbursement may be dependent on the status of the medical director. The wise selection of an excellent medical director can assure physician acceptance of hospice service and increase referrals.

The physician should possess special expertise in symptom management —especially pain control—and an awareness of the psychological impact of terminal disease. It is essential that she or he be able to work effectively with the hospice interdisciplinary team. In addition, the physician should have ready access to consultation in the areas of surgical–medical–rehabilitation expertise in the community.

The degree and type of involvement by the medical and nursing directors should be carefully worked out. And a formal statement of policy should be written so as to avoid confusion.

The Administrator

Both the nursing and medical directors will no doubt have an extensive health care background. Frequently, however, an administrator is necessary as well. Hospices are finally beginning to recognize that the complexities of reimbursement, personnel, accounting, and grant writing go beyond the normal areas of expertise of the care provider. The administrator is essential in overseeing the entire operation and keeping the hospice a viable fiscal entity. She or he should have appropriate training and experience in the management of health care services and should be experienced in working with health care providers and community agencies.

AFFILIATION WITH EXISTING RESOURCE PROGRAMS

The advantages of affiliation or cooperation with existing services and agencies are numerous. Organizations such as the American Cancer Society, American Red Cross, Meals on Wheels, American Federation of Women's Clubs, Junior League, as well as churches, synagogues and a variety of smaller programs can be included in responding to patient–family needs. Community hospice programs will succeed because of their willingness to cooperate with public and private home health agencies, nursing homes, and hospitals.

While the durable aspects of affiliation with some health care providers has become obvious, coordination with long-term care facilities is less developed.

Two basic factors support the contention that long-term care facilities need to be involved in providing hospice services. First, life expectancy is some 20 years longer than it was in 1900 (Allen, C., Brotman, H., 1981, p. 8). As medical science has decreased the death rate from acute infectious disease, people live to an age when chronic diseases such as stroke, heart attack, and cancer are more prevalent. Since chronic diseases require chronic care, many persons live in long-term facilities for several years before they die. Their homes are sold and families adapt to caring for them through the help of a nursing home.

Second, while many families are still in tact, the trends towards more working women, later marriage, more divorces, fewer children and greater geographic mobility mean considerable less family-centered care. The adult children of an 85-year-old woman, may themselves be 65 and in poor health.

Elderly individuals, as they approach dying, may not have the family and friends support system which is such an essential part of hospice care. Over 60 percent of women over 65 in 1981 were unmarried, widowed, divorced, or never married. (R. Sommers, 1982, p. 223) Of this group 43 percent live alone or with people who are not relatives. There is for these women, as well as for a large group of men, no one to take the responsibility for their care. These individuals who enter the long-term care facility following perhaps a stroke or a broken hip, will most likely remain within this system for terminal care.

The long-term care team should ideally have access to the training and basic conditions of a good palliative or hospice care program. There is a common argument that long-term care facilities will not, either because of philosophy or finances, provide complete hospice services. The institutional setting is a difficult one to personalize and individualize. Staff resources may be overextended making intensive support and time commitment for a dying patient almost impossible. But these arguments do not address the reality that people *will* die in these facilities and quality palliative care should be offered in the highest quality form it can be implemented. The difficulty of an ideal should not be used as an excuse not to attempt it. Many nursing homes provide skilled and sensitive palliative care and could contribute to our understanding of care for those alone and elderly. Much can be gained through cooperation between hospice and long-term care professionals that will ultimately benefit all their patients.

It can help financially to utilize local facilities, and interfacing with established home health agencies, visiting nurse associations, hospitals or nursing homes may facilitate reimbursement of skilled nursing services. A hospice may also fall under the umbrella of their certificate of need and licensing and thus bypass this costly and time-consuming procedure. (See Chapter 16 for methods of interfacing with an existing health care system.) It is important, however, that in any affiliation, the hospice maintain an autonomous administration (see also the Standards of Hospice Care, in Chapter 6).

STABILITY

The third stage in establishing a community hospice program is without end; it is ongoing and highly individual in character. It is generally agreed that qualities that contribute to hospice success are flexibility, persistence, and a sense of humor. A survey of 21 community hospices done through the E. McDowell Community Cancer Network, Inc. in Lexington, Kentucky revealed some interesting similarities among those hospices that were well supported by their communities and that had reached a stage of providing high quality care (see Table 13-4). No hospice program surveyed was without

Table 13-4. *Typical Characteristics of Successful Community-based Hospice Programs*

- The founding, or steering, committee had an accurate vision of the value of palliative care and the unflagging enthusiasm to inspire others to the cause. The committee presented the program as an additional health care service, not a "competitive attack on poor services."

- Key professionals, such as physicians, nurses, clergypeople, and agencies were included from the very beginning on the planning committee.

- Research was done early on community needs and available resources to determine the necessity for and feasibility of establishing a program. Clear goals were developed and written to define program services and the relationship of these services to those offered by other agencies.

- A broad-based program of public education was carried out through the media, speaker's bureau. Media persons were given factual material and interviews and encouraged not to "sensationalize" but to present accurately such issues as drugs, medical controversies, patient rights, and/or euthanasia.

- An executive committee was clearly defined. Individuals accepted leadership roles within such taskforces as education, patient care, bereavement, fund-raising and finance, and volunteers.

- By letters, speeches, and individual appointments official endorsement was secured from local professional associations.

- An education program intially drew on the best national resources available and then proceeded to follow a core curriculum adapted from an experienced, on-going program.

- The projected number of patients and geographic region to be served was realistically limited to staff and volunteer capabilities. An organized program of staff support was implemented before staff could begin to feel the effects of the stress inherent in the caregiving professions.

- Central to the administrative and professional components of the program are at least a small core of paid staff.

- Team composition and responsibilities are not compromised in the face of limited resources.

- Criticism is addressed openly with professional and educational lectures, reports, and individual conferences, and program weakness are acknowledged and marked for concerted attack. Critics are enlisted as part of an evaluative team.

Source: Blues (1980).

problems in at least one of the areas outlined in Table 13-4. And it must be admitted that much-needed programs had sometimes succumbed to disputes over agency control, professional role definitions—even the logo design to be used on letterheads. A strong characteristic, however, of programs that prosper is a constant concern, above all personal or institutional ambitions, for the quality of care provided to patients and their families.

No hospice should be developed without a funding plan. In the early development stages, many programs function with little or no funding. Some community hospices have grown up with a total treasury of less than $50.00 during this first stage. However, as mentioned earlier, few hospices operate efficiently without an administrator, basic office and telephone services, and educational expenses. This takes money.

Success in obtaining initial funding, before there are families to testify personally as to the hospice's value, will depend on community relations established through media, service organizations and clubs, and the materials developed and distributed. Each community will have special potential funds available, and most hospices are finding that grass roots sources are more approachable. It seems that organizations have more success in getting start-up funding through sources that actually see direct results from the services in their own community than from national foundations.

Funding can take three basic forms. *Philanthropic support* is provided by local foundations, individuals and memorials, churches, clubs, and other organizations. *Public support* is provided by governmental agencies such as the Administration on Aging, the National Institute of Mental Health, and the National Cancer Institute. Now that hospice is a somewhat established concept, these agencies have a particular interest in new methods for the delivery of quality care, innovative therapies, and evaluation and cost containment. A third area of funding is *reimbursement for services* through Medicare, Medicaid and, private, third-party payers such as Blue Cross. At the time of this writing, such payments are sometimes insufficient to cover hospice services, but they do provide ongoing funding for some of the nursing and medical care and will hopefully be funding many other components of hospice care in the future.

Any funding strategy, according to English (1980) should examine the following sources:

- Reimbursement and fee for service
- Shared services
- Federal government
- State government
- County–city governments
- Foundations
- Corporations-Associations

- Employee or union funds
- Other organizations, such as churches, societies, and clubs
- Private individuals
- General public

The effort to secure funding should be coordinated through both the finance and development committee and the research committee and directed in a unified way by a knowledgable administrator. If a single board member seeks and obtains a small grant from a particular source, that source may be unwilling to entertain a broader proposal (English, 1980).

REFERENCES

Allan, C., & Brothan, H. *Chartbook on aging in America.* Washington, D.C.: 1981. Whitehouse Conference on Aging, 1981, 8–9.

Blues, A. Caring for the terminally ill: The hospice movement. *Journal of Pastoral Counseling,* 1980, *15,* 28–33.

English, D. Can hospice be accomplished financially? (1978 Address to Catholic Hospital Association, St. Louis). In T.H. Koff, *Hospice: A caring community,* Cambridge, Mass.: Winthrop Publishers, Inc., 1980.

Gibson, M. How can it be accomplished financially? (1978 Address to Catholic Hospital Association, St. Louis). In T.H. Koff, *Hospice: A caring community,* Cambridge, Mass.: Winthrop Publishers, Inc., 1980.

Koff, T.H. *Hospice: A caring community.* Cambridge, Mass.: Winthrop Publishers, Inc., 1980.

Lunceford, J.L. Hospice in America. Paper presented at International Conference on Hospice, London, 1980.

Somers, A.R. Long-term care for the elderly and disabled. *New England Journal of Medicine, 307,* 4, 1982, pp. 221–225.

Wiegert, O., Blues, A., Wiegert, T. Community hospice programs: Factors to consider when planning to provide interfacing home and inpatient care options. *Journal of Obulatory Care Management, 4,* 4, 1981, pp. 47–57.

1. F	6. T
2. F	7. F
3. F	8. T
4. T	9. F
5. F	10. T

14

Integration of Hospice into the Acute Care System

Answer the following questions True (T) or False (F). Answers appear on the last page of this chapter.

1. *It has been clearly demonstrated that the only acceptable model for inpatient hospice care is a separate unit.*

2. *The long-term goals of inpatient hospices should focus primarily on the needs of cancer patients and cancer units.*

3. *A hospital's philosophy of care, goals, and objectives are major indicators of the possibility of developing a hospice program within that institution.*

4. *Hospice programs within hospitals can expect most of their funding to come from regular reimbursement channels.*

5. *Hospice educational efforts must be multifaceted, to include the general public; professionals throughout the hospital; the hospice team, including volunteers; and the patient-family.*

6. *In planning a hospice program, it is important to define the role of the hospital medical director in relation to the patient's attending physician and the rest of the hospice team.*

7. *The guiding strategy of a new hospice program should be to confront and challenge the staff providing fragmented care for the dying on the acute care wards.*

There is a danger...that terminal care may be seen as esoteric antiordinary medicine. It should be fully integrated into the best of medicine and recognized as a logical continuation of it when the focus on cure is no longer appropriate. *

T HE PRECEDING CHAPTER describes the groundwork for developing a community-based hospice. Because the same foundation is needed to begin a hospice within a hospital community, this chapter describes the same stages of building a hospice—formation, early development, and stability—while it focuses on the unique aspects of developing a program within the acute care system.

The long-range goal of establishing a hospice program within a hospital is not to draw boundaries around a select group of patients and a select group of staff who receive special privileges and resources, but rather to *integrate* the hospice concept into practice throughout the institution. Likewise, "the way must be kept open always for the patient to move, when appropriate, between the 'cure' system of the hospice and the 'care' system of the hospice, ensuring that nobody ever risks becoming locked into one or the other" (Saunders, 1981, p. 93).

FORMATION

A balance must be established between taking time to lay the strong organizational groundwork for hospice formation and the demands to begin patient services. Some organizational structure is best refined from the wisdom gained in starting to provide patient care within the hospital system, but basic foundations must be nailed down first or the structure will later crumble.

It usually takes four to six months to plan and implement an in-hospital hospice program. The program director needs to decide when it is appropriate to start providing patient services and then set that goal. It is difficult to start

---

*Saunders, C.M. The hospice: Its meaning to patients and their physicians. *Hospital Practice,* June 1981, *16,* 93–108.

providing services before team education and training is complete. The program director must evaluate the team's ability to respond adequately and then factor in the political impact of either waiting to start services or of beginning ahead of schedule. There is no right or wrong in making this decision. Rather, one must make the most prudent decision considering all the factors in one's own hospital setting. This is one example of the organizational development challenges that face a hospice program within a hospital.

Establishment of a Planning Committee

The hospice planning committee or task force should include people in power within the hospital system. Top administrative and medical staff including department heads should be reached through education and political process. A collaborative rather than a competitive spirit should be fostered: "What can we do together to address the needs of the terminally ill in our institution and community more effectively?" The goal is to gradually develop a broad powerful base of support and respect within the hospital community so that the hospice does not become the struggling project of just a few people with an "us against them" mentality.

The initial task of the planning committee will be self-education and then gradually the education of the entire hospital community. Many will be asking, "We have always cared for dying patients here. Why is a special program needed?" Educational efforts focus first on those in key policy-making roles, then on disseminating basic information hospital-wide, and then on the needs of individual departments and units.

The committee, or task force, must decide who will coordinate the planning activities. It is common for this person to be a nurse who is eventually hired as program director or coordinator. This person then embarks on the challenges of coordinating the formative stage of the program while resisting the demands for immediate patient services as discussed in the preceding section. Self-education and visits to operational programs prepare the director for the organizational tasks that lie ahead. The role demands the wearing of many hats in the formative stage: nurse, administrator, educator, politician, public relations expert, and sometime clerical worker, fundraiser, and accountant. Headaches may develop from the weight and balancing of all those hats; see Chapter 17 on stress reduction techniques for the professional.

Needs Assessment

Needs assessment within the acute care setting includes determining the needs of patients and the needs of staff. How many terminally ill people does the hospital serve? It is important to determine the annual hospital mortality rate, causes of death, and the areas of the hospital in which patients die.

Remember that the population of terminally ill people that the hospital serves includes those who die at home and in nursing homes; this number should also be estimated.

The target population for hospice services generally comprises persons with lingering, predictable dying courses rather than people who die of rapid, unpredicted deaths like those occurring in the emergency room, intensive care units, surgery, or obstetrics. Be careful, however, not to get boxed into considering services just for cancer patients. You might begin there, but assess the needs on cardiovascular, pulmonary, neurological, renal, and other services. One of the authors was assessing the patient population on one medical unit where the nurses claimed that none of their patients were in need of hospice because none were dying from cancer. The nurses did acknowledge, however, that perhaps 6 of their 30 cardiac patients were likely to die within the next year!

It is especially important to include within the overall needs assessment at the early formative phase an evaluation of needs as hospital staff perceive them. Do staff see a need for a hospice program? What do they see as patient needs and their own needs? What are their expectations? What are their educational needs? What about their interests, and how can they be involved and supportive of the program? Existing resource people and departments who already are offering components of hospice care such as grief counseling, pastoral care, and palliative physical care should be involved in all phases of planning. Creating a spirit of cooperation rather than territoriality is essential not only for the planning but for the ongoing success of the program.

Within the needs assessment an ongoing analysis can be started to examine those forces that support and those forces that obstruct the implementation of hospice within the institution (see Figure 14-1). This can be developed as an ongoing tool used both for analysis and for strategizing to strengthen supports and overcome obstacles.

Statement of Purpose

The planning committee states its philosophy and goals, which incorporate the explicit and implicit philosophy of the hospital community, national hospice standards, and the values and final decisions of the committee. The hospital philosophy of care can be enabling or it can be a major stumbling block. Review the hospital's and various departments' written philosophy statements. What kind of human needs is the institution as a whole committed to meet? Is the hospital committed only to acute curative medical care or to broader family and community services? Does the hospital have a stated commitment to care of the dying? For instance, the Medical/Moral Committee of a Medical Center describes the Center's approach and goals as follows:

Figure 14-1. Needs analysis of hospice within the institution

I. Forces that support implementation of hospice	(Strategy)
II. Forces that obstruct implementation of hospice	(Strategy)

To use this tool:

1. List all that comes to your mind under "forces that support," "forces that obstruct." It is not uncommon to find the same entry heading listed under both headings, e.g., nursing department "supports," nursing department "obstructs."

2. Define the conditions, people, and factors that generate support or lead to obstruction.

3. Brainstorm the possible alternatives for maintaining support and removing the obstructions.

4. Prioritize the alternatives and select those that promise the greatest degree of continuing support and resolution of obstruction.

5. Plan the implementation of alternatives in each column, building on what is positive. Recognize conflict and use it as a means to understand another's position. Strategy should include conflict management.

The Medical Center is dedicated to the care of the sick, injured and dying, offering all its human and technological resources to patients who come here for help. In most situations, this means that every possible effort is made to cure the sick, rehabilitate the injured, preserve life and restore good health. However, for those patients who are dying, the Center's goal is to assist them to die well rather than to prolong their lives. Helping the dying to live the end of their lives in a responsible and dignified manner is a goal equal in value to preserving life and restoring health.

Are social service, pastoral care, and primary nursing already organized to meet comprehensive holistic needs? Examine existing practices regarding bed utilization, family involvement, patient bill of rights, and decision making regarding code (resuscitation) status. How do the existing philosophy statements and the philosophy implicit in existing policies and practices support and/or contradict hospice philosophy? The committee must have beginning answers to these questions in order to plan and integrate hospice services into the hospital community.

The hospice program will eventually need to rely on support and collaboration among all the services: nursing, medical, social work, pharmacy, dietary, physical therapy, occupational therapy, pastoral care, and volunteer services. There are three shifts of nurses and, in a teaching hospital, there are both attending physicians and house staff. Each department and group has philosophies and practices that will be both supportive and obstructive.

The hospice program philosophy and goal statements incorporate national standards as defined by the National Hospice Organization (see Chapter 6). At this writing, the Joint Committee on the Accreditation of Hospitals (JCAH) had developed standards in collaboration with the National Hospice Organization. It has not yet been determined who will be the accrediting group.

The committee chooses the direction for the individual hospital. What is the patient population that will be served? What should be admission criteria? What model of hospital hospice program is best? Should there be a separate hospice unit or will the consulting team model be the best model?

A *separate hospice unit* offers the opportunity to create a total hospice environment that is supportive for both patient-family and staff. Such an environment can include more home-like patient rooms, family rooms, kitchen use, unrestricted visiting hours with family sleeping at the bedside, and the presence of children and even pets. Continuity of care can be well maintained, and staff can be educated to provide a high level of consistent palliative and psychosocial care. The team staffing the unit can develop a unified vision and collaborative supportive relationships. The Royal Victoria Hospital Palliative Care unit in Montreal is one prototype for this kind of unit; their manual is a useful tool for hospice unit development (Ajemian & Mount, 1980).

There are many challenges to the development and survival of a small in-hospital hospice unit. Consider admission criteria. What does transition to the unit mean for patients leaving units where they feel known and comfortable and have received active treatment? (And if the hospital has an oncology unit, how will the separate hospice unit relate to the oncology unit?) One would hope that image of active palliation would supercede the fear of a "death ward."

The smaller the unit, the greater the expense to the hospital. Can the unit be kept filled?

Another danger of operating a hospice unit within the hospital is the "little kingdom syndrome": given special resources and more nursing hours per patient, the unit may be resented by the rest of the hospital. This situation can be overcome by hospital-wide education and movement to integrate hospice concepts of care hospital-wide.

Finally, staff burnout threatens a small staff doing this intense work. Rotations, weekends, and vacations are difficult to schedule. To float staff through from other units poses challenges regarding their education to maintain high standards of palliation. These are just a few of the issues to be considered in planning a hospice as a separate unit.

The *consulting hospice team* within the hospital goes to wherever the terminally ill person is located in the hospital. Patients receive hospice services without transfering to a special unit and are able to be supported in the environment in which they entered the hospital. This arrangement can be particularly effective in reaching two groups of patients: those with newly diagnosed terminal conditions, and those with chronic disease on particular units (e.g., renal, neurological, cardiac) who are now considered terminal. A major advantage of the consulting team is the opportunity to educate the entire hospital community in hospice care, leading to improved care for all terminally ill patients and their families. The consulting team eliminates the "death ward" concept feared by many professional and lay people.

Challenges of the consulting team model include the difficulties of assuring consistent palliative care and maintaining a family-centered environment. Many different staff members influence the quality of care, and the challenge of their education, orientation, and inclusion in the collaborative planning process is immense. Another significant challenge is the acceptance by the medical staff of the hospice team nurse's role. In hospice, nurses make recommendations for pain and symptom management as well as other recommendations for care. These may or may not be well received. As the team's expertise becomes known and respected, this becomes less a problem and joint practice becomes more a reality.

Both the separate unit and the consulting team model present opportunities and challenges. In the best of all possible worlds, a hospital would be able to maintain a high-occupancy, separate hospice unit *and* a consulting team to integrate hospice care throughout the rest of the hospital units.

With the philosophy of care defined and the basic nature and model of the program clarified, long-term and short-term goals are defined. For example, following is the philosophy statement developed by the hospice task force of a Medical Center in Seattle during early development in 1979. Grounded in the philosophy, the long-range goals are defined. Short-range objectives are periodically revised for each goal. Examine the following hospice goals, with one example of derived short-range objectives.

A MEDICAL CENTER HOSPICE PHILOSOPHY AND GOALS

Philosophy Statement

The Medical Center believes in helping the terminally ill and dying to live the end of their lives in a responsible and dignified manner. This philosophy has provided the framework for the development of the Medical Center Hospice Program.

The main concern of the Hospice Program is the management of terminal disease in such a way that patients live as fully as possible until they die, and that their families live with them as they are dying, and go on living healthfully afterwards. Hospice care is based on symptom management, pain control, and support services that recognize the physical, social, emotional, and spiritual dimensions of living with dying. Patient and family participation in decision making regarding surroundings, companions, therapeutic management, and terminal care is recognized as essential and is encouraged. The Hospice concept of care emphasizes respect for individual life style and belief systems of each patient and family.

Program Definition

The Medical Center Hospice Program consists of a physician-directed, nurse-coordinated, interdisciplinary consulting team and trained volunteers. The team will work with the attending physician and primary caregivers throughout the hospital to provide hospice care to terminally ill and dying patients and their families who are referred to the program. The patient and family are considered the unit of care. The family is defined as those persons the patient considers to be his or her main support and primary caregivers. Family members are encouraged, but not required, to be an integral part of the care team.

The program provides both in-hospital care and the coordination of home care with existing community resources, with continuity and coordination of care between home and hospital readmissions and discharges. The program emphasis is on planning and coordinating home care for the patient, thereby extending the period of time in which the patient can safely, comfortably, and inexpensively as possible be cared for outside the hospital or other in-patient facility. If and when a patient does return to the hospital, continuity of Hospice care will be provided.

Education and support for the careproviders is an integral part of the Hospice Program. This includes bereavement care for the family and ongoing advice and service to the health care providers throughout the hospital.

Hospice services will be available 7 days a week, 24 hours a day, on an on-call basis.

Goals

I.   To help patients and families maintain their lives as fully as possible. To encourage and support participation in choices regarding therapeutic management, pain control, symptom management, terminal care, environment, and companions.

II. To assist the patient and family to live effectively while preparing themselves for death and bereavement.

III. To teach families to care for the patient and each other by identifying and responding to the physical, social, emotional, and spiritual needs they may have.

IV. To educate and support the professional and volunteer staff as they care for the terminally ill and dying patients and their families. Educational emphasis will be in the areas of pain control, symptom management, and support services, dealing with grief, loss, and dying.

V. To support the patient and family in their decision to remain at home and to coordinate home services when needed with existing agencies.

VI. To serve as a "back-up" to the home health care team and to make home visits when necessary to assist patients and families in their goal to remain at home.

VII. To provide continuity of hospice care when and if the patient is readmitted to the hospital.

VIII. To provide individualized bereavement care, the extent and length to be determined by factors prior to and following the death of the patient.

For example, under Goal IV is a secondary goal regarding the volunteer staff:

Goal: To maintain and develop the Hospital Volunteer Program to serve patients and families.

Objectives:

1. Continue to provide monthly educational and support meetings for present volunteers.

2. Continue to provide weekly support groups for volunteers.

3. Continue to supervise the activities and interaction of volunteers.

4. Expand the volunteers' role in bereavement follow-up.

5. Plan educational programs in bereavement training.

6. Explore collaborative training sessions with community hospice programs.

7. Provide one or two annual 30-hour "basic training" sessions for new volunteers.

8. Create a volunteer handbook.

Effective planning for implementation of goals includes realistic estimation of the time and resources needed to accomplish each short-term objective. Consider defining outcome criteria and how you will be accountable for the achievement of objectives. Do not underestimate the time and resources needed for education, orientation, on-call availability, and adequate staff coverage.

In addition to planning within the acute care system, the hospice task force and director need to be planning for the provisions of hospice home care services. A hospice program is only complete insofar as it provides continuity of care between home and hospital, so plannning for home care is essential. There are many questions to be considered. How and by whom will hospice home care be provided? Does the hospital already have a home care nursing team? If so, how will the hospital inpatient care services work with the home care team? Should there be a separate hospice home team, or is the present home care team ready to learn and expand to the role of hospice? How do the professionals understand the important role of volunteers? What are the educational needs of the professionals and volunteers? How will 24-hour coverage, 7 days a week be provided? Should the inpatient hospice director also direct the home hospice program? What channels for communication and accountability are appropriate between hospital and home teams? Obviously, adequate planning and coordination is necessary to achieve a smoothly running total program of inpatient and home services.

If the hospital does not provide home services directly, other questions arise. Should the hospital create a home visiting-nurse-type service in order to provide hospice services? Before deciding to take on this costly endeavor, it would be important for the task force to identify existing community resources. Is there already a hospice program or programs to provide home services? If so, how can services be coordinated with such existing services? If not, is there a home health services group like the Visiting Nurse Association that would be interested in expanding its services to include hospice home care? Can these models provide adequate home care hospice services? What will the relationship and responsibilities of the hospital be to the home group and vice versa? Will formal contracts be required?

After it is decided how to provide home services, guidelines must be established for referrals, feedback, and evalution of working relationships between the hospital and home teams. It is this joint effort that will enable patients and families to make the choices that best suit their needs, at home or in the hospital.

In planning a hospice program it is important to consider and include time and resources for liaison with the National Hospice Organization, regional and state hospice organizations, if they exist, and local hospice groups. This participation with other hospice groups can keep a hospice from developing in a vacuum and becoming myopic in its vision. Hospices can learn a great deal from each other and avoid others' mistakes, and together they can appreciate that different communities need to be creative in providing hospice services that fit their needs. No one hospice model is adequate to meet the needs of rural, metropolitan, and suburban hospice populations. Each hospice program must first commit itself to addressing the needs of its own community. Will or can the program be able to commit itself to broader responsibilities such as participating in writing national accreditation standards or state regulations for hospices? Will or can the program involve itself in working for reimbursement for hospice services? Will or can the program respond to the need for hospice care education by other groups in the community? The answers to these questions often depend on the leadership, vision, resources, and support available to and within the hospice team. The hospice program's consideration of these areas of external relationships is important in the long-range planning of the program.

Formation of a Board and Lines of Authority

The community hospice will find it advantageous to incorporate with an administrative board of directors and corporate by-laws, as discussed in the preceding chapter. A hospital-based hospice will need to decide whether to have an administrative board of directors or an advisory board. This decision needs to be carefully considered by the task force in conjunction with the hospital administrator. In most cases, an advisory board would be the choice since there probably already is an administrative board for the entire hospital. It is wise to create an advisory board whose membership represents all major patient care departments. Goals include examining long-range planning, program development, patient care issues, and the relation of the hospice program to the rest of the hospital. This advisory board can be a major means of integrating the hospice program into the hospital. Minutes of the meetings can be sent to the hospital administrator, medical director and other department heads to keep them informed. The advisory board picks up (implementation) where the task force left off (planning).

It is essential that the hospice program be placed on the hospital organizational chart. The consulting team model of hospice care should be a hospital-wide program, not the program of a single department. A clear line of authority, responsibility, and accountability should be established. Ideally, the director should not report to one department but should have an independent identity and the authority to report directly to the hospital administration, perhaps to an assistant administrator. This may not be possible in situations where good will and support is best maintained by coming under departmental organizational structure. Budget considerations also determine where the hospice program will fit into the hospital organizational chart.

Funding

Funding is first sought through the commitment of the hospital administration. Many hospitals have foundations—fund-raising arms—that will search for or raise monies to support the program. It is important to develop working relationships with regular hospital fundraisers and the public relations department rather than assume the burden of fundraising for your own program. Some advisory boards take on the function of fund-raising. The budget of the hospice program needs to be carefully planned, not only the start-up costs, but long-range costs, up to five years from start. There is no regular reimbursement mechanism for a consulting team hospice program. They must rely on the hospital's commitment to fund them and on community giving.

Separate hospice units will be reimbursed by an administratively determined charge per bed. Medicare reimbursement will be available as of November 1, 1983 for those hospice programs that can meet stringent criteria, including hospital and home care components that are administered jointly. The ingenuity and creativity that has made hospice care what it is today will be needed to respond administratively to the hospice care needs of tomorrow. As reimbursement for hospice care becomes a reality, the continued commitment of hospital and home care administrators will be needed to assure implementation of care that is best for the patients and families.

EARLY DEVELOPMENT

Review the task-oriented committees and other considerations identified in Chapter 13 as part of the early developmental stage. Several critical areas of program development are discussed here. We advise keeping the planning task force as advisors to the program director during this phase of development.

Education and Training

Working closely with medical and nursing education departments, hospice educational inservices must be planned and implemented on a hospital-wide basis. Include administration, administrative board, Foundation Board, all shifts of medical and nursing staffs, pastoral care, social services, pharmacy, dietary, occupational and physical therapists, volunteers, and other specialized services. Then there is the major ongoing task of educating the specialized hospice team for a separate unit and/or consulting service. Particular services, units, or staff (e.g., discharge planner, nurse clinicians, utilization review) may also be targeted for special training because they will be instrumental in referral and maintaining continuity of care for the hospice patient.

Education for the public is also essential at this time. Hospice literature is made available through the hospital and the community; publicity for the program is sought through speaking engagements, meetings, and media.

Lay Volunteers

Every effort should be made to work with existing hospital volunteer coordinators in the organization of a hospice volunteer program. Recruitment efforts identify a group of mature, committed individuals. Hospice volunteers function in an expanded volunteer role, requiring sound training and exceptional communication skills. The following tasks might be part of the "job responsibility" of a hospital-based hospice volunteer: relieving family members at the bedside of the patient; providing backrubs, ice chips, and small physical comforts to the patient; providing companionship, sometimes in silence, for the patient; writing letters, playing music, reading with the patient; bringing in things from home for the patient. A training program should include: an orientation to the hospital and home hospice services, protocol for the volunteer in relation to hospital staff, and lines of responsibility to the hospice team. These things should be taught in addition to the normal training for hospice volunteers. Hospital professionals will need time and education and bedside experience with the volunteer in the expanded supportive role to accept and appreciate their potential as part of the team providing comprehensive hospice care.

As soon as possible, the program director should have a coordinator of the volunteer program because volunteer recruitment, training, support, and communication with volunteers is a time-consuming responsibility. The quality of the volunteer component of the hospice program is crucial to its continued success.

Administrative Structure and Decisions

The interrelated roles of program director, nursing coordinator, and medical director will be clarified in the early developmental stage. (In many programs the program director and nursing coordinator are the same person.) This includes the line of organizational authority and relationship to other departments as already discussed. What role will the hospice physician assume in the medical management of hospice patients? That role should foster a positive working relationship, including education, with the patient's primary physician. How can an atmosphere of collaborative planning rather than authoritarian decision making be encouraged in policies and roles developed? This is also the time to define the roles of caregiving team members in relation to the patient and family, each other, and the program administration.

The program will make decisions at this time regarding what kind of medical records to keep that are different from the general hospital. A consulting team may need to keep some recording separate from the regular chart and to keep their own statistical information. Forms need to be developed to gather pertinent data for long-range planning.

Specific organizational structure for referral to home care agencies needs to be delineated. Orientation meetings, planned written and oral communication to assure continuity of care, and methods of evaluation must all be considered, as described earlier.

Office space and equipment needs must be adequately planned but not taken too seriously. Many of the best hospice programs started in poorly equipped, cramped quarters!

STABILITY

Stability is achieved when the program is providing well-defined services that are meeting its stated goals. In the context of the contemporary American economy and pressures within acute care medicine, hospice program administrators cannot relax on reaching program maturity. They will be expected to provide continuity with very limited resources. In maintaining funding commitments they will find themselves in stiff competition with other services. There are ongoing organizational stressors on top of patient stressors. The need for maintaining public relations throughout the hospital never ceases. The demand to expand patient care programs is great. It is good management to hold off on providing additional services if resources do not exist to do so. This involves *active waiting* rather than jumping in to do a poor job. Those who actively wait are actively assessing and strategizing to get what is needed in order to move ahead. Figure 14-2 uses the Needs Analysis Tool introduced in Figure 14-1 to demonstrate the application of hospice philosophy and administrative and management skills in analyzing one hospice program dilemma in the acute care setting. The guiding strategy for a continuing hospital-based hospice is to work diligently with the supporting services and gently but persuasively with the resisting forces in the common concern for patient welfare and excellent care.

Figure 14-2. Example of needs analysis*

I Forces that support implementation of hospice	(Strategy)
Some of the cardiovascular physicians and nurses ask the hospice team to address the needs of terminally ill cardiovascular patients and families and the professional caregivers.	Dilemma: The hospice team is already overcommitted—what should the team do? (Strategies incorporated into those listed below.)
Forces that obstruct implementation of hospice	(Strategy)
Hospice care team is understaffed to meet the need.	1. Assess number of hours needed to meet request.
	2. Budget in a position-hours to meet need and seek administrative support.
	3. Explain plan to cardiovascular team and plan for the future.
	4. Do not burn out the hospice team by starting services that overextend the present team.
	5. When staffed adequately begin to reach out to cardiovascular group.

Figure 14-2 (continued)

Some cardiovascular physicians and nurses are uncomfortable or opposed to hospice care.	1. Plan a series of educational meetings to discuss their concerns and to explain how hospice may complement their care. 2. Start with medical director, head nurse, nurse clinician. 3. Accept patient referrals and work closely with staff to achieve a sense of success on everyone's part. 4. Do not become unduly discouraged if first few cases are not "successful"—there will be rough edges.
Patients and families may be resistant to hospice, may feel they are "giving up" since they have been seeking acute cardiovascular care.	1. Gently respect process of patient and family. 2. Work with staff and patient and family in dealing with poor prognosis. 3. Help family plan for care; facilitate decision making in light of poor prognosis. 4. Introduce volunteers to give family a break.

*Adapted from Egan, Gerard. *The Skilled Helper.* California: Brooks/Cole Publishing Company, 1982, pp. 260–267, "Forced Field Analysis."

REFERENCES

Ajemian, I., & Mount, E. *The Royal Victoria Hospital Manual on Palliative/Hospice Care.* New York: Arno Press, 1980.

Breindel, C.L., & O'Hare, T. Analyzing the hospice market. *Hospital Progress,* 1979, Vol. 60, No. 10, p. 52–55.

Krant, M.J. Hospice philosophy in late stage cancer care. Journal of the American Medical Association, 1981, *245,* p. 1061–1062.

Meyer, K.A. The hospice concept integrated with existing community health care. NAQ, Community Outreach 1, 1980.

Mount, B.M. The problem of caring for the dying in a general hospital: The palliative care unit as a possible solution. *CMA Journal,* 1976, *115,* p. 119–121.

Saunders, C. The hospice: Its meaning to patients and their physicians. *Hospital Practice,* June 1981, *16,* 93–108.

Valentour, L.F. Hospice design keyed to program goals. *Hospitals,* 1980, Vol. 54, No. 4, p. 140–143.

Wald, F.S., Foster, Z., & Wald, H.J. The hospice movement as a health care reform. *Nursing Outlook,* 1980, *28,* 173–178.

RECOMMENDED READING

Breindel, C.L., & O'Hare, T. Analyzing the hospice market. *Hospital Progress,* 1979, Vol. 60, No. 10, p. 52–55.

Krant, M.J. Hospice philosophy in late stage cancer care. Journal of the American Medical Association, 1981, *245,* p. 1061–1062.

Meyer, K.A. The hospice concept integrated with existing community health care. NAQ, Community Outreach 1, 1980.

Mount, B.M. The problem of caring for the dying in a general hospital: The palliative care unit as a possible solution. *CMA Journal,* 1976, *115,* p. 119–121.

Valentour, L.F. Hospice design keyed to program goals. *Hospitals,* 1980, Vol. 54, No. 4, p. 140–143.

Wald, F.S., Foster, Z., & Wald, H.J. The hospice movement as a health care reform. *Nursing Outlook,* 1980, *28,* 173–178.

1. F	*5. T*
2. F	*6. T*
3. T	*7. F*
4. F	

15

Clinical Records and Research

Answer the following questions True (T) or False (F). Answers appear on the last page of this chapter.

1. *Clinical records are kept only as a tool for planning.*

2. *The initial plan of care should include goals and plans for palliation of each patient problem.*

3. *Patients-families should not participate in the recording of observations concerning patient physical or emotional status due to their less-than-objective perspective.*

4. *The validation of hospice program effectiveness is an important reason to collect data and complete research studies.*

5. *The beginning of research is frequently the identification of a problem.*

6. *Studies addressing questions concerned with naming establish interesting relationships among variables.*

7. *Relation-searching studies attempt to discover whether there are relationships among factors.*

8. *Studies addressing questions concerned with correlations determine those factors which cause certain conditions to exist.*

9. *Both setting and sample population should be representative of reality and should take into consideration a range of variables.*

10. *"Reliability" in instruments of measurement refers to the extent to which the measure will yield the same results for the same sample in repeated instances.*

What we learn from the dying applies to all of us during life. In a way it is the dying who are giving us a much better awareness of the gift of life. It is they who are our best teachers. *

BOTH CLINICAL RECORDS and clinical research are integral to learning from the dying and developing hospice care. Charting documents the dying experience and actions of the hospice team. It permits the examination of the caregiving process in writing. Research analyzes the processes and outcomes of caregiving to develop a solid theoretical base for hospice practices.

CLINICAL RECORDS IN HOSPICE CARE

The hospice patient record serves (1) as a tool for the individual nurse to review his or her observations and plan in a disciplined fashion; (2) as a communication channel between nurses and the rest of the professional team to identify assessments and ongoing plans; (3) as a legal document; (4) as a record for certification, accreditation, or quality assurance review; and particularly (5) as a means of documenting responses to palliative measures. Hospice–palliative care programs must develop recording systems that clearly identify common patient problems, actions taken to relieve these problems, and patient care outcomes. Careful charting enables chart review that retrieves information to develop and validate the expanding body of hospice–palliative care knowledge. Hospice records should be systematic and succinct.

Systematic and Succinct Documentation

Problem-oriented recording methods should be adapted to the needs of the individual program keeping in mind that recording tools should be

---

*Klagsburn, S.C. Hospice—a developing role. In Saunder, C. (Ed.). *Hospice: The Living Idea.* Philadelphia: W.B. Saunders, 1981.

thorough but should minimize the need for professionals to spend precious patient-care time writing volumes of material. Duplication of effort can be avoided by using carbon paper or photocopies or having clerical workers make copies.

The *data base* includes initial assessment information from all disciplines. Although ongoing nursing assessment should be comprehensive, as discussed in Chapter 4, the actual assessment tools included in the chart should be brief systematic outlines of areas to be considered. These permit individual judgment as to what is efficient and pertinent to record. Figure 15-1 is an initial physical data base and Figure 15-2 is a sample psychosocial data base.

A *problem list* is derived from analyzing the data. It is developed during initial assessment and continually expanded, with notation of when old

Figure 15-1. Initial physical data base

Identify landmarks of significant physical change:

Front   Back

I. Cardiovascular-Respiratory	V. Musculoskeletal
Subjective:	Subjective:
Objective:	Objective:
II. Gastrointestinal	VI. Neurological
Subjective:	Subjective:
Objective:	Objective:
III. Genitourinary & Gynecological	VII. Skin
Subjective:	Subjective:
Objective:	Objective:
IV. Fluid & Electrolyte	VIII. Other
Subjective:	Subjective:
Objective:	Objective:

Figure 15-2. Psychosocial data base: presenting problems

Coping Skills and Strategies

1. Patient-family's perception of illness and prognosis (denial-acceptance-need for preparation):

2. Ways of dealing with present crisis; history of coping strategies; recent and past losses:

3. General atmosphere of home environment:

4. Strengths, as identified by family:
   by counselor:

Social Network

1. Family members:
   Significant others:

2. Membership in community, church, or social–cultural organizations:

3. Amenability to outside help:

Spiritual Needs

1. Membership in church or organized religion:

2. Availability of church to family for support and assistance:

3. Expressed need for spiritual exploration:

4. Expressed need for memorial planning:

Resources Available

1. Financial (income and health insurance):

2. Need for additional caregiver and volunteer:

3. Need for patient advocacy within medical system:

4. Need for other social or legal services:

Patient's Stated Goals:

Family's Stated Goals:

---

*Designed by Polly Purvis, M.S.W., Hospice of Seattle. With permission.

problems are resolved. The hospice problem list should be an interdisciplinary undertaking whenever possible, focusing particularly on things the patient perceives as problems. In practice, this is often difficult to achieve because each discipline labels problems so differently. For instance, whereas the physician may state "Right hemiparesis 2° cerebral metastatis 2° oat cell ca of lung," the nursing diagnosis may read "Impaired physical mobility, altered cerebral perfusion, powerlessness," the social worker identifies the problem as "Anger over enforced dependency," and the patient says, "I can't get my damned leg to work right. How do you expect me to live like this?" Hospice team members need to work toward mutually understood language.

The *initial plan of care* includes goal statements and specific plans for palliation of each problem. Such a plan can be recorded in a variety of ways. It is vital, however, that nurses clearly document in the chart their progress notes and their specific plans for palliative intervention. This information should not exist only on an eraseable Kardex!

Progress records include both narrative notes and flow sheets. Flow sheets are particularly useful in documenting status of problems and response to palliative measures while minimizing nurse recording time; Figure 15-3 presents an example of a hospital hospice-unit flow sheet. Narrative notes are used in the nursing home and hospital only to record changes in patient status and plans. Home health nurses record narrative notes after each visit. Narrative notes that are succinct and systematic can also effectively follow several formats. The notes can be organized around a discussion of each active problem, or notes can be organized by systems or broad categories of patient need. In any case, notes using a "SOAP" format are usually best to document the care process: Such notes proceed from subjective (S) report by patient or family, to objective (O) data observed by professional, to the clinical assessment or analysis (A), to the plan (P) of care, which includes derived plans, stated outcomes, and documentation of interventions implemented. Following is a sample hospice home care progress note using the SOAP format in one broad category entitled "physical status." A program may, in the interests of brevity and conservation of writing time, choose not to SOAP on each problem but to examine them together during each writing.

6/6/83   Home visit

Physical Status. S: Report no right hip pain taking 2 tsp pain cocktail (5 mg methadone, 25 mg Vistaril) q6h. Concerned with increased sleeping, reduced ability to concentrate since started cocktail 4 days ago. Continued refusal to eat solids; "I can't force myself." Main intake soda pop and lemonade. No B.M. in 5 days despite 1 Colace 50 mg q.d. Coughing up small amount white sputum q A.M.
O: Walks upright without limp. Slow to respond to questions. Active B.T. Moist tongue, pink. BP 102/84, AP 98, R 18. Lungs cl. except rales at base. Palpable pedal pulses.
A: Good pain control finally. Analgesic causing decreased mentation. Anorexia-malnutrition. Not dehydrated. Constipated: needs better bowel regimen.
P: Continue at current cocktail dose and evaluate again in 4 days. Expect clearing of mental effect. Teaching and reassurance re: lesser mentation as temporary. Diet teaching re: high protein liquids. Explained anorexia as normal dying process—not to push him so hard to cause resentment-conflict. Explained pain cocktail causing constipation and need for regular bowel regimen. Recommended trying Metamucil 1 tsp p.o. BID and Colace 50 mg TID. Try MOM 30 cc tonight and Dulcolax suppos. 10 mg p.r. tomorrow if no results.

Figure 15-3. Sample hospice problem flow sheet

Problem	Date		
	6/7/83	6/8/83	6/9/83
Nausea-anorexia	Emeses x3 with full liquid meals. Began compazine 25 mg suppos. ½ hr. ac at 5 P.M.	o̅ emeses. Continuing compazine. Fluid intake 630 cc/day.	Emesis x1. Taking only sips of liquid. Continuing compazine q8h.
Insomnia	Observed not to sleep till 3 A.M. Awake at 6 A.M. Reports vivid dreams. Started use of relaxation tape at H.S.	Increased sleeping & lethargy. Unable to pay attention to relaxation tape.	As yesterday.
Dyspnea & Cough	T: 98.6 at 4 P.M. R: 24, ↓ B.S. at bases. Frequent cough with white sputum.	T: 101 at 4 P.M. R: 32 ↓ B.S. on right. Coarse rales on L. Frequent cough with yellow sputum. Started Ampicillin 250 mg po QID. Codeine 30 mg po q3-4h prn cough. O2 at 4 L/min. Continuous.	T: 101.2 at 4 P.M. R = 30. Otherwise as yesterday.
	6/7/83	6/8/83	6/9/83
Lower extremity edema	2+ to knee. Lasix 40 mg qd	unchanged	2+ to knee. Feet cyanotic. Continuing Lasix.

313

The *discharge summary* is written at death, transfer, or remission of a hospice patient. It includes a brief summary of major patient problems, interventions, and outcomes.

Documenting Psychosocial–Spiritual Care

As yet there appears to be no consensus among counseling professionals (nurses, social workers, psychologists, psychiatrists, spiritual counselors) as to desirable format or content for documentation of psychosocial–spiritual care. Practice should be determined by (1) the need to document psychosocial problems, counseling approaches, and outcomes; (2) ethical and legal constraints that require attention to confidentiality and concerns with libel when we describe the most private aspects of peoples' lives; and finally (3) the need to document psychosocial care for reimbursement purposes. Many find the SOAP format useful for recording systematic psychosocial progress notes, but some may find it forces a biomedical rather than a holistic model of the human psyche and spirit.

Since the psychosocial–spiritual dimension of care is so central to the hospice movement, documenting all the personal data collected and all the counseling strategies used becomes an insurmountable and questionable task. Charting should instead be a succinct summary of problems confronted and counseling strategies used. Table 15-1 identifies common psychosocial diagnoses and common counseling techniques. Greater detail regarding the complex interplay of family and individual dynamics, helping strategies used, and identification of goals and alternatives should be discussed in case conferences, even then maintaining careful confidentiality.

One strength of interdisciplinary hospice–palliative care is in the opportunity it offers for one-to-one case planning as well as for group conferences. The rich harvest of such meetings should be systematically recorded for each patient in retrievable minutes of each case conference. Major changes in plans should be noted in the chart.

Bedside Notes

An ongoing chart or journal at the patient's side facilitates continuity of care for many people. In the home this can include an organized medication–treatment record, individualized flow sheets, nursing recommendations, and observations regarding physical and emotional status. The record is best bound in a notebook rather than kept on different pieces of paper that are likely to be separated and mislaid. In both home and hospital, bedside notes provide a tool for communication between family members and caregivers

Table 15-1. *Common Hospice Psychosocial Diagnoses and Counseling Strategies*

Psychosocial Diagnoses

Anger
  ambivalence
  expression of hostility
  physical abuse, fighting
  verbal abusiveness

Confusion, disorientation

Contradictory patient goals

Denial, lack of understanding
  closed awareness—avoiding issues
  needs downplayed
  ignorance of feelings
  ignorance of disease
  reduced mentation—impaired
    decision making

Dependency, powerlessness
  patient loss of personal power
  dependent family or friends

Depression, hopelessness

Fear

Financial concerns

Grief reaction
  unexpressed
  immobilized
  identify coping mechanism

Immaturity, ineffective coping

Isolation
  cultural–language
  lack of social supports
  personal reticence
  emotional withdrawal

Lack of goals, no future planning

Exhaustion, overextension of caregivers

Self-destructive behavior
  suicidal thoughts

Stress-related symptoms

Unfinished business remaining

Counseling Strategies

Active listening
Advocacy
Conflict resolution
Coordination of team approach
Crisis intervention
Family counseling
Guided expression of feelings
*Guiding problem solving, decision
  making*

Networking
Orientation techniques
*Paraphrasing, summarizing,
  clarifying*
Relaxation, meditation, imagery
*Structured guidance when patient-
  family at a loss*
Teaching normal grief
Values clarification

who are present at different times and cannot confer directly. Family are encouraged to write down problems, observations, and suggestions. Some patients use the record to describe their own experience and to remember concerns and questions. For some it is a tool to maintain orientation and keep control of their own care. When the patient dies, this document can become part of the legacy for family members.

THE SCOPE OF NURSING RESEARCH

Research in Nursing Practice

The purposes of hospice nursing research are defined by the everyday practice of palliative care nursing. When a new patient is referred to hospice, a history must be taken, past charts and care plans reviewed, the family and patient consulted; this is *data collection.*

Next the facts and the observations are analyzed in order to assess status and define needs; this is *taxonomy,* or defining and naming. During these first two stages, many of the traditional forms of data collection may be used—questionnaires, scales, or charts of critical incidents.

Following diagnosis, a plan is formulated that carries with it the assumption that the actions taken will effect certain changes or have desired results. *Predictions,* based on a *hypothesis* of expected results, are made.

Finally, an *evaluation* must be made of whether or not the diagnosis has been correct and the treatment significantly effective. It is at this point that many of the researcher's most constant problems become troublesome.

- Was the original data valid?
- Have uncontrolled-for variables clouded the results?
- Can the results legitimately be generalized to other patient-care situations?

Research in Program Planning and Evaluation

The hospice program director confronts the same kinds of issues in his or her job of developing and maintaining high quality services. She or he should continuously collect data, formulate questions, propose improvements, assess outcomes, construct results, and arrive at conclusions and usable implications for future program changes.

This is the essence of scientific inquiry. It is a very valuable philosophy for all health care professionals to carry through their careers. While research cannot ever replace the personal satisfaction that comes from giving excellent patient care, what we learn from research provides the base of information from which we improve that case (Diers, 1974).

Donna Diers, in *Research in Nursing Practice,* comments on this very exciting time when the scientific examination of nursing practices is considerably ahead of that of other disciplines:

As we learn more about what in nursing brings about the desired effects for patients, the patient care gets better and better. When we know what in nursing practice works, we can design curricula to teach that, or invent nursing administrations to foster it.*

---

*From Diers, D. *Research in nursing practice.* Philadelphia: J.B. Lippincott Co., 1979, p. 4.

The Need for Applied Evaluation Research

Much practice and program evaluation, however, does not use the scientific method. The fact that something has been done a certain way for a long time is often thought reason enough not to change it. And changes, when made, may be based on an unexplained high-level decision, a report of new methods, an influential person's personal experience, or any of many external and subjective decisions. As a result, opinion as to whether the change was an improvement is often divided. Seldom is the attempt made to isolate causes of particular events or outcomes.

It is particularly important that, in a relatively new and expanding area such as care of the terminally ill, the most conscientious biomedical and social science methodology and criteria be used. Remarking that "Increasing demands for greater accountability are currently affecting the field of terminal care and hospice development," Robert Buckingham (1980, 158) lists six reasons hospice programs themselves should be evaluated:

1. To demonstrate to other groups that the hospice program is an effective health care program
2. To justify past or projected expenditures
3. To determine costs
4. To gain support for expansion of facilities
5. To determine future objectives
6. To determine program efficiency

The foregoing reasons are generated by recent developments in licensing, funding, reimbursement, and patient care expansion. The growing involvement of the federal government and the additional interface with a variety of community agencies and institutions make such documentation essential.

IDENTIFYING RESEARCH PROBLEMS: STEPS IN CLINICAL RESEARCH

Interest in research usually begins with an identified problem. In nursing this may be a nursing practice problem. When people confront a problem, they tend to react out of habit in one of several different ways:

1. They may become angry or merely annoyed, depending on how other things are going that day.
2. They may try to find someone else to deal with it.
3. They may become curious and think about alternatives but do nothing.
4. They may become curious, define alternatives, and begin to design a research project.

In other words, the perspective one has on a problem, can, but does not always, include the option of really studying it and solving it. The tendency to be curious and to direct that curiosity into a valid evaluative project is an attitude—a habit—that can be learned. In the practice of palliative care there is a great deal to wonder about and to study, because good terminal care is, in some ways, a pioneering effort. Many previously held myths are being shattered, and traditional care procedures are being questioned and changed. It seems as if the changes are toward better patient care, but do we honestly— and scientifically—know that they are better? Or are they, even in their improvements, as good as they could be with more analysis?

Careful consideration of a problem and the development of a theory can serve many useful purposes. Theory may generate a hypothesis for testing, it may be useful as a description of a set of phenomena that had previously seemed to be independent, it can be a base from which to design and plan, and it can serve as an aid in learning. Theory frequently ties together observations one has made, feelings one has had, and behaviors one has either been a part of or witnessed. Theory can explain why certain things are commonly done or identify practices that are needed but often overlooked.

The steps in undertaking clinical research can be outlined as follows:

• *Identify the problem.* Is there a connection between individual incidents and a general condition? Is the problem of significance to merit analysis? Can the situation be improved through study? Is it within the researcher's area of authority and expertise to study?

• *State the problem.* Can the study be narrowed to the extent that it is a manageable study? Can its relationship to the larger–general practice be stated? Can the question be focused in such a way as to make it clear what the parameters are?

• *Describe the significance of the problem to practice and theory.* What- who is affected by the problem? How great is the difference between the present state, and what would result from improvement? Are there other problems that result from the existence of the original problem? Is this problem only a part of some larger problem?

• *State the questions that must be answered in order to understand the problem.* What are the two (negative-positive) sides of the issue? What factors create or affect the problem? Can many questions be listed from which the most relevant ones can be drawn? Are they answerable through research?

• *What data must be collected in order to answer the relevant questions.* Are the data available? What will be the cost in time, energy, money to collect the data? Do you have access to both the data and the necessary resources? In what forms will the data be collected?

• *Formulate the study and state the hypothesis.* Can you predict various outcomes from the study and state these as hypotheses?

The next few sections introduce the methodology of clinical research. Those who will be involved in the design, implementation, and/or analysis of research data can find valuable in-depth discussions in modern nursing and research texts and in extensive articles (see, e.g., Abdellah & Levine, 1965; Dickoff, James, & Semradek, 1975; Diers, 1979; Wald & Leonard, 1964; Wandelt, 1970). The journal *Nursing Research* also provides current comprehensive monthly accounts of research in the nursing field.

The first step, identifying the problem, carries with it the assumption that hospice nursing has as its aim the improvement of patient and family care. Research problems will then center around improving clinical knowledge and clinical judgment, which will result in improved clinical practice and, ultimately, better patient care.

There are basically four categories of scientific questions:

1. Questions concerned with naming
2. Questions concerned with existing relationships
3. Questions concerned with correlations
4. Questions concerned with cause and effect

We will look at each of these categories next.

QUESTIONS CONCERNED WITH NAMING

Research in the area of description, which provides names, or labels, for categories can be extremely important. It is often a descriptive study and the labels it produces that heightens awareness of a new field or an increased scope of practice. Elizabeth Kübler-Ross's stages through which a dying person passes were effective in demonstrating a common experience, within individual parameters, that could be understood and supported. The identification of levels of stress has greatly advanced preventative, stress-reduction therapy. Behaviors, attitudes, beliefs, physical responses can all, through various classification systems, becomes predictable and therefore more manageable. Descriptive studies and naming constitute the most basic type of research and, as useful means of characterizing the important aspects of a situation, they are frequently the first step in other research designs.

In descriptive studies the research questions are posed. What does a nurse who deals daily with dying patients and families begin to feel about his or her own mortality? In what ways do families deal with a patient who speaks openly of his or her death? The source of information may be many observations, over time, and in a variety of settings. Concepts are developed as new experiences, reactions, or responses are recorded. When it becomes evident that in every possible situation, responses are replicating already recorded data, it can be assumed that there will not be whole new categories of responses, and the observation stage arbitrarily ends. Actually, it is almost never certain when such studies should be concluded, and in a sense they are always left open to additional insights.

Considerations that should always be carefully evaluated are as follows:
- *The setting.*   If the setting is unique, such as a hospice unit, it may be the setting itself that is the issue. It is difficult to argue that the observations may not have wide applicability in hospitals or nursing homes. If the settings are varied, such as each patient's home, it may be difficult to screen out important and different variables at work in one setting but not in another.
- *The population sample.*   It should be demonstrated that the sample is representative of the population to which the results will be generalized. The fuller the sample is of members who will contribute widely diverse responses, the more certain the researcher can be that there will not be many other unexplained patterns of response not observed. For example, in a situation where children's anxiety levels are being described following visits to dying parents, it would be an obvious omission to use as a sample only relatively young children visiting their mothers. The question is always: is the sample an accurate and a large enough chunk of reality from which to draw conclusions?
- *The study design.*   The study design comprises (1) the instruments for data collection, (2) the process of data collection, and (3) the processing and analysis of data. Forms used to collect data include a variety of forms, surveys, charts, and narratives. It is important that such written records be somewhat consistent and uniform. Over time—and studies are often pursued over as much as a year or two—as data accumulates, perceptions may change, and interpretations can unwittingly be altered if the data are not stated objectively. The sheer amount of data can become overwhelming if the data are not organized. Topics, date, time, and setting should be noted, or coded, in some relatively simple way. Data collection can take place through interviews, observation, patient reporting, the literature, or retrieval of information from existing records. The process and analysis of data does not involve the test of hypotheses. Generally there is no statistical proof involved. The final step in analysis of a descriptive study will be the interpretation of the data in order to formulate concepts and categories. At this stage of the study it is particularly helpful to have a group of colleagues open to discussion of shared experiences and implications.

QUESTIONS CONCERNED WITH
EXISTING RELATIONSHIPS

Questions in this group suggest that there may be relationships among the factors one has chosen to study. If, for example, there are categorical or describable levels of anxiety among children visiting dying parents, then what other factors may relate to those categories? Examples of such factors are age of the child or of the parent, sex of the child or of the parent, setting of visit, preparation of child or of parent for visit. The purpose is not to predict a response within a certain situation, but to discover what factors do relate to the theory.

For example, it might be of value to determine what actions of nurses or physicians seem to be associated with willingness of dying patients to discuss their fears and apprehensions. In discussing the effectiveness of hospice home care teams it might be wise to determine what factors in the home are related to effective care, such as telephone service, comfort of environment, or safety and adaptability of bathroom. A study of relations among team members might also yield interesting results.

Data Collection

Data are collected in much the same way as in descriptive, or naming, studies. The literature should also be carefully surveyed for relevant associations. Theory may be discovered where there was none before. The whole concept of pain has evolved through awareness that it is not purely a physiological phenomenon but relates to the spiritual, psychological, and social dimensions as well.

Research Design

Studies of relationships are only as good as the research questions on which they are based. The who, what, when, where of each situation should be outlined. For example, in determining what social factors are related to difficulty in managing pain, some of the research questions might be, Who is in pain? When are they in pain? What type of pain do they describe? How often and under what circumstances are they in pain or not in pain? The settings and sample should be as comprehensive as the population to whom the study addresses itself. The larger the number of possible relationships and variables, the larger the population should be. As with descriptive studies of any kind, the whole range of instruments can be used; the guiding principle of collection should be objectivity. A conscientious recording of all raw data is advisable. If data are collapsed into categories (such as "adult," "child," "relative-friend") rather than recorded precisely (e.g., "Male, 12, son") the raw data will not be there if there is a need later to redetermine categories.

Data Analysis

Data analysis consists primarily of comparing cases in order to identify the presence of factors relating to that data. Several kinds of relationships should be noted:

- Something occurs in the presence of a specific person, object, or event.
- Something does not occur in the presence of a specific person, object, or event.
- One factor changes as another factor changes.

The goal of answering questions about existing relationships is to suggest hypotheses and thus to make possible continued research to explore correlations and cause-effect relationships.

Questions Concerned with Correlations

Studies concerned with the relationship that exists among factors are said to be *correlational.* Such studies assume that the first two levels of research have been carried out and that (1) factors have been named and/or categorized, and (2) relationships among such factors have been hypothesized. This assumption can be confirmed through research or the literature.

Correlation means that factors occur together or change together. Correlational studies make no statement about the possible causative effects of any factor. Correlation is said to be *positive* if the factors change together in the same direction (e.g., the *greater* the amount of time the dying patient spends alone, the *greater* his or her stated amount of pain) or *negative,* if as one factor increases, the other decreases (e.g., the *more* time the patient stays involved in meaningful activity, the *less* pain medication is required to maintain an acceptable comfort level).

It is important to note that in correlational studies, the existing situation is not altered or manipulated in any way. The data are collected in the natural situation, and the analysis determines whether the predictions about relationships are in fact correct. The real strength of the correlational study lies in its confirmation or negation of a hypothesis and the evidence it provides about the probability that the relationship found is not accidental.

Examples of hospice-related research problems that would be good candidates for correlational studies are as follows:

- In what ways do inpatient hospice patients behave differently from home-care hospice patients?
- Are inpatient hospice patients' perceptions of the effectiveness of hospice care significantly different from home-care hospice patients' perceptions of effectiveness of care?
- Do families of hospice inpatients feel differently about their involvement from families of hospice home-care patients?
- Do patients with body changes related to the reproductive system react differently to the diagnosis of terminal disease than patients without such changes?
- Do patients of different ages-sex react differently to the need to adapt to increasing physical deterioration?
- In what way does respiration vary with constant intravenous infusion of morphine and regularly scheduled oral morphine?
- How do patient's life-long coping styles correlate with physical aspects of their death?

In all of these examples, the research deals with differences. Such studies are particularly valuable in situations where factors cannot be manipulated by introducing a presumed cause in order to study its effect.

Research Designs

The design of a correlational study may be retrospective, prospective, or cross-sectional.

In the *retrospective* design, one event has happened prior to the other and the researcher must look back at historical data to gain information. A retrospective study would need to be done, for example, in order to compare number of days in hospital among patients who have died in hospice home care or in hospital home care programs. The *prospective* study, looks forward in time for its data. An example of such a study might be a comparison of the use of hospice services among patients with and without young dependents. One would first determine the number of dependents and perhaps characterize their level of dependence. One could then compare this information with future requests for and use of services.

The *cross-sectional* design is perhaps the most familiar of all designs. Quite simply, it involves measuring two factors at the same point in time in order to determine whether the factors are associated. For example, one might study the opinions of the hospice music therapy program held by patients of different ages, sex, or ethnic group. People could be asked to rate their satisfaction with the hospice music therapy program, and these ratings could then be compared to the demographic data. The results might show that those of certain ages, sex, or ethnic group seem to find music therapy more effective than those of a different age, sex, or ethnic background.

Correlational studies begin with a formally stated hypothesis or prediction of correlations. For example, "youth hospice patients (under 18) will express greater satisfaction (statistically defined) with the hospice music therapy program than the young adult group (19–29)." This hypothesis is called a *directional hypothesis* because it predicts the direction of the correlation as well as its existence.

Both setting and sample population should be representative of reality and take into consideration a range of variables. Needless to say, a study of expressed appreciation of music therapy among patients would not be representative of the general public if done at the Infirmary at Wolftrap (a conservatory for talented young musicians).

Data collection and the instruments used should be consistent, objective, and unbiased by the researcher's belief in the direction of the hypothesis. Also, one must not be tempted to assume that one factor's presence with another implies a causal relationship. For example, although there may be a high correlation between socioeconomic group and throat cancer, if alcoholism is so strongly associated with both factors then it may be the more important variable.

QUESTIONS CONCERNED WITH
CAUSE AND EFFECT

There are studies that allow us to draw conclusions about cause and effect. These studies subject the relationships established in correlational research to an analysis of whether one factor actually causes another to occur. Three things are essential in order to infer a causal relationship. First, the two factors in the hypothesis must vary together as they do in correlational studies. Second, the time order must be such that the factor inferred as the cause must precede the factor presumed to be the effect. Third, other possible causes, or variables, must be controlled through techniques such as *randomization.* Randomization includes the assignment of subjects to groups in such a way as to assure that each subject has an equal chance of being assigned to the experimental or control group. Two variables are usually considered. One, the *independent variable* is introduced at some point in time and its effects on the other variable, the *dependent variable,* are measured. Measurements to be compared are taken before and after the independent variable is introduced. A second matched group is measured at the same points in time but is not exposed to the independent variable. For example hospice nurses might be measured for ability and comfort in discussing religious issues with patients. One group is then randomly assigned to attend a seminar dealing with such issues; the second group does not attend. Finally, both groups are again tested. All other factors being equal, a greater change in the *treatment group* (the one that attended the seminar) than in the control group (the one that did not attend) could be attributed to the exposure to the seminar.

As with all the previously discussed research designs, setting and sample must be representative of what is real and natural. The process of assigning individual subjects to the control or treatment groups must be random and unbiased. For example, people who might choose, on their own, to participate in the treatment group (attend the seminar) might share a variable (some characteristic such as interest in and enthusiasm for the topic) that would be a more direct cause of their improvement than the content of the seminar.

Research findings are described as *supporting* or *not supporting* the hypothesis. To say that a hypothesis is "supported" means that the probability that the change happened by chance is less than some predetermined level, such as 1 percent or 5 percent. The reader interested in pursuing the complexities of creating the appropriate design, collecting valid data, and subjecting that data to statistical analysis should consult a text devoted to research such as Diers's *Research in Nursing Practice* (1979).

Nursing, as a practice profession, is also involved in developing new and better systems of care. (Lindeman, C, 1974) The designs that address changes that can bring about desired improvements are often called *prescription studies.* In these often massive projects the particular problem is painstakingly analyzed, using all available literature, as well as survey and research methods. Goals are then set for the improved system. All elements of patient need, institutional concerns, and other constraints of time, personnel, and resources are considered. Key results that will mark change are selected. The "prescription" is "filled," and the results are then measured. Such studies are complex, intricate, and often uncontrollable, but their effect on real-life practice is perhaps the greatest of any research.

MEASUREMENT

Measurement is that system of quantification used to provide evidence of the degree to which a hypothesized relationship exists. It is wise to select a measurement that is close to the research concept it is to measure. According to Wolfer (1973), problems occur in this area when individuals use one or another of the following:

• Physical measurements (heart rate) to measure a psychological state (fear). How is it possible to determine that the increase in heart rate is not due to excitement or physical exertion?

• Indirect measures of a state, such as relying on charts, recorded observations, or staff behavior to determine patient state.

• Scales that use extreme or absolute categories that almost no one chooses (e.g., "In my life I have [always, sometimes, never] been painfree").

• Measurements that impose an order on things that are not ordered (e.g., such as male, female or ethnic groups).

• Measurement of a self-reported attitude used as a measurement of actual practice (e.g., accepting the report of nurses that they would discuss a patient's sexual problems with him or her instead of measuring how many actually do discuss the topic).

Measurement instruments can also be evaluated on the basis of the following five criteria:

1. *Reliability.*   The extent to which the measure will yield the same results for the same sample in repeated instances, or the extent to which two measures agree.
2. *Validity.*   The extent to which the measurement measures what it is supposed to measure.
3. *Appropriateness.*   The extent to which the measure fits the sample. (A survey in English would not fit a Spanish-speaking population, perhaps even those for whom English is a second language.)
4. *Sensitivity.*   The extent to which the measurement measures the variation and degrees of what is measured. (Requests for medication as a

measure of patient pain may measure whether pain does or does not exist in the patients who do request medication, but this measure does not address the differences in individuals' pain.)

5. *Meaningfulness.* The extent to which the measure reveals anything useful, applicable, or important (Mendenhall, 1979).

HUMAN RIGHTS IN RESEARCH: THE NUREMBURG LAWS

The rights of human subjects are of great importance in research. Standards of ethics in experimentation and clinical research, based on the Articles of the Nuremburg Tribunal (Katz, J., 1972), emphasize that voluntary consent must be informed, that the research must have value and necessity, and that it must be well documented and planned, and that it must not cause unnecessary physical and mental suffering and injury. Furthermore, any research involving human subjects should not involve risk greater than the importance of the problem and it should be conducted with the highest skill and care, in the best possible facility for patient safety. No experiment should ever be implemented when there is knowledge in advance that it may cause death or disabling injury. The patient must also have the right to terminate the experiment, and the scientist has the responsibility to terminate the experiment if there is reason to believe that continuing will cause the subject injury, disability, or death.

PRIVACY AND CONFIDENTIALITY

It is generally agreed that reports of research should never contain information that can be used to identify individuals. Although confidentiality is generally protected in research through the use of initials or numbers to refer to cases, confidentiality is sometimes breeched when names or patient records are used in raw data or in video or audio tapes, or when patients are discussed by name in professional and even casual conversations among researchers or practitioners. In more recent years, being allowed access to and use of data have also been dependent upon the researchers' ability to guarantee the same human rights to confidentiality or privacy (McElveen, 1975).

PUBLICATION OF RESEARCH RESULTS

Conclusions, in order to be of value, must be shared. Reports of research should include a description of hypotheses, design, data, and analysis procedures. Findings should be described by conscientious researchers who should also use all available evidence and reason to make some suggestion as to how the results may affect future practice and as to the possibilities for additional research.

There is a great need for nursing practice research and for publication of such research (Martinson, 1982). Nursing professionals—practitioners, educators, and researchers—should feel the obligation to share the knowledge gained from their studies. Interesting studies should be integrated into classroom presentations of theories and concepts. The dissemination of research results may be facilitated by conferences and seminars. Publication, however, remains the most extensive means of disseminating research results. An excellent list of nursing journals and their publication policies appears in an article in *Nurse Educator* (McClosky, 1977), and an editorial in *Nursing Research* reports a number of additional options for getting nursing research into print (Carnegie, 1977).

REFERENCES

Abdellah, F.G., & Levine, E. *Better patient care through nursing research.* New York: Macmillan, 1965.

Buckingham, R.W. Evaluation of hospice programs. In T.H. Koff (Ed.). *Hospice: A caring community.* Cambridge, Mass.: Winthrop Publishers, 1980.

Carnegie, M.E. Editorial avenues for reporting research. *Nursing Research, 1977, 26,* p. 83.

Diers, D. *Research in nursing practice.* Philadelphia: J.B. Lippincott Co., 1979.

Dickoff, J., James, P., & Semradek, J. Designing nursing research: eight points of encounter, Part II. *Nursing Research, 1975, 24,* 84–88, 164–176.

Klagsbrun, S.C. Hospice—a developing role. In Saunders, C. (Ed.). *Hospice: The Living Idea.* Philadelphia: W.B. Saunders, 1981.

Lindeman, C.A. *Delphi survey of clinical nursing research priorities.* Boulder, Colorado: Western Interstate Commission for Higher Education, 1974.

Martinson, I.M. *The crisis of the dying child.* Presented at families in Crisis Workshop, Portland, Oregon, Institute for Health Care Education, Oct. 2, 1982.

McClosky, J.C. Publishing opportunities for nurses. A comparison of 65 journals. *Nurse Educator, 1977, 2,* 4–12.

McElveen, P. Critical issues in access to data. In M.V. Batey (Ed.). *Communicating nursing research.* Boulder, Colorado: WICHEN, 1975.

Mendenhall, W. *Introduction to probability and statistics.* (5th ed.). Belmont, California: Wadsworth Publishing Co., 1979.

Wald, F.S., & Leonard, R.C. Toward development of nursing practice theory. *Nursing Research, 1964, 13,* 309–313.

Wandelt, M. *Guide for the beginning researcher.* New York: Appleton-Century-Crofts, 1970.

Wolfer, J.A. Definition and assessment of surgical patients' recovery and welfare. *Nursing Research, 1973, 22,* 394–401.

1. F	6. F
2. T	7. T
3. F	8. F
4. T	9. T
5. T	10. T

16

Understanding One's Own Feelings About Death

Answer the following questions True (T) or False (F). Answers appear on the last page of this chapter.

1. *Caregivers experiencing burnout can often trace their distress to a previously unresolved grief.*

2. *Many people have never confronted their own mortality and are uncomfortable in the presence of death.*

3. *Daily exposure to death statistics and to news of life-threatening disasters has made people better able to handle the death of a loved one.*

4. *Because modern families are more divided geographically, there is less of a support system available when someone is dying.*

5. *It increases one's fears of death to reflect on experiences when his or her impressions of the dying process were formed.*

6. *Describing the way one would want to die and how one would like to be remembered heightens awareness of one's own mortality.*

7. *No one can ever completely understand how someone else feels about dying.*

8. *Most traditional religions provide comfort and security in the knowledge of the usefulness of life and the hope of life's continuation.*

9. *Many patients do not fear death as much as dying alone or in great pain.*

10. *"Compassionate detachment" is not possible; one must truly feel all the dying patient feels to be helpful.*

The doctor or nurse who has evaded the fact of his/her own death can have nothing to say to someone who can no longer evade. Whatever he says will be a lie—symbolized by excessive heartiness of manner, by empty denials and assurance, or by vague dissembling. *

I N CARING FOR THE DYING PATIENT, we are asked to understand and respond. Yet this presents a real problem, because if to understand another person in his or her life requires that we experience the same situation, then we are without a frame of reference. For most of us, prior to our professional career, will not have dealt with a potentially irreversible, life-threatening illness.

RECOGNIZING THE ISSUES

Most dying is done now in hospitals or institutions, often behind a drawn curtain. One of the reason for the increased fear of death today may be that so few people ever actually see it happen. Almost no one is familiar with death. If death were less a stranger to all of us we might be better able to live with the thought of death as a necessary backdrop against which the importance of life's experiences are emphasized. Still, we must, in order to share feelings with the patient, deal with dying at least at the level of recognizing our own fears and anxieties. A number of literary works address this issue and might well be read and discussed as part of this section on understanding ones own feelings about death. They include: dying is fine, but Death, e.e. eummings; Is My Team Plowing, A.E. Housman; *Of Time and the River,* Thomas Wolfe; The Death of Ivan Ilych, Leo Tolstoy; *A Death in the Family,* James Agee; Death of a Hired Man, Robert Frost.

---

* From Epstein, C. *Effective interaction in contemporary nursing.* Englewood Cliffs, N.J.: Prentice-Hall, 1974.

EXPERIENTIAL EXERCISES

A state of "compassionate detachment" is a necessary beginning to effective professional care. The ability to be comfortable enough with one's own death not to deal constantly with it each time one is confronted by another's death is the key to genuine and helpful response. As important as a social and cultural framework is understanding one's own reactions to death or the patient who is dying, of even greater importance is the personal confrontation with one's own learned reactions to and beliefs about death.

The questions and exercises presented in Figures 16-1, 16-2, and Appendix 16-1 are helpful in enabling hospice staff to become more aware of personal beliefs and to begin understanding life-long fears of death. Do not skip (or avoid) these materials. They may be more important than all the reading one could ever do about general beliefs and feelings on the topic of death.

The questionnaire in Figure 16-1 takes about 20 minutes to complete. It will require personal responses, and answers should be confidential. The

---

Figure 16-1. Questionnaire on dying

Try to choose one best response to each question. Some questions clearly present an opportunity for discussion or for multiple choices as to answer, but select the concept that most closely agrees with your belief. You will have a chance for discussion following completion of the questionnaire.

1. I remember that when I was a child my family talked about death

   a. openly, including me
   b. openly, in front of but not including me
   c. as if it were taboo
   d. only when I wasn't present
   e. rarely or never

2. My first encounter with dying was with

   a. grandparent/great-grandparent
   b. parent
   c. brother or sister
   d. pet
   e. friend
   f. other family member
   g. hero
   h. someone close to a friend or to a family member but not to me

3. When I was a child, my concept of what happens after death was that one

   a. went to heaven or hell
   b. went to sleep
   c. stopped breathing and moving
   d. joined nature
   e. disappeared mysteriously
   f. no concept

4. Today, I believe that after death one

Figure 16-1 (continued)

    a. has a spiritual after-life
    b. sleeps eternally
    c. is non-existent

    d. cannot know what will happen
    e. joins with the universe, nature, life's energy
    f. no concept

5. I think about my own death

    a. almost every day
    b. frequently

    c. once in a while
    d. almost never or never

6. My main reason for not wanting to die is that I'd

    a. be unsure of the kind of afterlife I would have.
    b. be unable to provide for my family.
    c. not be able to complete my plans

    d. die with pain.
    e. not have control over what would happen to people I care about.

7. Some people believe that we can will ourselves to start dying. I believe this

    a. substantially

    b. partially
    c. not at all

8. Thinking about dying makes me

    a. angry
    b. afraid
    c. uncomfortable

    d. depressed
    e. happy to be alive
    f. other

9. If my physician knew that I had a terminal disease, I would want him or her to tell me.

    a. True

    b. False

10. If my physician did not tell me of my terminal diagnosis, I would want a nurse to tell me.

    a. True

    b. False

11. If I knew I was terminally ill, I would want to talk about it to

    a. no one
    b. my mate
    c. close family

    d. clergy
    e. physician
    f. nurse
    g. a close friend

12. If someone I really cared for was terminally ill and wanted to talk about it, I would feel

    a. awkward
    b. willing and comfortable

    c. honored
    d. very sad

13. The thing I dread most about the dying process is

    a. pain
    b. mental deterioration
    c. being someone I wouldn't like

    d. dependency
    e. fears about afterlife
    f. sadness of loved ones

Figure 16-1 (continued)

14. I find the sight of a dead body

   a. revolting
   b. frightening
   c. disconcerting
   d. satisfying
   e. natural

15. When there is a funeral for someone I care about I

   a. usually do not go
   b. go but dislike it
   c. am pleased to go
   d. go if it is convenient

16. When people begin talking about death in a casual situation I

   a. feel anxious
   b. feel embarrassed
   c. think it is too personal
   d. am interested in their ideas
   e. am bored

17. The illness that I would least like to have is

   a. heart disease
   b. cancer
   c. diabetes
   d. kidney disease
   e. arthritis
   f. multiple sclerosis
   g. stroke
   h. other _____

experience of completing the survey should serve as a basis for small group discussions and a sharing of values about dying and death. The soliloquies in Appendix 16-1 provide a sensitive and thought-provoking exercise which should trigger good discussion about individual perspectives on death. One's personal perspective can be analyzed by completing the questionnaire in Figure 16-2.

The Caregiver

Perhaps one of the most difficult parts of supporting and caring for dying patients is to feel without being overwhelmed, to care without being overcome, to participate without losing identity. When caregivers are reliving some experience of their own, possibly some unresolved grief situation, they are likely to be of little use to the patient or family. If the grief is for the caregivers themselves and for the past, if they are caught in a stage of denial, anger, or guilt, then the patient's sorrow becomes only a reflection of their own unresolved emotion. It is not unusual that when caregivers evidence definite signs of stress or burnout, they can often trace such reactions to their inability to handle the intensity of the presence of death. In order to enter into the grief of others without despair, one must have first dealt with his or her own grief.

The prototype of the hospice professional is the caring, sensitive person who assists the peacefully acceptant dying one. The nurse who does not

Figure 16-2. Reflection as a source of understanding

1. Speculate about your own death. What will be the cause? How old will you be? What will the place and circumstances be? Who will be affected by your death? What will the funeral be like? What will the bereavement process be for those close to you?

2. Describe the way, if it were up to you, that you would prefer to die. Describe the way, if it were up to you, that you would least like to die.

3. You have just learned that you will die in a matter of months. Write a letter to someone with whom you want to share this.

4. Write the eulogy you would prefer.

5. Describe the way you react, the masks you wear, the things you say, when talking with someone who has just lost a loved one.

6. How does your interest in hospice care fit into your responses to death?

7. Write about the times in your life when you have been closely associated with death or dying. This reflective journey back through life may help you focus on experiences that possibly formed your present attitudes. Try to remember your original emotions as honestly as possible.

8. List as many as you can remember of the fantasies and fears you have held in your life. It will be easy to list the movies, books, stories, and jokes that were sources of fear but try also to get at the deep-seated fears. To admit such fears—those fears to which our gut reaction is far greater than our rational response tells us is appropriate (darkness, snakes, etc.)—is to begin to weaken them. Understanding may explain their relationship to the way we protect ourselves from the fear of death.

recognize the unrealistic demands of this image may suffer a great deal of confusion and guilt. Attitudes toward the dying patient and his or her family and friends are as varied as our attitudes toward every other individual person with whom we interact. People die pretty much in the manner in which they have lived. They may be kind and considerate, brave, or profoundly philosophical, or their behavior may be selfish, demanding, miserly, vindictive —a whole host of generally unpleasant characteristics, heightened by physical discomfort and emotional confusion.

Some dying patients are extremely difficult to care for, and we may need to rotate responsibilities for such individuals. Although most patients who die cause sorrow in those around them, difficult patients may elicit from those who have to cope with them a sense of relief at their passing. It will be the nurse's hardest task to assimilate all these feelings. These feelings must not be denied but must be recognized as human response to another's very human behavior.

The Historic Perspective

Anxiety about the confrontation with death has found expression and resolution in the testaments of every religion. In Al Koran, Chapter 75, this fear of the unknown is addressed, "Man would ever deny that which is to come. He asks, 'When will this day of Resurrection be?' But when mortal eyes are utterly darkened, and the Moon eclipsed; when the Sun and Moon are brought together—on that day man will ask: 'Whither can I flee?'" And in Muslim tradition, the resurrection is confirmed in the recitation by those around a dying person of the prayer, "All glory to Him who controls all things! Unto Him you shall all return" (Baqui, 1979, p. 1).

Judeo-Christian literature confirms the promise of comfort and hope for immortality of the soul in Job, 19:25–27 RSV: "I know that my Redeemer lives and He will stand at last upon the earth. And after my skin has been thus destroyed then from my flesh I shall see God: Whom I shall see on my side, and mine eyes shall behold and not another." (See also Levenstein, 1979, p. 3.)

Death has been central to the psychologists' search for meaning of self. Freud states that the unconscious does not recognize its own mortality and that it is impossible to imagine our own death. He recognizes that even as we attempt to do so, we think of ourselves still present as spectators. (Freud, 1915) This Freudian view suggests that what we are most anxious about concerning death is that which we cannot *know*. Recent observations have revealed a source of fear different than one of physical destruction. It is now thought that the greater fear is of helplessness and abandonment; a fear of the destruction of self, of individual identity. Levcton (1954) labels this *ego chill,* "a shudder which comes from the sudden awareness that our non-existence is entirely possible" (p. 70).

The American culture, in general, has been death-denying. Our culture has assiduously ignored the fact of death, offering us little chance to become comfortable with it. In this connection it is interesting to contrast traditional children's rhymes and tales with some of their more modern variations. Humpty Dumpty, originally unable to be "put together again" has a different ending in the modern *Space Child's Mother Goose,* which happily removes considerations of death:

> *Humpty Dumpty sat on a wall.*
> *At three o'clock he had his great fall.*
> *The King set the Time Machine back to two.*
> *Now Humpty's unscrambled and good as new.**

Throughout the years, a number of revisions to *Little Red Riding Hood* have also made this tale more palatable. Originally "eaten all up," Little Red Riding Hood in 1948 was still eaten but was saved by a woodsman who

---

*From Winsor, F. *The space child's Mother Goose.* New York: Simon & Schuster, 1968, p. 41.

chopped open the wolf and saved her. By 1957, the woodsman was bursting in to save Riding Hood before the wolf could even get to her. But the advantages of putting the death question out of the sight of children have not gone unchallenged more recently. In the past decades our changing view of death as a part of the life cycle and something to be dealt with openly has brought to popularity such beautiful and creative books as E.B. White's *Charlotte's Web*.

In the meantime, there exists a generation of people who avoid the topic of death at all costs. These people always avoid relationships with people who might die, and one cannot discuss a will with them. They minimize separation and project the future without a hint of mortality.

WHY CAN WE NOT DEAL WITH DEATH?

Feifel (1965) believes that six conditions underlie the difficulties the American culture has in dealing with death. The first is *urbanization*. Because people are moving away from nature, except for recreational purposes, they are not witnessing the life–death cycle.

Second, *separation of the aged and ill* from the general society has hidden death and dying. The elderly and those near death are often moved into nursing homes or hospitals. Because we now anticipate such separation, it increases the fear of death as a lonely and abandoned experience.

Third, *the nuclear family* has grown smaller and is often isolated. Increasingly three definite situations result as families in one geographic area comprise a nuclear unit and extended family relatives are scattered across the country: there is less family support to help care for someone who is dying; few people see relatives die; and, after a death, the remaining family is far more alone.

Fourth, the *secularization of religion* has removed the cushion against the impact of death offered by many religious beliefs in their emphasis on the meaningfulness of death and promise of a future and immortality. The loss for many people of such religious answers has made the question of death much harder to cope with.

A fifth unsettling factor, according to Feifel, is *advanced medical technology*. The illusion created by modern science is that human beings are in control of death, or at least that they can stall the inevitable. We are left with the bio-ethical dilemmas presented by euthanasia, differing definitions of death, and the living will.

Feifel's last condition is *death desensitization*. The almost daily exposure to both the news of mass death (e.g., plane accidents, guerrilla attacks, foreign invasions, riots) and the possibility of nuclear attack or accident has numbed us to the significance and value of human life. Such mass death has made almost insignificant the individual death. In fact, it is a minor 6 o'clock news story if only a couple of people are killed by a sniper. A whole village has to be wiped out before it seems important.

Even more extraordinary than the foregoing, according to Feifel, is that the group to which care of the dying has been entrusted—the health care professions—deny death more than the general populace. Evidence of this denial is seen in the avoidance of the dying patient's room. In defense of their behavior, hospital staff may suggest that it is unwise to "upset" the terminal patient by discussions. In fact, it is more often the staff who become awkward and nervous. Patients seem willing, even relieved, to share their dying experiences with others. Kübler-Ross (1970) reports that of the dying patients she worked with, only 2% rejected the opportunity to discuss their dying.

No one denies that it is extremely difficult for anyone to resolve the threat of the end of self within the framework of everyday existence and productivity. Robert Jay Lifton (1972) experienced this decreased ability to cope with the face of death. After days of emotionally draining interviews with victims of the Hiroshima disaster, Lifton reports that he developed a protective detachment. Through this confrontation with story after story of death and despair he was bombarded with evidence of his own vulnerability, and out of defense he turned off the confrontation.

Lifton's mode of detachment is also known as *distancing*. One creates distance between an emotion-arousing event or situation and one's own responses in order to maintain the objective attitude necessary to make a scientific contribution. Distancing, which is a means of ordering the chaos of life's unpredictability, should not be confused with *denial*.

PSYCHOLOGICAL WAYS OF ADDRESSING DEATH'S INEVITABILITY

There are many attitudes toward death in the American culture. In one way or another, these attitudes do address the inevitability of death.

Death-Defying Attitudes

The death-defying attitude is rooted in our heritage. We have long regarded as virtuous those who have stubbornly fought and were willing to die for religious causes, nationalism, political ideologies, and freedoms. A negative kind of death-defying can be seen in the person who dares or tempts death by sustaining a highly dangerous, "dare-devil" life-style.

Another kind of death defying can be seen in those who, like many physicians, view disease as an enemy and themselves as warriors in that battle. An example of this popular mind set would be the "war against cancer." Great honor and respect are accorded those in the healing professions who, many would agree, "snatch patients from the jaws of death."

Death-Desiring Attitudes

To desire one's own death is considered somehow un-American. Yet is is far more common in our culture than we admit. A death-desiring attitude is found in many who are severely debilitated, disabled, and unhappy. The elderly who are ill, living on fixed low incomes, and without family love and support comprise a large group who might welcome a release from living.

Death-Accepting Attitudes

A whole range of attitudes place death in perspective as a part of the continuity of life—a part that is essential to regeneration, to existence. Death may be seen as a conclusion, passage, or beginning but always as a natural part of the life process. The death-accepting attitude describes, through metaphor, the stream becoming a river, flowing at least into the sea, or merging into the greater being.

This view is comforting in the case of the life lived fully or a 'timely' death at an advanced age. There is also the peace that comes from the knowledge of one's place in what Thomas Berger, in *Little Big Man* (1964) calls the "universal circle" where all things of nature know no separation. The narrator, Little Big Man, tells of his climb up the mountain with the aged Chief, Old Lodge Skins.

The chief recounts his life's experiences, his regret that his tribe has suffered so at the hands of the white people and the belief that his people will live on through their qualities of strength and bravery. When they reach the summit the ancient chief throws off his blanket and yells the great battle cry of the Cheyenne. "Come out and fight!" he was shouting. "It is a good day to die!" (Berger, 1964, p. 444).

The understanding and acceptance of Little Big Man for this closing of the universal circle then concludes. "He laid down then on the damp rocks and died right away. I descended to the treeline, fetched back some poles, and built him a scaffold. Wrapped him in the red blanket and laid him thereon. Then after a while I started down the mountain in the fading light" (Berger, 1964, 444–445).

Death-Continuation

Another view of death is based in fear, not of physical death but of ceasing to exist—that beyond death is nonbeing. The issue becomes one of "giving meaning" to death. The solution to this, for many, is a religious one, through the transcendence of physical death. "For whosoever will save his life shall lose it, and whoever will lose his life for my sake shall find it" (Matthew 16:25) is seen as assurance of "life-being" after death. Life thus gains meaning as a doorway to a more important afterlife.

INVOLVEMENT OF SELF
WITH THE DYING PERSON

To help the dying, one must first face his or her own mortality. Only in this way can one avoid rejecting the dying person out of fear or traumatically fusing oneself with him or her. In this way one does not deny the death or react with such blinding sensitivity that all objectivity and ability to help is lost.

As interest in death and dying has reawakened, attitudes of acceptance have occasionally been dangerously distorted. Detachment has sometimes been escalated by professionals into total detachment through extreme distancing and depersonalization. The barriers of professionalism cause the person to become "an oatcell of the lung"—dying to become a "series of stages." Death is external to the patient, held at bay by the successful therapy or, if it does occur, it is not the medicine that is to blame—it "always happens in a certain percentage."

Nurses are often taught not to discuss serious issues or personal matters with a patient. Their role models, and even didactic sessions, encourage a professional, efficient briskness. The ability not to become emotionally involved is frequently seen as a sign of maturity. Yet nurses, social workers, and therapists see patients often when the patient is at a personally vulnerable stage. The possibilities are almost endless for a relationship to develop (Littlefield, 1982). C. Murray Parkes (1978) has said, "I do not think we can avoid this issue. Human relationships are dangerous. When we get attached to our patients we begin to suffer with them and we may even become involved to the point where we are overwhelmed by our own distress and become useless to them. Although this is true, I do not think it justifies the extreme distancing which is encouraged in many teaching hospitals" (p. 55).

THE POSITIVE SIDE OF DEATH

It is often useful when confronting a condition like death, that is difficult to accept, to consider how things might be if that condition were not inevitable. It may be a bit of a rationalization, but it is important to recognize the significance of the very positive aspects of death. The very fact that man cannot escape death, real or symbolic, means that life must be constructed with full realization of that fact. Peter Kostenbaum (1972) points out that acceptance of this inevitability allows a person actually to begin living—free of the debilitating threat of an unknown mortality and free of the indecisiveness and lack of courage caused by the threat of symbolic death. There is actually a real vitality in the realization of death. Kostenbaum emphasizes that this recognition that we won't live *forever* spurs us to achievement and concentration on essentials. In essence, he is saying, we need death in order to savor life. It encourages us to waste no time in seeking and finding fulfillment. It strengthens the bonds of love and fondness to know that our time is precious.

Ernest Becker, in *The Denial of Death* (1973), also sees death as a primary motivating force in the actions and reactions of human beings. Becker writes that the avoidance of the futility of death may take the form of noble actions for peace and goodness, which allows a "heroic transcendence" of death (p. 136).

Death points up the impermanence of everything but our integrity and the constancy of our principles. This is all we really own. The idea of death helps us to gain a perspective that is both noble in recognizing what is truly important and humorous in the recognition of what is irrelevant and foolish (Kostenbaum, 1972).

When one is confronted with the challenge of caring for the dying patient, many questions about the whys, hows, and whens of disease and death arise. It is normal to experience these questions in relation not only to the patient but to oneself. A nurse or any health care professional is not immune to experiencing fear, frustration, or even a sense of fatalism when confronted with these questions. It is very difficult to accompany someone on the road to death, to "be with" the person. But nursing and supportive care can greatly smooth that path if both clinical and emotional maturity are shared with the patient. And it should be remembered that although demanding of inner resources, working with dying patients does provide many opportunities for personal growth and self-awareness. It is a constant lesson in the value of sensitivity and of setting priorities to a fulfilling life. For, over time, the significance of the quality of a life well led may far outweigh the spectre of dying (Mount, 1980). The interest on any caregiver's investment of emotion is often an immense satisfaction in having fulfilled the patient's needs for closeness at a time that is potentially frightening and lonely.

REFERENCES

Baqui, M.A. *Jewish and Muslim Teachings Concerning Death* (occasional paper). South London Mosque: St. Joseph's Hospices.

Becker, E. *The denial of death.* New York: Free Press, 1973.

Berger, T. *Little Big Man.* Greenwich, Conn.: Fawcett Publishing, 1964.

Blues, T. *Soliloquies,* unpublished, 1978.

Epstein, C. *Effective interaction in contemporary nursing.* Englewood Cliffs, N.J.: Prentice-Hall, 1974.

Feifel, H. The function of attitudes towards death. In *Death and dying: Attitudes of patient and doctor.* New York: Group for the Advancement of Psychiatry, 1965.

Freud, S. Thoughts for the times on woe and death. *Collected Papers* (Vol. 4), London: Hogarth, 1915.

Katz, J. *Experimentation with human being.* New York: Russell Sage, 1972, p. 305–306.

Kostenbaum, P. The vitality of death. *Omega,* 1972, *2,* 269–271.

Kübler-Ross, E. *On death and dying.* New York: Macmillan, 1970.

Levenstein, M. *Jewish and Muslim teaching concerning death.* St. Joseph's Hospice Publication, *Occasional Paper,* London, 1975, 3–5.

Leveton, A. Time, death and the ego-chill. *Journal of Existentialism,* 1954, *6,* 69–80.

Lifton, R.J. On death and death symbolism: The Hiroshima disaster. *Psychiatry,* 1972, *27,* 191–210.

Littlefield, N.T. A brief relationship. *American Journal of Nursing,* 1982, *9,* 1395–1399.

Mount, B., & Voyer, J. Staff stress in palliative hospice care. In B. Mount & I. Ajemian (Eds.). *Royal Victoria Hospital manual on palliative hospice care.* New York: Arno Press, 1980.

Parkes, C.M. Psychological aspects. In C.M. Saunders (Ed.). *The management of terminal disease.* London: E. Arnold, 1978.

Russell, B. *Portraits from Memory.* New York: Simon and Schuster, 1956.

Winsor, F. *The space child's Mother Goose.* New York: Simon and Schuster, 1968.

White, E.B. *Charlotte's Web.* New York: Harper and Row, 1952.

1. T	*6. T*
2. T	*7. T*
3. F	*8. T*
4. T	*9. T*
5. F	*10. F*

Appendix 16-1. *The Dramatic Soliloquy as a Source of Understanding*

The following soliliquies can be read in class by a narrator and four readers. It is best if these people are seated front center and thus visible to the class. Each reader, in his or her turn, should stand and read. Time should be allowed for discussion following the total presentation.

Prologue (read by the narrator)

The soliloquy is an ancient dramatic convention, employed by the dramatist to convey a character's innermost thoughts and feelings. The character, alone on stage, speaks directly to the audience but as if the audience were not present. It is always understood that when a character speaks in soliloquy, whether that character is a noble hero or a villain of the deepest dye, he speaks the truths of his heart so far as he knows them. In the following soliloquies there are no heroes or villains, merely some ordinary people who, as all of us must often do, are trying to deal with a difficult aspect of life.

The Woman

I can't decide what's worse—to have to die, or to have to live among these silences. I thought it would be a relief to get home, away from the hospital, away from "How are we today, Mrs. Richardson," and that baby-talk praise the first time I could walk to the bathroom. And Dr. Weaver, talking to the wall about radiation treatments to stop the cancer from going any further. But it's no different here. I thought it would be fine to put a dress on again, until I saw how it hangs on me. And how I wish I could take that picture off the mantel, the one of Ed and Tim and me taken only a year ago last Christmas. I recognize my husband and my son, but who is that healthy, smiling woman holding her boy in front of her with her husband's arm around her shoulders? I can't stand to look at her and know she's gone. All that's left is this pale, thin ghost with an aching back that Doane's Pills and radiation therapy aren't going to stop.

But I can't take the picture down. They'd notice. We can't have that. There's been some agreement not to notice.

Ed's been so helpful, doing the laundry, cleaning the house. I know I should love him for trying to help, and I hate myself for resenting the things he does as if to keep away from me. Why can't he look at me anymore, or hold me so I know I'm a person and not a broken thing you have to keep around? Why can't I be grateful for the chance to act out my role as the wife whose husband is helpful and considerate and who keeps their boy from bothering her while she gets better?

Because the doctor didn't remove my heart and brain and soul with my uterus, I know I'm dying. Their silences and empty talk and my weakness have told me that. We all know. So why do we pretend? Why do I let them take themselves away from me before I'm gone? I've got so much I want to say, so much I want to do. I have to talk to Ed about Tim and try to bring them closer together. They'll need each other when I'm gone. And Ed needs to know it's all right if he marries again, for a man needs a wife, and a boy a mother. I want him to understand that it's all right, that it will make me feel better if I can think they won't be alone. I want to talk to Tim about growing up. I'd like to teach Ed something about cooking—where everything is. For all the things he's done in taking care of everything, the kitchen's not been his domain, and I don't want them eating out all the time. I'd like to make a will, even though I want everything, except a few keepsakes for my sister, to go to Ed and Tim. But I'd like to be able to have it written down, to have some say in what becomes of what I have. If I could do these things I'd get my love back for them. I know I would. Oh God, if I can't have my life, then please give me my husband and my son before I die. I want to tell them how sorry I am for what they're going through and how it's all right to be sorry for me and even to cry a little.

But they don't look at me. How awful and ugly I've become. They won't touch me. They won't talk to me.

Oh, I know deep down I'd do the same, the way I avoided talking to Mother after the first heart attack. I'm no better. And that's the whole trouble. I talk now about taking a trip when I'm well again. But I can't stand it. I don't have it in me to forgive them, and I don't have the strength to die alone. I need to live and die among them, not alone. It takes so long. It's such a waste.

What's worse? To have to die, or to have to live among these hateful silences? What difference does it make? I'm doomed to both.

The Man

I always thought I'd be the first to go. Well, actually, I never really thought about it at all until the doctor told me Ellen would die. It was just something you understood about the proper order of things.

And then I learned that it hadn't worked out the way it should have, and I suddenly felt responsible, as if I'd done something wrong, or not done something I should have. All I knew, when he told me, was that I couldn't tell her, not then; and I felt a little guilty about that, for not knowing how and for fearing I'd break down. And so I was glad when Dr. Weaver seemed to agree that it might be best to let her believe she'd recover, at least for a while. Why make things even worse?

Of course, I knew the time would come when she'd have to know anyway, but it's sort of funny when you think of it—I remembered when I was a boy growing up and wondering when my father would tell me about sex, which I was learning about anyway from my own body and the other kids and books. But I wanted him to talk to me about it anyway, especially when I had my first wet dream and was so scared of what my body had done in my sleep, without my knowing or willing it. I don't like things I can't control. But he never did talk with me, my father. And so I grew up anyway, and I knew he knew, and he knew I knew, and it all seemed okay, though there was always something missing between him and me.

I thought it might be like that—that Ellen would eventually know and we wouldn't have to talk about it at all. And maybe it is best, after all. Maybe she doesn't really want to know. Every time I ask her how she feels she says fine and turns back into the newspaper or her sewing or the TV. She talks about a trip to Florida when she's strong enough to travel.

The trouble is, even if she doesn't want to know, I've just got to talk to somebody. I can't seem to manage this alone. I wish Tim were old enough to understand. But what's going to happen to us? How can I take care of him by myself? It's not right for a boy to be without a mother. I've always taken care of anything. I've worked hard, and planned, and saved. I bought this house and built the garage myself. I would have had the furniture paid off next year if all this hadn't happened. I thought I'd bought enough insurance, but now I'll have to use some of what we'd been saving for Timmy's education.

Everything's going wrong. Things are happening that I can't control anymore. You'd think she'd say something. Doesn't she worry about Timmy coming home to an empty house after school? She knows I can't get off work that early. And what will I do with him? He's never really talked to me, always to his mother. I had it figured we'd be close when he got older, when we could do things together, go to ball games or whatever.

Oh, I don't know why I'm taking this out on her. It's not her fault, but it's all going wrong and I'm just plain scared and I can't even look her in the eye. There's so much to think about. So much to talk about. How can I tell her now? Why didn't the doctor tell her? I could see he wanted me to do it. But he's the doctor isn't he? He should know about these things. How to do it. What to say. And now he looks at me in a funny way, as if it's all my fault. But how can I tell her now? She'd blame me for trying to deceive her when I told her she'd be all right, like its supposed to be, like in the picture on the mantel? What did we do wrong?

The Boy

Bobby says he heard his mom tell his dad that my Mom has cancer. But I said you get cancer from smoking cigarettes and Mom doesn't smoke. Bobby says you can catch it from somebody, like measles. Bobby doesn't know everything. But cancer is what you die of. Is Mom going to die?

I know Mom's sick. She's so thin and white. I'm afraid to look at her. It's scary. I could ask her if she's going to die, but Dad says not to bother her while she's getting well from the hospital. He says she needs her rest and peace and quiet.

Still, I wish I could ask her, like when I asked her where Dad took Tinker and didn't bring him back when Tinker got sick. She said Tinker had to be put to sleep and it didn't hurt. She said Tinker was better off asleep than hurting. She called being dead, "asleep." But it can't be asleep when you don't wake up, if you sleep forever. How long does forever go on?

I asked Dad what's wrong and he said Mom had stomach trouble. That's where I came from, her stomach. Maybe I hurt her when I was in her stomach. Why can't Dad be sick? But Dads don't have babies. It wouldn't be too bad if Dad died because he never talks to me like Mom used to. I've seen people die on television, but it always happens right away, like when they got shot and sometimes they talk to somebody bending over and then they close their eyes.

If you can catch cancer from somebody else I might get it from Mom. But I don't want to die. Maybe that's why Dad won't let me be near Mom too much.

The Doctor

I don't know. Maybe I should have insisted that Richardson tell his wife the truth. A little push would have done it. In some ways it would have been easier than for me to give her the full prognosis. It sometimes steadies them when they know.

But it wasn't up to me to tell her, to face those questions: How long do I have? Why me? What did I do? What's going to happen to my children? Isn't there anything you can do? Sure, I understand the fear, the hysteria. I'd be scared stiff too. That's just the trouble. I can't react to these questions and still do my job. I can't go around being scared and feeling like a failure. Don't they understand that I've done everything I can do? That there are limits? Why don't they come in earlier? Dammit, I could tell that Richardson wanted me to do more of the explaining for him. But I did tell her—she just doesn't want to hear. It's almost as if by not listening to me it isn't really happening. I tried to explain so she'd understand but I'm a surgeon, not a social worker. God knows I've got feelings too, but I can't spend all my time brooding every time I lose a patient. I can be sorry; I'm always sorry, but I'm only a doctor, and that's what they never understand. That a doctor is not a savior.

I sometimes think that the myth of the doctor that got started somewhere and won't let go is to blame for all of this. The myth of the kindly, white haired physician sitting next to the bed of the feverish child, bringing him through the diptheria with love and kindness and the magical contents of a little black bag. Well, the little black bag sure as hell won't get rid of the carcinogens in the air we breathe and the water we drink and the preservatives we eat—the whole damn cancerous environment.

What am I getting so angry about? I've got to settle myself down, and realize all over again that there isn't anything I can do. I'm just a doctor and I've got feelings too. But I can't let them get the better of me. I can't do my job if I have to keep admitting how helpless I am.

The Neighbor

I see her sometimes when Ed takes her to the hospital for radiation therapy, and once last week when she was in her yard hanging some blankets on a line to air them out. I saw how she strained to lift them, and I wanted to go over and help, to ask, even, how she's feeling and if there's something I can do. But how do you face that face? That awful pallor, those hollow eyes? I don't know why I watch her through the windows. Some morbid curiosity? Am I no different from the ghouls who gather round auto wrecks? Maybe. But I think I can feel in myself a dreadful but very human curiosity to see what one rarely sees in a neighborhood anymore. Old people are taken to nursing homes to finish out their lives, and those of us who don't make it to the nursing homes die in hospitals. We don't die in our own beds. There are no more funerals in homes. We've made death invisible. But something in us needs to be reminded of our mortality, and so we sneak peeks at it—from a safe distance, of course. Our detachment costs us dearly, for we can't ultimately detach ourselves from death. What we accomplish by our denial of it is to separate ourselves from one another. One out of four of us, they say, will get cancer. But what we forget is that four out of four of us will die. As the poet said, after all the diseases go the way of the passenger pigeon and the great auk, there will still be plain old death.

There must be a way to make it real again, to bring our mortality back into our lives, so we can confront it and speak of it and learn to accept it as part of the nature of things. I'm tired and ashamed of peeking at it through curtains.

How different, how wonderful it would be if I could see Ellen as a person, a woman, a neighbor, a friend. As a person who is dying and not as Death itself. To make her a human being again, to walk up to her and look her in the eyes with a smile of greeting, to say, "Hi, Ellen, glad to see you again. Can I help with anything?" How wonderful, how easy, and how impossible it seems. But there's got to be a way.

T. Blues, 1978

17

Professional Stress and Distress

Answer the following questions True (T) or False (F). Answers appear on the last page of this chapter.

1. *A mature hospice nurse will be able to perform his or her professional role without experiencing stress.*

2. *The high expectations of nurses working with the dying are easily achieved through the hospice movement.*

3. *Nurses with high self-esteem will be able to meet all the patient's needs.*

4. *Some nurses work with the dying in order to resolve their own fears of death and loss.*

5. *It is normal for a nurse in a new hospice program to experience feelings of intense powerlessness and sadness during the first year of work.*

6. *Recurrent pain in your back or neck can be a barometer of stress in your life.*

7. *One difficulty of caring for the dying is that dying persons are essentially powerless to meet their own needs.*

8. *The compassionate hospice nurse values work activities over home life.*

9. *Running promotes relaxation for some people, whereas total silence and absence of activity can achieve the same effect for others.*

10. *The hospice organization needs to encourage cost efficiency without wearing the individual nurse out from overextension.*

Do we keep our lives uncluttered with things and activities, and avoid commitments beyond our strength and light?—Pacific Yearly Meeting of the Religious Society of Friends, 1973.

L IFE IS A PROCESS of ongoing adaptation to change. Stress can be defined as a demand for adaptation that either results in growth or, if excessive, threatens physical and emotional health. This chapter describes the stresses inherent in working with the dying and explores personal and organizational ways of responding to those stresses to avoid staff burnout. *Burnout* is defined as deterioration of individual well-being, with loss of compassion. McElroy (1982) has reviewed the literature on cancer nursing and burnout.

STRESSES OF HOSPICE WORK

Working with terminally ill people makes some unique demands. Performing this work full-time and in a hospice or palliative care program increases the kinds of stress to which one will be subject. Table 17-1 lists some of the common work-related stressors that are discussed in this section.

The Patient Population

One of the most difficult problems in working with the dying is the constant need to establish and then relinquish relationships with people. And the grief and pain of others touches the grief and pain in ourselves. Staring into the face of our own grief and death has been discussed in Chapter 16. The powerful experience of death and dying is a daily companion to the hospice nurse. No matter how committed one is to the value of comforting care, it is terribly difficult to accept the reality that no one in our entire caseload is likely to get better.

348

Table 17-1. *Work-Related Stressors*

- Daily confrontation with death and loss
- Daily confrontation with physical and psychosocial suffering
- Idealized expectations of achievement
- Being under close scrutiny and feeling the need to win support for the hospice movement
- Economic insecurity
- Ambiguous job description
- Work overload
- Evolving identity and philosophy
- Intense small-group dynamics
- Demanding, broad-spectrum needs of patient and family
- Challenges to values
- Unconscious personal agendas
- Need to express intense feelings
- Limited power as nurse
- Crisis and change in home and social life
- Threat to personal relationships of overextension at work

In addition to compelling us to face grief and death, the intensity of dying patients' daily circumstances is highly stressful to the nurse witness. We observe multiple symptoms out of control that we must struggle to manage. We must face irreversible deteriorating bodily changes: puffing up, discoloration, distortion, weight loss that may make people look like Auschwitz victims. In addition, we are sometimes confronted with the end-of-life harvest of all that has been unhealthy and unloving in a person's lifetime. That is, we are often witness to family squabbles, divisive or nonexistent communication, lack of reconciliation, ignorance and denial, self-destructive behavior, poverty, and oppression. Occasionally this opportunity for witness is inspiring and nurturing, as we are fortunate to be at the side of those integrated and wise human beings who have achieved reconciliation and meaning in their lives, and can share this with us.

The Mission of the Program

The nurse who is working with the dying as a part of a developing hospice program or agency is susceptible to the vulnerabilities unique to the hospice movement. These include glorious written and spoken ideals that place lofty expectations on the nurse, often without established practical mechanisms for achievement. Nurses in a new program place high expectations on themselves, in addition to those imposed by the agency. Nurses expect themselves to achieve "good deaths" for their patients, as described in the literature, but in a new program the path to this goal—given limited personal, agency, and community resources—has yet to be cleared. Meanwhile, the nurses know that their care and "success" with each case is under intense scrutiny by fellow professionals and by the community. Often agency practices, such as death counseling and the use of high-dose narcotic regimens, are quite controversial in the professional community. Each home case may be considered an opportunity to win primary physician understanding and support; each hospital admission may be an opportunity to "convert" new staff members as they see how comfortable hospice patients can be. Suddenly we are supposed to be public relations experts!

Lack of clear goals and structure within an evolving program is a tremendous opportunity to be a pioneer, but the way of the pioneer is often unknown and constantly changing. Source of salary may be uncertain from month to month. High expectations of achieving the "good death," coupled with the promise of 24-hour availability to patients and families, leads many professionals to work extended overtime hours, often without reimbursement. In the beginning of a program, it is not uncommon for a single nurse to make himself or herself available 24 hours a day, 7 days a week! Many nurses must wear multiple hats such as administrator, fund raiser, bookkeeper, nurse, and housekeeper. Because the job description is ambiguous, the job itself is highly stressful in its developmental stage. The hospice movement and the subprofession of hospice nurse are still emerging. Underlying premises and directions are still hotly debated: "The hospice movement must proceed through various ideological battles as the field struggles to define itself" (White, 1981). Our identity is subject to change.

William White describes the hazards of working within a small hospice program that becomes a close social network, increasingly cut off from others and trapped in complex interpersonal dynamics within the group. The leadership is often idealized, and staff may self-righteously judge outsiders (White, 1981). Those outside the hospice group may feel growing resentment at the assumption that they cannot do for the patient what hospice can.

The Individual Nurse

A person's ability to adapt effectively in a role that includes care of the dying within a hospice program is determined by multiple factors. Primary is a sense of personal and professional self-esteem and self-direction, as opposed to a tendency to derive one's identity and worth from others' approval. Education determines effectiveness by providing an adequate knowledge base and an understanding of the use of a goal-centered nursing process. Nursing education also generally has emphasized that "nurses meet all the patients' needs." This ideal is unrealizable in actual practice. Many nurses begin hospice practice in the hope that now they *will* finally be able to somehow meet all their patients' needs. Growth in the caring role demands self-examination and adaptation in philosophy regarding health, healing, and caregiver responsibility to "make everything better." The person must be willing to question many old assumptions that have provided past security in practice.

Individual adaptability is determined significantly by the nurse's motivation to work in this role and his or her awareness of self. Vachon (1978) lists some of the unconscious needs and hidden agendas that can lead one to work with the dying and can affect the nature of that work: attraction to the avant-garde aspects of the death and dying movement; need to control dying and suffering and thus feel mastery over them; a sense of religious or humanistic calling; previously unresolved issues of personal grief and loss; anticipation of a life-threatening illness in oneself. And, according to Vachon, nurses often hope to displace their feelings of personal inadequacy and powerlessness. Thus self-awareness is integral to an effective hospice nursing role. The nurse needs to become conscious of his or her own agendas as they interface with patient, family, team, and agency directions. She or he needs to recognize personal stressors and coping behavior. Indeed, the nurse's prior patterns of coping with stress is another indicator of coping effectiveness in the hospice nurse role. The ability to verbalize feeling and conflicts and to adapt behavior to changing circumstances is central to avoiding hospice role distress.

Some dilemmas inherent in the contemporary practice of professional nursing increase stress in the hospice nursing role. In hospice care, there is increased demand and opportunity for independent clinical judgments and for collegial interdisciplinary relationships. However, the nurse generally still suffers from lack of power in contrast to the physician with organizational mandate. In practice, the nurse becomes the primary health care professional for the dying person and his or her family. Officially, however, the nurse's involvement is usually secondary and delegated by the physician's signature on orders and on treatment plans. Until the nurse's role as a primary provider is accepted and made legitimate, his or her whole plan of care is controlled by the physician's pen. Indeed, the nurse's ongoing challenge to work as a colleague and not a subordinate to the physician who nevertheless is in command adds stress upon stress.

Another indicator of individual coping effectiveness is the personal life-style of the nurses—the events and rhythm of his or her personal life as they affect and are affected by work. When home and social life is besieged by developmental and situational crises and changes, it can be very difficult to maintain, in an effective manner, a work life that demands ongoing adaptation to change. Nurturing relationships and personal activities must be developed and sustained to prevent severe hospice work distress.

COPING WITH DISTRESS

Distress is inevitable in adapting to work with the dying. There are many ways, however, to encourage individual and professional well-being and to prevent burnout.

The Adaptation Process

Bernice Harper (1977) has described a predictable normal process as the health professional adapts to working with the dying for the first time. During the first 3 months, according to Harper, the process of intellectualization is predominant; nurses focus on cognitive understanding of the multiple aspects of their new job. Between 3 and 6 months, nurses experience their first real involvement with patients and families and their suffering. Feelings of helplessness and anger emerge. Between 6 and 9 months nurses are likely to experience depression, as they identify closely with the patient's tragedy. Harper expects "emotional arrival" somewhere between 9 and 12 months; she characterizes this time as one when the nurse is freed from overidentification with the patient, from guilt, and from depression. Between the first and second years the nurse develops deep compassion, with accompanying self-awareness and solid professional expertise.

Each professional adapting to hospice work will progress through this type of adaptive process at his or her own rate, lingering in some stages and moving quickly through others. Some will be stuck at intellectualization or overidentification, and all regress there at times. How can we maximize healthy adaptation during these first years and maintain our "deep compassion" and enthusiasm over the long haul?

Self Awareness

Working with the dying demands insight and the willingness to explore oneself. Working with the dying also offers tremendous opportunities for growth in self-awareness and understanding of life. Feelings and perceived needs and values require ongoing exploration.

Feelings are explored through one-to-one attentive listening, in groups designed for mutual support, and occasionally in written journals. Group expression works well as trust is developed, but many "private people" continue to prefer expression with one trusted individual, perhaps combined with writing. Unresolved personal pain and loss bring constant reminders in hospice work; Chapter 16 enables the reader to explore personal history and reactions regarding death itself. It is vital that the nurse become aware of whatever conflicts have been unresolved and of the destructive coping mechanisms that may have been utilized to keep such conflicts out of awareness. Some may choose professional counseling to heal old hurts. Vachon's (1978) work reminds us of the need to recognize our personal agendas in choosing hospice work, agendas that may be related to those unresolved personal problems and feelings of inadequacy.

In seeking to become aware of feelings, it is extremely useful to learn to recognize one's own bodily warning signs as negative feelings begin to well up. Is there a churning of the stomach, a tightening in the jaw, perspiration, slight dizziness? These may progress to a Pandora's box of complaints ranging from headache, neck ache, back ache, stomach ache, diarrhea, insomnia, recurrent respiratory infections, and on to that growing list of serious stress-related diseases, many of which are terminal! In contrast, it is well to learn to be aware of one's bodily sensations when one is rested, at peace, and enjoying life. Then you can describe how you would like to feel, and identify how far "out of kilter" you have moved under stress.

Finally, it is extremely important to continually scrutinize beliefs as they are affected by hospice work. Examine values about health and healing and dying, about responsibility for helping patients and families feel better. Steiner (1973) suggests that when caregivers perceive their patients as helpless and needing to be taken care of, rather than caring for themselves, the caregivers themselves tend to feel powerless and victimized. "Rather than feeling satisfaction and joy in helping others, they experience frustration having to work against difficult odds, a sense of bottomless responsibility, and heartbreak over failure.... For good therapy to take place it is essential...that the person seeking help be seen as a complete human being capable of taking power over their life" (Steiner, 1973, p. 21). The nurse who attempts to take over the burdens of others will be burdened and burned out. The nurse who makes clear contracts with patients-families to help them in areas that they choose, with the patient and family having clear final responsibility for choosing to help themselves or not, will be far better off. And goals for care must be realistic and achievable (see Chapter 4).

Even with a clear sense of realistic responsibility, hospice nursing still often demands more giving than getting and as a result, there is an energy deficit that must be filled. Figure 17-1 presents a stress and burnout self-exam tool that may be helpful in self-assessment. It is advantageous to go through this self-examination periodically. Modify the tool so as to include your personal indicators of building stress, or to make the tool as applicable to the circumstances of your specific team or agency.

Ability to adapt effectively to work-related changes is also influenced by the numbers of changes in one's personal life that are demanding adaptation. The Holmes Stress Scale lists life changes in order of their demand and threat to emotional and physical health (Wyler, 1971). This scale reminds us that even changes that appear to be wholly positive, such as outstanding achievements or holiday festivities, put stress on our adaptive capacities.

Figure 17-1 Stress and burnout self-exam

1. *Personal Involvement Checklist*

_____ Canceling personal activities due to work

_____ Regularly receiving one or more patient calls in an evening

_____ Routinely spending longer with patients than planned

_____ When demands build up, tending to do things myself rather than ask for help

_____ Performing a helping–therapy role for needy people outside of work

_____ Main focus of conversation with own family-friends is work and patients

_____ Family or friends are distressed about preoccupation with work

_____ Main source of personal satisfaction and self-esteem is work

_____ Social contacts are diminished

_____ Increased family problems

2. *Frustration Checklist*

_____ Difficulty in communicating with patient-family

_____ Difficulty in communicating with team member

_____ Team conflict over goals for patient

_____ Patient and/or family in denial

_____ Unable to help patient-family with distress

_____ Unclear work expectations

_____ Practice being criticized

_____ Always giving support, seldom receiving

_____ Unable to function effectively

_____ Growing distance between self and patients

_____ Angry with patients and families

3. *Feelings Related to Being Overextended*

_____ Feel overwhelmed by own flaws

_____ Feel guilty if I say "no" when asked to help

_____ Feel overwhelmed with patient needs and amount of work

_____ Feel I'm not doing a good job

_____ Feel crabby, resentful, sarcastic

_____ Feel exhausted

_____ Feel lonely and isolated

_____ Feel behind in all my responsibilities

_____ Indulging in alcohol, food, cigarette or other chemical excesses

_____ Feel unmet need to talk about intense work experience

_____ Cannot slow down

4. *Physical health*

_____ Sleep disturbances

_____ GI disturbances

_____ Back pain

_____ Recurrent extended respiratory infections

_____ Headaches

_____ Other

Table 17-2 presents some of the most stressful life changes listed by Holmes and his associates in decreasing order of impact. Use of the entire Holmes tool may be helpful in self-assessment.

Self-Care

"Give from your own excess, not from your essence," Taft (1982) says. We must live fully in a life-affirming way. We must find ways to be filled up and *nourished;* to care for our own spirit, heart, and body. This includes slowing down to hear our inner voice, to find our center, to be still. It includes

Table 17-2. *Some Items from Holmes Scale*

Death of spouse	Retirement
Divorce	Change in health of family member
Marital separation	Pregnancy
Jail term	Sex difficulties
Death of close family member	Gain of new family member
Personal injury or illness	Business readjustment
Marriage	Change in financial states
Fired at work	Death of close friend
Marital reconciliation	Change to different line of work

Source: Modified from Wyler, A.R., Masuda, H., and Holmes, T.H. Magnitude of life events and seriousness of illness. *Psychosomatic Medicine,* 1971, *33,* 115–122. With permission.
Note: The entire Holmes Scale contains 42 items, of which the first 18 are shown here. Items are assigned scores in decreasing values (e.g., "Death of Spouse" is scored 100, "Divorce" 73, etc.), and to obtain a total "life-change" score, one scores every item each time it has occurred within a given period of time.

good people, play, laughter, taking time for small joys. Table 3-3 in Chapter 3 lists "energy sources" that we can recommend to ourselves as well as to patients and families.

Feelings need affirmation and release. The most effective channels for such release go by way of sharing with peers, either as individuals or in a group setting. Relations with family and friends are at risk if we expect such people to absorb the heaviest portion of our needs to debrief and discharge emotion. Acting out distress by means of physical activity, such as chopping wood or hoeing up the weeds in our garden when the "weeds of life" are harder to remove is very effective for some of us. Finally, our bodies need good food, rest, activity, and loving.

Hospice staff need to learn *stress reduction techniques* to maintain spiritual, emotional, and physical balance in the face of the sheer intensity of this work. Many excellent books describe ways to live peaceably with the stresses of life. The works of Hans Selye (1974) and Kenneth Pelletier (1977) are a good place to begin a more detailed exploration. Meditation, relaxation, imagery, and autogenics, described in Chapters 7 and 8 as helpful in breaking the cycle of stress for patients, can be equally helpful to us. When you feel drained at the end of the day, lie down and switch the tape recorder to your own voice, soothingly directing you to be "calm and quiet" and perhaps head for ten minutes to a peaceful meadow in your mind. Or you may find vigorous physical activity to be the most effective stress-reduction technique. Instead of imagining a meadow, you may choose to get out and jog in one!

Personal limit setting is pivotal to developing self-care ability. Set clear *boundaries* between your professional and your personal lives. Limit responsibility to what seems reasonable, considering your personal "strength and light." Remember that you cannot do everything *now* and you cannot do everything *alone. Beware of making promises you cannot keep.* Read Smith's *When I Say No I Feel Guilty.* Recognize patients' central responsibility for their own welfare. A few patients and their families have intense dependency needs that can be consuming. Recognize your own limits and identify them clearly. The nurse who gives help should rightly expect fair compensation from patient, agency, and/or insurance; and whatever gift of self or in kind that patient-family may choose. One patient gives us rhubarb from the garden; another gives us a blessing at the end of each visit. This maintains some balance in the helping relationship and empowers the giver.

ORGANIZATIONAL STRESS REDUCTION

"Dysfunctional responses to professional stress can be viewed as a symptom of system dysfunction in the same manner that emotional problems of individuals can be viewed as a symptom of dysfunction in the nuclear family system" (White, 1981, p. 319). For this reason, it is essential to assess organizational effectiveness in maintaining vitality and minimizing stress in staff members, to develop organizational strategies to minimize stress and burnout, and to identify methods to support the stressed individual team member.

Organizational Problems

The organizational system requires scrutiny when a significant number of staff are experiencing unacceptable levels of stress. Some symptoms of agency-wide stress include frequent tardiness, absenteeism, staff turnover, increasing interpersonal conflict, scapegoating of individuals, blaming organizational problems on an external enemy, and decreased quality of care (White, 1981). Organizational stressors common to developing hospice programs have been described earlier. Among the many challenges are lofty ideals, often without practical mechanisms for achievement; intense scrutiny; lack of clear structure; work overload and multiple roles; economic insecurity; ideological battles; and intense team relationships. Although some of these difficulties are inherent and almost unavoidable when a program is still young, accumulating stress can be minimized by deliberate personnel policies and strategies.

Organizational Strategies

Team members should be hired selectively, encouraged to use each other supportively, granted flexible working conditions, helped to limit overextension, trained in productive time management, and recognized with reasonable benefits and affirmation. Screening prospective team nurses is a demanding process. If a nurse is well matched to the hospice role a great deal of stress can be avoided. Those selected for interview should be screened first by a critical review of resumes for strong professional credentials and experience.

Applicants should be interviewed by several team members, preferably one representing each discipline active on the team. LaGrand (1980) proposes special scrutiny to determine ability to adapt to stressful work circumstances and lists the following guidelines:

- Careful analysis of the motivation to serve others
- Analysis of personality characteristics and job compatibility
- Indication of ability to relate well to others and be sensitive to the human needs of specific situations
- Past history in meeting high-stress problems
- Realistic goal-oriented work habits
- Analysis of physical condition, vitality, and energy levels

As a framework for job interviewing, it is useful to describe some sample clinical and other work-related circumstances and ask the applicant to analyze the situation described and indicate what action she or he would take. The sample situational questions that follow might elicit information that would help determine an applicant's psychosocial assessment skills, empathy, respect for individual choice, limit-setting skills, need to pursue a personal agenda, and existing skills in personal stress reduction.

- Janette Martin is a 22-year-old associate degree nursing student who has taken a leave of absence to care for her 24-year-old husband, a carpentry apprentice, who is choosing to die at home of pulmonary metastates secondary to his long battle with malignant melanoma. It is 5:30 P.M., following an extensive home symptom-management and grief counseling discussion that began at 3 P.M. You prepare to leave and Jan says, "Oh, won't you please stay. I'd feel so much better if you could stay until my mother-in-law comes at 10:00 P.M." How would you respond?
- Joe McNally lives with his oldest daughter. Following the failure of his last chemotherapy to induce any change in his hepatic metastases, he has taken to bed and refused to take solids. He refuses to see his parish priest anymore; "Let the devil take me, I don't give a damn!" Joe will not see his physician, who has desperately made a hospice nurse referral. What would be your goals at the first visit?
- You have just spent two hours with a middle-aged man who has been sobbing and rocking in severe pain. You were unable to control the pain with the drugs easily available and finally had to hospitalize him for relief. How would you feel? How do you think the rest of your day or evening would go?

It is important to describe stressful situations that will elicit the kinds of answers most relevant to working in *your* particular program. Real incidents from the past, with names changed, often provide the most useful responses upon which to base the decision to hire a prospective candidate.

The hospice program's need to encourage cooperative decision making and support (see Chapter 5 on interdisciplinary teamwork) runs contrary to the conventional working relationship, in which each isolated individual professional struggles to prove his or her worth and competence in competition with others. True cooperative relations take time to grow and are possible only when individual team members possess self-esteem and thus have no need to put down others. Nurses should be encouraged to share difficult tasks and difficult patients and to "trade off" those difficult tasks and patients if needed. They also need to be encouraged to trust each other with favorite patients rather than experience the mixed blessing of being the pivotal caregiver for a patient and feeling obliged to be available night and day for him or her. Team support groups should be encouraged and attendance required during "on-duty" time. It is not supportive to be asked to go to an evening support group *on your own time* after putting in a 9-hour day.

A flexible work schedule is critical to long-term survival of hospice team members. Permit long weekends, leave, and vacation time. The nurse needs time to grieve, to relax, perhaps to work with a less intense caseload. Some of us wish we could occasionally be transferred to the newborn nursery for a month! It is very difficult to build this kind of flexibility into a standard 40-hour-a-week job. On call time adds evening and weekend hours. Some agencies hire special evening and weekend "on call" nurses to lessen the burden on the regular team. Other programs hire part-time nurses to minimize burnout, often primarily due to budgetary constraints. The challenge of so-called half-time hospice nurses, as we have learned from personal trial at Hospice of Seattle, is to avoid being available *half of each hour* through the day and night!

The agency needs to help nurses stop their overextension to avoid problems of compensating overtime and in order to maintain a functional, healthy staff. This is in contrast to so many organizations who try to get more and more work from less and less staff. This produces burnout, ill will, and rapid turnover. Team members need to help each other to recognize overextension and develop individual as well as team limit-setting plans. Examples of team strategies could include an agreement among nurses to trade off responsibilities *before* overtime threatens to accumulate or a policy decision not to give out personal phone numbers and to rely only on a beeper for emergencies. A helpful strategy may encompass *whatever enables the individual nurse to create a reasonable boundary between personal and work life and enables personal life to be energizing and not constantly interrupted.*

Accompanying a concern for team overextension is the contrasting concern for effective management of time and for maximal efficiency in carrying out the multiple tasks of developing a hospice program while trying to demonstrate excellence in handling a caseload of dying people. The stress of having constant exposure to death cannot be allowed to become an excuse for poor performance and inefficiency. Time management workshops are helpful. The team needs to provide time for pause and pondering, for periodic opportunities to scrutinize administrative developments and patient care outcomes. A team that is focused on seeing as many patients as possible in as little time as possible will not have time to synthesize knowledge and experience and thus to gain wisdom in action. Chapter 15 discusses responsibility for the development of new knowledge.

Hospice teams need to prepare themselves to be highly skilled in dealing with stress and conflict and thus to help alleviate these problems in patients-families, as well as in their personal–professional lives as hospice team members. Staff should be encouraged to integrate imagery, meditation, massage, and countless other healing and relaxing approaches into their lives in a manner compatible with their personal styles. We should not be preaching what we do not practice ourselves. Conflicts among family members and conflicts within the hospice team are among the most unsettling realities to be faced in this work. Conflict resolution is skill that is integral to maintaining peace and balance. Amidst the warring human family, there is finally a growing body of knowledge and increasing numbers of people are becoming experts in mediation and reconcilation. Hospice team members need to secure training in this area.

Finally, organizational structure needs to build in rewards and recognition for the hospice nurse whenever possible. There should be commitment to make pay and benefits competitive. Inservice and continuing education opportunities should be ongoing. Effort should be made to secure recognition from the community and fellow professionals. The atmosphere must be one of mutual regard and affirmation. As the hospice ages, questions will be raised regarding justification and necessity of special supports, involvement in decisions, flexibility, and benefits for the hospice staff while at the same time demand for maximum productivity mounts. Succumbing to the pressures of such inquiries and demands causes a syndrome of whole-agency burnout symptoms characterized by loss of compassion and poor quality care, staff turnover, and staff conflicts. To reach out in caring to the sick, staff nurses must be valued and supported. Those health care agencies with stable productive staff are always those with active nurse participation in decision making, responsiveness to staff personal needs, and active reward for high-quality work performance.

Responding to the Distressed Individual

The overstressed individual team member needs help from other team members in recognizing and dealing with the problem as well as from those in a coordinating, supervising role. The coordinator must clearly define his or her role and availability in this area. Among staff, there should be continuous mutual monitoring of individual and organizational signs of stress and burnout. Some stress and distress is a normal and expected process that must be faced in the ongoing adaptation of each team member and the team as a whole. Those in a coordinating role are responsible to point out individual signs of stress, overextension, and setting unattainable goals. Coordinators arrange supportive help for the individual to determine underlying causes of increasing stress. The coordinator responds to the immediate respite needs for the stressed individual and then plans, with that person, strategies to decrease organizational stressors and enhance personal and professional supports (White, 1981). One agency responded to a nurse's growing stress as described in the following vignette:

Case Example: Preventing "Burnout"

The interdisciplinary team noticed that the 3-year veteran nurse in the group, Carolyn Martinellie, was becoming increasingly sarcastic and cynical, making patients the brunt of her jokes. She was repeatedly attacked by a "flu bug" that prevented her from attending support meetings. Three of her neighbors were currently seriously ill at home, and she had frequently been called by them in the wee hours of the morning. Her daughter was newly divorced and had moved home, with her 3-year-old son, to live with Carolyn and her husband. Carolyn was constantly working overtime hours at hospice.

The team chaplain and the team nurse's aide had separately brought to the nursing coordinator their concern that Carolyn was "burning out." They both would have preferred to discuss their concern with Carolyn herself at a support meeting, and they felt she was avoiding them. She was also "too busy" to join them for coffee and talk.

The coordinator made an appointment with Carolyn "to discuss your heavy workload." In the meeting they began to explore Carolyn's increasing symptoms of distress and her experience of mounting personal and professional burdens. Together they planned for immediate respite so that Carolyn could take off for a 4-day weekend at a friend's cabin where there was *no phone*. The coordinator organized other nurses to assume Carolyn's on-call responsibilities for the next two weeks. Carolyn agreed to ask her daughter to seriously consider joining a local single mothers' support group to help herself and relieve some of Carolyn's emotional overload.

In two additional sessions, Carolyn and the coordinator evolved long-term plans. They asked the team to change the time of their support group so that Carolyn would find it easier to attend. Carolyn resolved to tell her neighbors that she simply could not respond to their phone calls after 8 P.M.

In addition, Carolyn's caseload was modified to exclude patients in their 20s and 30s, whose care she found most stressful to deal with personally. She traded these cases with another nurse who found patients in denial to be a much greater burden. Carolyn's daughter gradually regained her self-esteem and sense of independence and made a decision, with the support of her single mothers' group, to move to a nearby apartment with her son. Carolyn made an ongoing resolution to enjoy a 2½ day weekend once a month alone with her husband.

It is difficult work to hold the bodies and look into the faces of the dying day after day. Nurses who are periodically overwhelmed with such intensity will be comforted and able to move forward if they have friends and colleagues standing patiently beside them and if the organization maintains a supportive flexible work environment as described. When the organization has done its best, however, to maintain burnout-prevention strategies and a nurse is still frequently unavailable or unable to take his or her share of patients and workload, she or he dearly needs assistance to either practice personal strategies that work toward higher performance or resign gracefully. We do not help each other by lowering standards.

REFERENCES

Harper, B. *Death: The coping mechanism of the health professional.* Greenville, S.C.: Southeastern University, 1977.

LaGrand, L. Reducing burnout in the hospice and the death education movement. *Death Education,* 1980, *4,* 261–75.

McElroy, A. Burnout - A review of the literature with application to cancer nursing. *Cancer Nursing,* 1982, *5,* 211–217.

Pelletier, K.R. *Mind as Healer, Mind as Slayer. A Holisitc Approach to Preventing Stress Disorders.* New York: Dell, 1977.

Selye, H. *Stress without distress.* New York: Signet, 1974.

Smith, M. *When I Say No, I Feel Guilty.* New York: Bantam, 1975.

Steiner, C. The rescue triangle. *Issues in Radical Therapy,* 1973, *1,* 20–24.

Taft, T.K. *Strategies for staff support.* Discussion at Basic Symposium on Care of the Terminally Ill, Seattle, February 25, 1982.

Vachon, M.L.S. Motivation and stress experienced by staff working with the terminally ill. In G. Davidson (Ed.). *The Hospice.* Washington, D.C.: Hemisphere, 1978.

White, W. Managing personal and organizational stress in the care of the dying. In *Hospice Education Program for Nurses.* Washington, D.C.: U.S. Department of Health and Human Services, 1981.

Wyler, A.R., Masuda, M., & Holmes, T.H. Magnitude of life events and seriousness of illness. *Psychosomatic Medicine,* 1971, *33,* 115–122.

1. F		*6. T*	
2. F		*7. F*	
3. F		*8. F*	
4. T		*9. T*	
5. T		*10. T*	

CODA

*To those who confront the difficulties of implementing the ideal hospice
program, yet continue to strive to do so—*

In *Through the Looking Glass*, the White Queen says, "I will give you something
to believe. I am just 101, five months, and a day."

"I can't believe that!" said Alice.

"Can't you?" the White Queen said in a pitying tone. "Try again. Draw a long
breath and shut your eyes."

Alice laughed. "There is no use trying," she said. "One can't believe in impossible
things."

"I dare say you haven't had much practice," said the Queen. "When I was your age
I always did it for a half-hour a day. Why, sometimes I believed as many as six
impossible things before breakfast."

Index

A

Coping
  with distress, 352–356. *See also* Distress,
      coping with
  individual
    assessment of, 57
    ineffective, as nursing diagnoses,
        134–135t
Correlations, research questions concerned
    with, 322–323
Corticosteroids
  in pain control, 166
  in symptom relief, 120–121
Cough as nursing diagnosis, 130–131t
Counseling-spiritual concerns committee,
    purposes and responsibilities of, 284
Crisis intervention with family, 258–262
Cross-sectional design for correlational
    study, 323
Cultural background, assessment of, 58
Cure system, 5–6
Cyanosis in approaching death, 183

D

Dalmane, 118
Darvon, dosage, effectiveness and
    limitations of, 168t
Data in research on existing relationships
  analysis of, 321–322
  collection of, 321
Data base in clinical records, 310, *311*
Death
  approaching
    bleeding and, 188–189
    infection and, 187–188
    pain and, 188
    predictable changes in, 179–187
      in breathing, 181–182
      in circulation, 183
      in consciousness, 183–184
      death rattle as, 182–183
      disorientation as, 184
      fluid rejection as, 180–181
      food rejection as, 180–181
      maintenence in, 181
      oliguria as, 181
      recognizing last days in, 186–187
      restlessness as, 185
      in vital sign, 185–186
    seizures and, 189
    signs of, 186t

causes of, 178–179
dealing with, by children, developmental
    stages in, 268–269
desensitization to, American attitudes
    toward death and, 336–337
fears surrounding, 35–36
feelings about, understanding own,
    329–346. *See also* Feelings about
        death, understanding own
finding meaning in, for family, 257–258
imminent, recognizing, 186–187
inevitability of, psychological ways of
    addressing, 337–339
losses preceding, facing, 32–34
positive side of, 339–340
self-willed, 16
Death-accepting attitudes in addressing
    death's inevitability, 338
Death-continuation in addressing death's
    inevitability, 338–339
Death-defying attitudes in addressing
    death's inevitability, 337–338
Death-desiring attitudes in addressing death's
    inevitability, 338
Death rattle
  in approaching death, 182–183
  as nursing diagnosis, 132t
Death vigil, 189
  in coma, 190
  diagnosis of death in, 194–195
  dying person in, 189–190
  environment for, 190
  for immediately after death, 195–196
  location of, 192–194
  spiritual journey and, 191–193
  waiting for death in, 190–191
Decadron, 120
  in pain control, 166
Decision making
  cooperative, in organizational stress
      reduction, 358
  for dying person, 36–40
  in integration of hospice into acute care
      system, 304
Decisions social, 229–234. *See also*
    Teamwork, social decisions in
Decubiti as nursing diagnosis, 142t
Dehydration in approaching death, 180
Deity, concept of, assessment of, 59
Deliquency as grief reaction, 207–208
Delta-9-tetrahydrocannabinol for vomiting,
    119

Demerol, dosage, effectiveness and limitation of, 168t
Denial
  in grief process, 34, 203
  patient, professional honesty and, 21–22
Depression
  in grief, 204
  as nursing diagnosis, 134–135t
  pain and, 149
Desensitization, death, American attitudes toward death and, 336–337
Developmental stages in dealing with death by children, 268–269
Dexamethasone, 120
  in pain control, 166
Diagnosis, terminal, 31–34
Diagnostic conclusions, assessment of, 59–61
Diary in self-discovery, 37
Diazepam, 118
  for pain control, 167
Dihydromorphone, dosage, effectiveness and limitations of, 168t
Dilaudid, dosage, effectiveness and limitations of, 168t
Dioctyl calcium sulfosuccinate for constipation from narcotics, 171
Dioctyl sodium sulfosuccinate for constipation from narcotics, 171
Diphenhydramine, 117
  in combined drug regimens, 165
  for pain control, 166
  for terminal cardiopulmonary failure, 179
Directional hypothesis for correlational study, 323
Discharge planning, hospice team in, 49
Discharge summary in clinical records, 314
Disorientation
  in approaching death, 184
  as nursing diagnosis, 145
Displacement in patient-physician relationship, 14–15
Distancing, 337
Distress, coping with, 352–356
  adaptation process in, 352
  self-awareness in, 352–354
  self-care in, 354–356
Distressed individual, responding to, 359–361
Divine will as religious concern, 212
Documentation, systematic and succinct, in clinical records, 309–314

Dolophine, dosage, effectiveness and limitations of, 169t
Doxepin, 119
  for pain control, 167
Drugs
  adjunctive, for pain relief, 166–167
  dependency on, no fear of, in terminally ill, 163–164
  regimens for, combined, for pain relief, 164–165
  in symptom relief, 117–121. See also Pharmacological symptom relief
Dulcolax for constipation from narcotics, 171
Dying child, care of, 123–127. See also Child(ren), dying, care of
Dying role, transition from, sick role to, 40
Dysphagia as nursing diagnosis, 131–132t
Dysphnea as nursing diagnosis, 130t

E

Education
  in integration of hospice into acute care system. 303
  and training committee, purposes and responsibilities of, 284–285
Ego chill in response to death, 335
Elavil, 119, 120t
  for pain control, 167
Electrolyte imbalance as nursing diagnosis, 140t
Elimination, bowel, alteration in, as nursing diagnoses, 132–133t
Emergencies in symptom control, 122–123
Emotional factors affecting grief reactions, 209–210
Emotional reactions to loss and grief, 206–207
Empowering dying person, 36–43
  decision making in, 37–40
  discovering others in, 37
  strengthening identity in, 36–37
Endorphins in pain control, 149
Energy sources for dying person, 39t
Environment, modification of, in pain control, 154–155
Evaluation, initial, and decision for admission, 47–48
Executor, selection and duties of, 230
Expectation, realistic, for helping dying person, 43

Percodan, dosage, effectiveness and
limitations of, 169*t*
Percoset, dosage, effectiveness and
limitations of, 169*t*
Pharmacological pain relief, 162–174
adjunctive drugs in, 166–167
combined drug regimens in, 164–165
drug dependency and, 163–164
intrathecal morphine in, 172–174
narcotics in, 167–174. *See also* Narcotics
oral drugs in, 164
"pain cocktail" in, 165–166
in prevention of symptoms, 162–163
principles of, 162–166
Pharmacological symptom relief, 117–121
antianxiety agents in, 117–118, 120*t*
antidepressants in, 119, 120*t*
antiemetics in, 118–119, 120*t*
corticosteroids in, 120–121
Pharmacologist and hospice team, 77
Phenergan, 117
for pain control, 166
Phenothiazines
for pain relief, 166
for symptom relief, 117–118, 119, 120*t*
Philosophy statement of medical center
hospice, 298–299
Physical care of dying child, 126–127
Physical changes, assessment of, 50–54,
55–57*t*
Physical factors affecting grief reactions, 208
Physical measures in pain control, 156–157
Physical mobility, impaired, as nursing
diagnoses, 135–136*t*
Physical therapist and hospice team, 78
Physician
hospice, in hospice team, 73–74
and patient, relationship between,
honesty in, 12–16
primary, in hospice team, 73–74
Physiological reactions to loss and grief,
205–206
Plan of care, initial, in clinical records, 312
Planning committee, establishment of
in establishing community hospice,
277–278
in integration of hospice into acute care
system, 294
Positioning in pain control, 156
Prednisone, 120
in pain control, 166
Preparatory grief, 199

Prescription studies, 324–325
Pressure in pain control, 157
Pressure sores as nursing diagnosis, 142*t*
Privacy in research, 326
Problem list in clinical records, 310–312
Problem-solving
reduced, as nursing diagnosis, 145*t*
support system in, 238–239
Prochlorperazine, 118
for pain control, 166
Program, planning and evaluation of,
research in, 316
Program definition of medical center
hospice, 299
Progress records in clinical records, 312, *313*
Progressive relaxation in stress reduction,
114–115
Promethazine, 117
for pain control, 166
Propoxyphene hydrochloride, dosage,
effectiveness and limitations of,
168*t*
Providence as religious concern, 212
Psychiatrist and hospice team, 78
Psychoactive drugs, adverse effects of, 120*t*
Psychological factors
affecting grief reactions, 209
individual, grief reactions conditioned by,
217
Psychosocial assessment, 54, 57–59
Psychosocial care, documentation of, in
clinical records, 314, 315*t*
Psychosocial diagnoses for hospice patients,
61*t*
Psyllium for constipation from narcotics,
171
Publication of research results, 326–327
Pulmonary failure, death from, 179
Pulse, changes in, in approaching death, 185
Purpose, statement of, 278–279
in integration of hospice into acute care
system, 295–298

R

Radiotherapy, palliative, in pain control, 158
Randomization in study of cause and effect,
324
Realistic expectation for helping dying
person, 43

S